MW00576050

Score Higher on the

UKCAT®

Fourth Edition

Special thanks to those who made this book possible:

Simone Abbou, Matthew Callan, Louise Cook, Rupali Dikkar, Scarlet Edmonds, Joanna Graham, Brian Holmes, Katie Hunt, Bharat Krishna, Mia Olorunfemi, Marianna Parker, Teresa Rupp, Nimesh Shah, Rachel Swain.

UKCAT® is a registered trademark of the UKCAT Consortium, which was not involved in the production of, and does not endorse, this product

This publication is designed to provide accurate information in regard to the subject matter covered as of its publication date, with the understanding that knowledge and best practice constantly evolve. The publisher is not engaged in rendering medical, legal, accounting, or other professional service. If medical or legal advice or other expert assistance is required, the services of a competent professional should be sought. This publication is not intended for use in clinical practice or the delivery of medical care. To the fullest extent of the law, neither the Publisher nor the Editors assume any liability for any injury and/or damage to persons or property arising out of or related to any use of the material contained in this book.

Published by Kaplan Publishing, a division of Kaplan, Inc.
750 Third Avenue
New York, NY 10017

10 9 8 7 6 5 4 3 2 1

ISBN: 978-1-5062-2447-3

TABLE OF CONTENTS

How to Use This Book

Welcome to Score Higher on the UKCAT, Fourth Edition

One test stands between you and a place at the medical school of your dreams: the UKCAT.

No matter how strongly you perform in your GCSEs and A-levels, you are likely to find the UKCAT incredibly challenging. Most students who apply to study medicine get top results in their other exams, and are used to surpassing any academic challenge they have encountered. Such students make up virtually the entire UKCAT cohort, and so the UKCAT is designed to differentiate among this cohort of highly capable and resourceful students.

Most UKCAT test-takers do very little to prepare for the exam, and each year countless students find that Test Day comes as a rude surprise. They have never sat an exam that they were unable to finish, or in which they were unable to understand fully the nature of the questions being asked. Sadly, these students are unable to get a place studying medicine because of their poor UKCAT results, and must wait another year before taking the test again. At Kaplan, we have helped hundreds of students in this situation over the past few years, and they always tell us the same thing: they wish someone had told them they could prepare for the UKCAT.

You have everything you need to score higher on the UKCAT—let's start by walking through what you need to know to take advantage of this book and the Online Centre.

Your Book

There are two main components to your *Score Higher on the UKCAT* study package: your book and your Online Centre. This book contains the following:

- Detailed instruction covering essential skills for Verbal Reasoning, Decision Making, Quantitative Reasoning, Abstract Reasoning and Situational Judgement
- Time-tested and effective Kaplan strategies for every question type
- Two full-length practice tests, with answers and explanations

Your Online Centre

Your Online Centre lets you access more than 700 additional practice questions to reinforce your UKCAT skills and improve your speed and accuracy. Online resources include the following:

- A third full-length practice test (Mock Online Test)
- The UKCAT Score Higher Question Bank, with 400 practice questions
- The UKCAT Short Test, with more than 60 practice questions
- Test updates (available in June for the upcoming UKCAT), so you will be informed about any late changes or developments that could affect your UKCAT preparation

All the online practice tests and questions simulate the UKCAT interface you will experience on Test Day.

Getting Started

1. Register your Online Centre.
2. Take a UKCAT practice test to identify your strengths and weaknesses.
3. Create a study plan.
4. Learn and practise using this book and your Online Centre.

Step 1: Register your Online Centre

Register your Online Centre using these simple steps:

1. Go to **kaptest.co.uk/ukcattest**.
2. Follow the onscreen instructions. Please have a copy of your book available.

Access to the Online Centre is limited to the original owner of this book and is nontransferable. Kaplan is not responsible for providing access to the Online Centre to customers who purchase or borrow used copies of this book. Access to the Online Centre for this edition expires on 30th April 2019.

Step 2: Take a UKCAT Practice Test

It's a good idea to take a practice test early on. Doing so will give you the initial feedback and diagnostic information that you need to achieve your maximum score.

You can use the Diagnostic Test (Chapter Two of this book) as your first practice test. This Diagnostic test, which includes all five sections of the UKCAT, will give you a chance to familiarize yourself with the various sections and question types. It also allows you to accurately gauge the pacing required for each section, so you can identify the sections requiring the most practice.

Mark the answers in this book as you complete the Diagnostic Test. You may wish to use scrap paper to make any notations or calculations, just as you would use the noteboard on Test Day. You may also use a calculator with the basic arithmetic functions (not a scientific calculator). After completing the Diagnostic Test, check your answers against the Answer Key at the end of the test. Count up the number of correct responses in each section, and add these totals to the Scoring Table. Use the Scoring Table to find your approximate scores. Make a note of these scores, as they will serve as a baseline for your performance on subsequent practice tests.

Review the explanations for every question to better understand your performance. Look for patterns in the questions you answered correctly and incorrectly. Were you stronger in some areas than others? This analysis will help you target your practice time to specific concepts.

Step 3: Create a Study Plan

Use what you've learned from your diagnostic test to identify areas for closer study and practice. Take time to familiarize yourself with the key components of your book and Online Centre. Think about how many hours you can consistently devote to UKCAT study. We have found that most students achieve top scores with three to four weeks of committed preparation before Test Day.

Schedule time for study, practice, and review. One of the most frequent mistakes in approaching study is to take practice tests and not review them thoroughly—review time is your best chance to gain points. It works best for many people to block out short, frequent periods of study time throughout the week. Check in with yourself frequently to make sure you're not falling behind your plan or forgetting about any of your resources.

Step 4: Learn and Practise

Your book and Online Centre come with many opportunities to develop and practise the skills you'll need on Test Day. Read each chapter of this book and complete the practice questions. Depending on how much time you have to study, you can do this work methodically, covering every chapter, or you can focus your study on those sections and question types that you find most challenging. You will inevitably need more work in some areas than in others, but know that the more thoroughly you prepare, the higher you will score on Test Day.

Initially, your practice should focus on mastering the needed skills and not on timing. Add timing to your practice as you improve fundamental proficiency. Use the UKCAT Score Higher Question Bank in your Online Centre to build mastery of individual question types and to improve your pacing. As soon as you are comfortable with the question types and strategies, take and review the additional full-length practice tests in your book and Online Centre.

If you would like additional resources to help you prepare for the UKCAT, visit us at **kaptest.co.uk/UKCAT**.

Thanks for choosing Kaplan. We wish you the best of luck on your journey to UKCAT success.

Assessing the UKCAT

LEARNING OBJECTIVES

In this section, you'll learn to:

- Identify the sections of the UKCAT
- Explain how the UKCAT is scored
- Explain the advantages of question triage

Doctors cannot help patients get better without first completing an assessment, to ensure that they fully understand the issues and symptoms their patients are presenting. It is essential to adopt the same mindset when preparing for the UK Clinical Aptitude Test (UKCAT), which serves a very different purpose than any other exam you have taken, and presents very different challenges than you are likely to have encountered on any previous exam.

As part of your initial assessment of the UKCAT, you will complete the Kaplan UKCAT Diagnostic Test (Chapter 2), which will help you to understand the issues with question format and timing in each section. First, let's take a few minutes to consider the fundamental logic of the UKCAT.

Why sit the UKCAT?

The basic reason to sit the UKCAT is that it is required for admission to more than two dozen medical and dental programmes in the UK. The 26 universities that require the UKCAT for medical and dental admissions are known as the UKCAT Consortium, the test-maker responsible for the UKCAT since its inception in 2006. Most universities in the UKCAT Consortium require the UKCAT for undergraduate admissions, though a few require the exam for postgraduate admissions. Check the test-maker's website (www.ukcat.ac.uk) for a current and complete list.

Some UK universities, including Oxford and Cambridge, require a different exam called the BMAT (www.bmat.org.uk) for medical admissions. Depending on which universities you plan to apply to, you may have to sit both the UKCAT and the BMAT.

How important is the UKCAT?

There is a further reason that the UKCAT is an essential part of the medical and dental admissions process: most programmes that require the UKCAT will use your results to determine which applicants are invited to interview. The most common approach is to set a 'cut-off' score: applicants with UKCAT results above the cut-off are invited to interview; those with UKCAT results below the cut-off are not. In this sense, then, your UKCAT result will likely be 'make or break' for getting into a medical or dental programme.

Most programmes that use a cut-off score are rather discreet about the fact that they do so, and as a result it can be difficult to find out exactly where they draw the line between scores that get invited to interview and scores that are out of luck. Anecdotal evidence from many students who have been through the admissions process

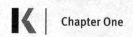

recently reveals that the cut-off score is usually right around the average mark on the UKCAT, which is currently a total score of 2540, or an average of 635 in each section. To ensure that you score higher than the cut-off score, you will want to try and score above average on the UKCAT. The good news is that it is very possible to do so, but you will need to invest time in learning Kaplan's top tips and putting them into practice. In order to secure a medical or dental interview, it is essential to prepare for the UKCAT, and to do your absolute best to get the highest score possible on Test Day.

What does the UKCAT test?

The UKCAT is not a test of content that you studied at GCSE or A-level, and it has been designed with a very different format and timing than those exams. As such, the UKCAT will require a very different approach. The UKCAT consists of five sections, each of which tests your ability to provide the most correct answers in a very short time.

Here is a brief overview of the task, number of questions and timing in each section.

Verbal Reasoning: You must assess statements by finding relevant information and making inferences from a reading passage. You must answer 44 items in 21 minutes.

Decision Making: You must apply logical, sequencing and numerical skills to a wide range of question types. You must answer 29 questions in 31 minutes.

Quantitative Reasoning: You must find relevant data and complete basic calculations (most involve arithmetic, algebra and/or geometry). You must answer 36 questions in 24 minutes.

Abstract Reasoning: You must find patterns or progressions in sets of shapes, and match new shapes to existing patterns and progressions. You must answer 55 items in 13 minutes.

Situational Judgement: You must determine the most pressing issues in a clinical or educational scenario, and evaluate a series of possible responses to the scenario. You must answer 68 items in 26 minutes.

As you can see, the UKCAT will not require you to use any content that you learnt in school, with the exception of a few basic formulae (e.g. those involving percentage, mean, speed and geometry) in the Quantitative Reasoning section. Most of the work required to answer correctly in most sections is particular to the types of questions on the UKCAT. Thus, you will need to learn the workings of the various question types, so you can improve your speed and accuracy at answering individual questions and in working through each section.

Timing is also a significant challenge on the UKCAT. You have about a minute to answer each Decision Making question, and 30 seconds or less to answer each question in the other four sections. This timing is much quicker than you will likely have experienced on any exam you have sat previously. It is very common for students to be unable to finish one or more sections of the first UKCAT test paper they sit, so don't be alarmed if this happens to you on the Kaplan UKCAT Diagnostic Test. Just be glad that you are not one of the many unlucky students each year who have the experience of being unable to finish whilst sitting the actual UKCAT. Sitting the realistic practice tests in this book will be essential in preparing yourself for the timing and 'endurance' factors of answering 232 questions in 2 hours on Test Day. You can obtain a further practice test free of charge at www. kaptest.co.uk/ukcattest. Each additional practice test you sit will enable you to improve your timing, give you more opportunity to practise Kaplan's top tips and allow you to make mistakes. Remember: any mistake you make whilst practising for the UKCAT is one you can avoid on Test Day.

The test-taking format is a further challenge in that the UKCAT is taken on a computer at a testing centre. You can find a complete list of UKCAT testing centres on the UKCAT website, along with a tutorial and demonstration of the test-taking interface. The UKCAT Consortium also provides three full-length practice tests and a small selection of practice questions for each section in the computerised interface, which are available for free on the UKCAT website. You are strongly advised to work through these tests and questions, but you should do so after completing the chapters in this book. Don't worry if you have worked through the official computerised practice tests and practice questions already. If you haven't, you will get more out of them once you have learnt Kaplan's top tips and completed the paper-based practice tests in this book. It is essential that you become familiar with the exact appearance and functions in the test-taking interface. These include the option to move back and forth between questions, to flag questions for review and to review questions (whether flagged, unanswered or all questions) at the end of a section. The computerised interface also includes an onscreen calculator, which you will want to practise using so you can be prepared for Quantitative Reasoning.

How is the UKCAT scored?

The first four sections of the UKCAT are each scored from 300 to 900. According to the test-maker, most people who sit the UKCAT score between 500 and 700 in each section. Scores above 700 in any section are considered difficult to achieve, and very impressive indeed. According to data provided by the UKCAT Consortium, the average score is just above or below 600 in each section.

Your results are tabulated by the computer, and you will be given a printout when you leave the testing room. Don't lose this printout, as there is a charge to obtain a replacement copy. Your results are automatically sent to the universities you select on your UCAS form; for this reason, you must sit the UKCAT in the year when you are applying for admission. Scores do not carry over from one year to another, and you can sit the UKCAT only once per year.

Although the scores are scaled from 300 to 900, the actual scoring is very simple. You get a mark for each correct answer. There is no negative marking, so you do not lose any marks for incorrect answers. You do not gain or lose any marks for questions that are left unanswered. Leaving many questions unanswered in one or more sections is the most common mistake made by UKCAT test-takers on Test Day. Doing so virtually ensures that you will score well below the average in at least one section, which will make it difficult to pass the cut-off score required for interview.

Situational Judgement scores are given from Band 1 to Band 4 (highest to lowest), depending how many of your answers match those determined by the panel of medical experts. You get full marks for choosing the correct answer, and partial marks for choosing an answer that is close to the correct answer. The exact details of the partial marking have not been disclosed by the UKCAT Consortium, but this means that you have a good chance of getting some marks for each Situational Judgement question, so long as you mark an answer.

How do you get top scores?

The first tip, if perhaps a somewhat obvious one, is to mark an answer for every question. You may not be comfortable with marking answers for questions you have not actually attempted. However, it is possible that you may find yourself running out of time as you get to the end of one or more sections, despite your best efforts in preparing for the UKCAT, as the timing is so tight. If you have a few questions you are unable to work out properly, it is better to mark an answer and gain a chance of picking up the marks than to leave them blank and have 0% chance of picking up the mark.

Verbal Reasoning and Abstract Reasoning questions have three or four answer choices. Decision Making and Situational Judgement questions have four answer choices. Quantitative Reasoning questions have five answer choices. Consider the odds of guessing correctly when guessing blindly—as compared to guessing strategically—in the following table.

Number of answer choices	Odds of correctly guessing blindly	Odds of correctly guessing strategically, after eliminating 1 answer	Odds of correctly guessing strategically, after eliminating 2 answers
3	33%	50%	100%
4	25%	33%	50%
5	20%	25%	33%

When you can eliminate one or more answer choices, guessing strategically gives you a much stronger chance of answering correctly and picking up the mark. The odds of guessing blindly are not bad, particularly when there are only three answer choices. Still, you should only guess blindly if you are running out of time and at risk of leaving questions unanswered.

You can minimise blind guessing by following the next tip: maximise your marks with question triage. Since you have so little time to answer each question, the UKCAT can challenge you by presenting you with a few questions in each section that take far longer than the average timing per question to answer properly. For instance, you might see a few questions in the Quantitative section that would take 2 or more minutes to solve using straightforward maths, rather than the 30 seconds allotted. If you take the time to answer one such question by doing the straightforward maths, and spending 90 seconds more than you have, then you will effectively have ensured that you are unable to answer 3 questions later in the section. Unless you were on the final Quantitative set, you could be sure that there would be at least 3 more questions that you could reasonably answer in 30 seconds each. Answering those 3 questions would earn you 3 more marks, whereas answering the one long question picks up only a single mark. Since there are fairly few questions in each section that are meant to be very time-consuming, you must triage these questions. Rather than following the usual timing, spend no more than 10 seconds on one that appears to be very time-consuming. Make a strategic or blind guess, mark an answer, flag the question for review and move on. You will need to practise for triage—and to build up your confidence in deploying triage as a test-taking strategy—but students who do so usually score well above 700 in most (if not all) sections of the UKCAT.

The reason for this has to do with the exact correspondence of the number of correct answers in each section to the scaled scores from 300 to 900. Based on extensive feedback from students who have sat the UKCAT, we have prepared a scoring table which you can find at the end of the two practice tests in this book (on p. 100 and p. 420). If you check the scoring table, you will notice that you can score 700 or above by answering approximately three-quarters of the questions in a section correctly. A score of 700 in a section would place you in the top 10% of UKCAT test-takers—a phenomenal achievement, and one you can attain without answering all the questions in a section correctly.

All the questions in the UKCAT have been written for a certain objective level of difficulty. If you think of question difficulty as a continuum from easy to medium to hard, most questions will be in the 'medium' range on the continuum, with a few towards the extremes of 'easy' and 'hard'. Time-consuming questions (i.e. those that take more than the allotted time per question to answer) are always objectively at the 'hard' end of the difficulty continuum, and the test cannot give you very many of these in any one section. Triage can thus help you maximise your marks in each section, by spending the time allotted on the easy and medium questions, which should certainly account for at least three-quarters of the total. Maximising your marks on these questions will be essential to earning a high score.

The final tip for getting a top score on the UKCAT is to make the most of this book. Learn the test formats and tips for each section. Practise for strategy as well as pacing. This book is loaded with Kaplan timed practice sets, which will allow you to practise triage, while also deploying Kaplan's top tips and ensuring that you answer every question before time is up. Review the worked answers for every question you attempt while practising, so you can ensure that you are getting the right answers for the right reasons, and in the fastest time possible.

When you are ready to begin your UKCAT preparation, set aside a couple of hours and sit the Kaplan UKCAT Diagnostic Test in Chapter 2. Be sure to review all the worked answers soon after the test—ideally the same day, or the next day. Many UKCAT test-takers never sit a full-length practice test, so you will have a huge advantage over the competition after finishing the next chapter.

Score Higher Online

Full details of the 2018 UKCAT will be published on the UKCAT website in May 2018. The details in this book are based on the 2017 UKCAT; normally, the changes from year-to-year are relatively minimal. You should check the UKCAT website (www.ukcat.ac.uk) in May to confirm the current test specifications. Check your Online Centre in June for information on test updates, including any guidance on how to modify this book for the most up-to-date UKCAT prep.

Kaplan UKCAT Diagnostic Test

Diagnostic Test General Instructions

You have 2 hours to complete the Kaplan UKCAT Diagnostic Test. You will need the following items:

- This book
- A pen or pencil to record your answers
- Scrap paper for any scratch work and notations
- A timer (such as one on your watch, mobile or computer)
- A calculator with basic functions (i.e. not a scientific calculator or mobile phone)

Time each section strictly, so you can practise under test-like conditions.

On Test Day, you will have an additional minute to read the directions for each section. That minute cannot be used to answer test questions, so it has not been included here. Time yourself using the timings given once you turn each instructions page and start work on each section.

Answer the questions as quickly and accurately as possible. There is no negative marking, so you are strongly encouraged to mark an answer for every question in each section.

Pace yourself so you can attempt all the items in each section.

Record your answers on a sheet of paper, and check them against the explanations in Appendix B once you finish.

N.B. You cannot write on the test paper on Test Day, because the test is taken on a computer. Be careful not to get into the habit of writing on the practice questions in this book. Make any notations, eliminations or other markings entirely on scrap paper, and not directly on the questions themselves.

Your score on Test Day corresponds to the number of questions you answer correctly. You can find your equivalent score on the scoring table at the end of the test.

When you are ready to begin the Diagnostic Test, turn the page and read the directions for the first section.

Section 1: Verbal Reasoning (22 Minutes)

This section contains 11 passages, each of which is followed by four items. Most items will be questions, each with four answer choices. Your task in a Verbal question is to select the best answer from the options given.

Other items will consist of a statement, with the answer choices True, False and Can't tell. You must assess the statement based on the passage. Select True if the information in the statement is stated explicitly in the passage or a valid inference from the passage. Select False if the information in the statement contradicts what is stated in the passage. Select Can't tell if there is not enough information to determine whether the statement is True or False.

Answer all 44 questions in Section 1, selecting one of the possible answers and circling the letter corresponding to the appropriate answer in your test paper.

When you are finished with this section, you may use any remaining time to review your work in this section only. Once you proceed to the next section, you may not return to this section.

You will have 22 minutes to answer the questions. It is in your best interest to select an answer for every item as there is no penalty for wrong answers.

Set your timer for 22 minutes, turn the page and begin the section.

Since the first confirmed sighting in 2006, an increasing number of Pizzly, or Grolar, bears have been spotted in northern regions of Canada. It has been known for some time that grizzly bears, also known as brown bears, can produce fertile offspring with polar bears; indeed, the two species have often been mated in captivity. Historically, however, instances in the wild have been highly unusual. The rising temperature in recent years is thought to be responsible for brown bears travelling further north, bringing them into contact with polar bears on the northern coastline.

Recent research has demonstrated that all of today's polar bears are descended from prehistoric (and long since extinct) brown bears that lived in Ireland. Female brown bears of this very ancient species interbred with a similarly prehistoric species of polar bear during the last Ice Age, which ultimately wiped out the earlier, non-hybrid polar bears. Scientists were able to prove that today's polar bears maintain a direct hereditary line to the prehistoric brown bears of Ireland using mitochondrial DNA. An offspring's mitochondrial DNA is identical to its mother's, and can be used to trace maternal ancestry back through the generations. Bones and teeth from about a dozen female brown bears that lived in Ireland 100 to 380 centuries ago – during the last Ice Age – match the mitochondrial DNA found in polar bears today.

Polar bears and brown bears are usually known to favour very different behaviours and climates. Polar bears eat a diet composed exclusively of meat and fish, and excel at swimming and hunting prey, in the cold, icy seas that are their required habitat. Brown bears live in the forest and eat a diet that includes carnivorous options, along with plants and berries.

Of course, Ireland is far too warm for polar bears today, though its climate would have cooled considerably during the Ice Age, bringing the prehistoric polar bears into contact with the ancient brown bears that would join them in creating the polar bear as we know it today.

1. Which of these statements about brown bears cannot be true?
   A. They are known to eat plants and berries.
   B. They eat only meat and fish.
   C. They favour a habitat with trees.
   D. They prefer a habitat that is not watery or icy.

2. The ancestry of polar bears has been traced to prehistoric brown bears in Ireland because the two types of bears have:
   A. identical mitochondria.
   B. the same mitochondrial DNA.
   C. mothers with similar traits.
   D. an unbroken chain of paternal genes.

3. In the last Ice Age, it must be true that:
   A. Iceland's climate cooled.
   B. Ireland's climate warmed up.
   C. Iceland's climate warmed up.
   D. Ireland's climate cooled.

4. The author would be most likely to agree with which of the following assertions?
   A. Some bears survived the Ice Age.
   B. Mating between species is a common occurrence.
   C. No bears survived the Ice Age.
   D. There are no examples of successful mating between species.

Sarah Bernhardt was a French stage and early film actress, known in her day as 'the most famous actress the world has ever known.' She was educated at the French Conservatoire, the Government-sponsored school of acting at that time, from the age of 13, and made her debut as a member of the French national theatre company Comédie-Française in 1862. Bernhardt did not really become recognised, though, until 1868, when she performed the role of Anna Danby in Alexandre Dumas' play *Kean* at the Odéon Theatre in Paris.

Bernhardt's fame grew further in the 1870s, and she enjoyed a decades-long career as an actress across Europe and the Americas. Among her most famous roles were Zanetto in the verse play *Le Passant* by François Coppée, which she played by special request before Napoleon III, and the title role in Voltaire's *Zaire*, performed after her return to the Comédie-Française in 1872. Bernhardt was also well known off-stage for her strange habits and complicated personality. The novelist Alexandre Dumas, son of the author Alexandre Dumas (who wrote *Kean*) and author himself of *The Three Musketeers*, described Bernhardt as a notorious liar, and she was widely rumoured to sleep every night in a coffin, rather than a bed. Little is known about her biography or early life; her birth certificate was lost in a fire when she was young, and she fabricated new birth records in order to prove citizenship for the French Légion d'honneur. Even though her past is largely inscrutable, her work has been immortalised on screen, in art and in photographs; her image appears in a number of paintings by the famous Art Nouveau painter and decorative artist Alphonse Mucha. She was a pioneer in film, playing Hamlet in the short film *Le Duel d'Hamlet* in 1900 and starring in eight motion pictures and two biographical films. Today, she is best remembered as a serious dramatic actress, for the work that earned her the nickname 'The Divine Sarah' in the late nineteenth and early twentieth century.

5. All of these statements regarding Sarah Bernhardt's career are true except:

   A. She never appeared in films.
   B. She played the role of Hamlet.
   C. Her career spanned two centuries.
   D. Her career spanned multiple continents.

6. An unusual fact about the novelist who wrote *The Three Musketeers* is that:

   A. his father was also a novelist.
   B. he and his father were not actually French.
   C. he and his father had the same name.
   D. his father was France's best-known actor.

7. The author suggests that Sarah Bernhardt's personal history:

   A. was entirely fabricated.
   B. was based in unfounded rumours that she was a vampire.
   C. is more or less unknowable.
   D. is irrelevant to her reputation.

8. According to the passage, in the 19th century the French government:

   A. fully funded the French national theatre.
   B. invested heavily in early films.
   C. supported the work of Art Nouveau painters.
   D. subsidised a theatre training scheme.

The Town and Country Planning Act, passed in 1947, established the national system of town planning and development still in use across the UK today. The act outlined laws governing ownership, construction, and development of property across the UK, administered on the local level by 421 Local Planning Authorities. The system is plan-led, meaning that all development of properties in the UK must begin with a development plan, public consultation and planning permission.

Over time, the Town and Country Planning Act has become a particularly effective vehicle through which the Government has been able to achieve its objectives for climate control, reduction of carbon emissions and housing access, among other initiatives. In addition, the act makes provisions for the protection and maintenance of listed buildings, those that carry architectural or historical interest. Owners of such structures can be required by law to keep these buildings in good repair, and must receive listed building consent before they are able to make any alterations that would affect the structure's character or appearance.

Fifty-nine years after its institution, the Town and Country Planning Act was revised, and the Development Plan formerly required by the law was replaced by the Local Development Framework. The change was designed to increase community and public involvement and also to help promote such government initiatives as energy efficient transportation, highway safety, housing supply, and natural preservation. Today, planning applications must also include a Design and Access statement, which describes the proposed design and the process by which it was determined, the extent of public engagement and the ways in which the proposed development adheres to the relevant principles of good design. The Design and Access statement is one way in which the government creates planning policies with an eye to broad public interests, rather than the private interests or profitability of a single individual or corporation.

9. It must be true that the Town and Country Planning Act:

    A. has not changed fundamentally since it became law.
    B. is concerned with preservation as well as construction.
    C. no longer requires a Local Development Framework.
    D. applies only in England and Wales.

10. According to the passage, which of these assertions must be false?

    A. Listed buildings can be refurbished.
    B. Listed buildings have some architectural or historical relevance.
    C. Listed buildings can never be repaired.
    D. Listed buildings cannot be altered without consent.

11. A planning application in the UK today must include:

    A. some evidence of engagement with the public.
    B. a Development Plan.
    C. consent of the local council.
    D. a study of projected impact on local roads.

12. The author would most likely agree that town planning:

    A. cannot impact the housing supply.
    B. can reduce carbon emissions.
    C. cannot improve highway safety.
    D. should only apply to publicly-owned property.

All testimony taken by the commission must be transcribed in the language in which it is given. The possible languages for testimony to the commission are English, French, Arabic or a tribal language.

All testimony must also be summarised in either English or French. Summaries of testimony may be prepared in the field, or at the commission's head office in Strasbourg. Due to a lack of trans-lators who speak both Arabic and French in the field, all testimony transcribed in Arabic can only be summarised into French at the head office. No-one at head office speaks the tribal languag-es, so all testimony taken and transcribed in a tribal language must be summarised in English or French by translators working in the field.

All summarised testimonies will be translated into the alternate language (English or French), before being indexed with all other summaries in the same language. The alternate translation of summaries and indexing of summaries must be completed at head office.

13. No-one at head office translates Arabic.

    A. True
    B. False
    C. Can't tell

14. A testimony may be taken, transcribed and initially summarised entirely in English.

    A. True
    B. False
    C. Can't tell

15. Testimony taken in a tribal language must be transcribed in French.

    A. True
    B. False
    C. Can't tell

16. Summaries of testimony taken in Arabic must be completed in Strasbourg.

    A. True
    B. False
    C. Can't tell

The foundations for United Nations Educational, Scientific and Cultural Organization (UNESCO) World Heritage Sites were laid almost a quarter of a century before the first locations were recognised in 1978. In 1954 the government of Egypt decided to construct the Aswan High Dam. The dam's resulting reservoir would flood a part of the Nile Valley that contained invaluable cultural and historical sites from ancient Egypt and ancient Nubia. Per a 1959 request from the Egyptian and Sudanese governments, the then Director-General of UNESCO, Vittorino Veronese, petitioned member states to lend support and donate funds to preserve the historic sites. As a result, several notable temples were salvaged and relocated, hundreds of sites were excavated and recorded, and thousands of artefacts were recovered.

Hailed as a success, the campaign led to UNESCO's preparation of a draft convention for the protection of humanity's significant cultural heritage. In 1965, the United States' White House called for the collective preservation of historical sites and natural sites with the establishment of a World Heritage Trust. The trust would encourage international cooperation to protect "the world's superb natural and scenic areas and historic sites for the present and the future of the entire world citizenry." A single text encompassing the conservation of cultural and natural wonders was agreed upon and the Convention Concerning the Protection of the World Cultural and Natural Heritage was signed during UNESCO's General Assembly in Paris on 16 November 1972. It came into force three years later, on 17 December 1975.

Today, there are over 1,070 World Heritage Sites in 167 countries. The United Kingdom itself has 26 cultural, four natural, and one mixed site – as well as a threatened site: Liverpool's Maritime Mercantile City. One of the world's largest trading centres in the 18th and 19th centuries, the Maritime Mercantile City had a pioneering role in the development of modern dock technology, transportation, and port management. While it was declared a cultural World Heritage Site in 2004, the World Heritage Committee – the governing body that enforces the Convention – listed the Maritime Mercantile City as in danger in 2012. Liverpool Waters, a proposed redevelopment scheme of the docklands north of the city centre, would significantly alter the skyline of the city as well as fragment and isolate the distinctive dock areas.

17. The United States called for the preservation of natural sites as well as cultural sites because:

A. the United States had an abundance of superb natural sites.
B. it wanted both to be preserved for future generations.
C. a natural site in the United Kingdom is threatened by a redevelopment scheme.
D. member states were more likely to donate funds to protect natural sites.

18. According to the passage, which of the following statements about Liverpool's Maritime Mercantile City is true?

A. It is one of the world's largest trading centres.
B. Liverpool's skyline is changing as a result of its redevelopment.
C. The area made innovations in transport, technology and management within harbours.
D. Maritime and mercantile history is no longer considered valuable by the World Heritage Committee.

The foundations for United Nations Educational, Scientific and Cultural Organization (UNESCO) World Heritage Sites were laid almost a quarter of a century before the first locations were recognised in 1978. In 1954 the government of Egypt decided to construct the Aswan High Dam. The dam's resulting reservoir would flood a part of the Nile Valley that contained invaluable cultural and historical sites from ancient Egypt and ancient Nubia. Per a 1959 request from the Egyptian and Sudanese governments, the then Director-General of UNESCO, Vittorino Veronese, petitioned member states to lend support and donate funds to preserve the historic sites. As a result, several notable temples were salvaged and relocated, hundreds of sites were excavated and recorded, and thousands of artefacts were recovered.

Hailed as a success, the campaign led to UNESCO's preparation of a draft convention for the protection of humanity's significant cultural heritage. In 1965, the United States' White House called for the collective preservation of historical sites and natural sites with the establishment of a World Heritage Trust. The trust would encourage international cooperation to protect "the world's superb natural and scenic areas and historic sites for the present and the future of the entire world citizenry." A single text encompassing the conservation of cultural and natural wonders was agreed upon and the Convention Concerning the Protection of the World Cultural and Natural Heritage was signed during UNESCO's General Assembly in Paris on 16 November 1972. It came into force three years later, on 17 December 1975.

Today, there are over 1,070 World Heritage Sites in 167 countries. The United Kingdom itself has 26 cultural, four natural, and one mixed site – as well as a threatened site: Liverpool's Maritime Mercantile City. One of the world's largest trading centres in the 18th and 19th centuries, the Maritime Mercantile City had a pioneering role in the development of modern dock technology, transportation, and port management. While it was declared a cultural World Heritage Site in 2004, the World Heritage Committee – the governing body that enforces the Convention – listed the Maritime Mercantile City as in danger in 2012. Liverpool Waters, a proposed redevelopment scheme of the docklands north of the city centre, would significantly alter the skyline of the city as well as fragment and isolate the distinctive dock areas.

19. According to the passage, which of these statements must be false?

   A. Liverpool Waters poses a risk to a World Heritage Site.
   B. The ideas behind the World Heritage Trust came into force 10 years after the initial proposal.
   C. The United States is no longer a member of UNESCO.
   D. UNESCO was not formed until 1978.

20. The author would most likely agree that:

   A. the majority of natural World Heritage sites are in the US.
   B. Liverpool is at the forefront of modern technology.
   C. natural areas were officially recognised as World Heritage sites in 1972.
   D. innovation and progress are not always beneficial.

The last few winters in the UK have proven especially harsh. Each winter seems to bring several major snowfalls of 5 to 8 inches in 24 hours; most of the UK is not equipped for such 'blizzards'. Only a few local authorities in England have snow ploughs, as gritting lorries are usually sufficient for snowfalls of 3 inches or less. Unfortunately, gritting salt is not effective during snowfalls with larger accumulations, with the consequence that thousands of schools have had to shut, sometimes for a week or even longer, until the snow has melted, because there is no other way of clearing the roads and pavements.

Many people have suggested that the UK must plan better and invest in appropriate winter equipment, so the country does not continue to stop working and traveling whenever there is more than a few inches of snow. Some countries with very harsh winters, such as Norway and Sweden, view road safety as a shared responsibility of all drivers (rather than purely a matter of state spending) and require all cars and lorries to switch to studded tyres during fixed dates each winter. Other countries that experience frequent blizzards in winter, such as the USA and Canada, invest in mechanised equipment that can clear airport runways quickly, dig out snow that has settled around planes parked at boarding gates and 'de-ice' planes so they are safe to fly in the harshest of winter conditions. Sadly, there is no such equipment at major British airports such as Heathrow, where a blizzard in December 2010 required hundreds of planes that were parked at passenger gates as the snow fell to be dug out by hand, resulting in severe flight delays for five days and costing the airlines and the British economy to lose tens of millions of pounds.

Alongside blizzards, there have been several instances of severe rainfall and flash flooding throughout the UK in recent years, such as Storm Desmond, which affected 16,000 homes in Cumbria during December 2015, and flash flooding in Cornwall in the summer of 2017, with a month's worth of rain falling on a single day in August. This heavy rainfall can be equally disruptive without effective preparation and planning: Storm Desmond is estimated to have cost the country £500 million.

21. The author would least likely agree with which of these assertions?

   A. A storm in 2015 incurred costs of £500m.
   B. Winters in the UK have been much snowier in the last few years.
   C. Snow ploughs are only effective at combating snowfall of 3 inches or less.
   D. The UK experienced a blizzard in 2010.

22. Gritting salt works best when:

   A. applied to roads before snow falls.
   B. used in combination with studded tyres.
   C. supplied from North America or Scandinavia.
   D. fewer than 3 inches of snow accumulates.

23. The passage suggests that Heathrow does not have:

   A. any of the equipment found at American airports.
   B. all the same equipment as Canadian airports.
   C. a plan to deal with passengers in a blizzard.
   D. a method of clearing snow from parked planes.

24. The most severe consequence of heavy snow in the UK mentioned in the passage is that:

   A. children missed a day of school.
   B. pavements were especially slippery.
   C. financial losses in the tens of millions were incurred.
   D. Heathrow had to hire American de-icing equipment.

Kathleen Mansfield Beauchamp Murry, better known by her pseudonym Katherine Mansfield, was born in 1888 in New Zealand. The daughter of a prominent banker, she moved to London in 1903 to attend Queen's College, where she trained as a professional cellist. She would go on to become one of the early 20th century's most significant short story writers, best known for writing in which she explored alienation, mental illness and disruption. Some of her short stories, such as 'The Garden Party,' 'The Daughters of the Late Colonel' and 'The Fly,' continue to be taught in schools and universities today.

Though she lived only 34 years, Mansfield had an active and tumultuous life. She was close to many important members of the literary community in London in the early 20th century, including such notable writers as Virginia Woolf and D.H. Lawrence. She was engaged several times, and, in 1909, married George Bowden, a singing teacher, whom she left just hours into their marriage. This hasty marriage and divorce particularly distressed her parents, who sent her away to a spa town in Germany later that year. Though a very difficult time in Mansfield's life, her time in Germany was enormously influential on her writing. It was here that she was introduced to the work of the late Russian playwright Anton Chekhov, who would become one of her most important literary inspirations.

Mansfield was incredibly prolific while she was in Germany. Returning to London the following January, she published more than a dozen short stories in A.R. Orage's socialist magazine *The New Age*, though she had managed to publish only one story and one poem in the previous fifteen months she'd spent living in London. Her time in Germany also set the foundation for the first published collection of her stories, *In a German Pension*. The collection was well received by critics in the UK and inspired her to submit a short story, "The Woman at the Store" to John Middleton Murry's magazine *Rhythm*. The two would marry in London in 1918, a year after Mansfield was diagnosed with tuberculosis. Though Mansfield sought treatment abroad in her later years, her illness prevented her from ever returning to her home in New Zealand. She died in 1922 in France, while seeking treatment.

25. Chekhov lived in Germany for a time.

    A. True
    B. False
    C. Can't tell

26. Of all the arts, Mansfield achieved greatest recognition for her accomplishments in music.

    A. True
    B. False
    C. Can't tell

27. Mansfield was a prominent socialist.

    A. True
    B. False
    C. Can't tell

28. Mansfield was married and divorced in the same year.

    A. True
    B. False
    C. Can't tell

Light travels faster than anything else in the universe, but it still has a finite, relatively constant speed: 299,792,458 meters per second, when travelling in a vacuum. This finite speed means that we can derive a unit of distance from the speed of light: a light-year is the distance that a particle of light can travel in a year. It also means that the further away a source of light is, the older the light will be when it eventually reaches an observer. Accordingly, many of the distant stars in the night sky may already have ceased to exist – what we are actually seeing is simply the light they emitted millions of years ago.

We first began to understand light in this way during the nineteenth century, when a number of different scientists undertook experiments to calculate the speed of light to a high degree of accuracy. One of the most famous of these scientists was Michel Foucault, a Frenchman who developed a system of rotating mirrors that allowed him to measure the discrepancies in time between different channelled beams of light. Foucault's system allowed him to measure the speed of light as 298,000,000 m/s, a far more accurate reading than had previously been achieved. Foucault's method was later expanded to an even larger scale in the U.S. in 1926, bringing the measurement to an unprecedented level of accuracy.

One of the first people to recognise the implications of the constant speed of light in a vacuum was a German scientist called Felix Eberty. In 1846 he published a book called 'The Stars and World History', which used the recently discovered fact of the speed of light to imagine the possibility of looking into different points in the history of the earth. This short work – perhaps one of the earliest works of science fiction – imagined what would be possible if humans were able to travel away from Earth faster than the speed of light and then look back upon it. By varying their distance, he wrote, they would be able to vary the age of the light that reached them, and therefore see events on the surface of the earth hundreds or even thousands of years ago.

It is now generally accepted that nothing can travel faster than the speed of light, so Eberty's notion that humans could 'outrun' light and then look back upon the earth remains a fiction. But his ideas were very influential in their time. Albert Einstein, the physicist who famously developed the general theory of relativity at the start of the twentieth century, later cited 'The Stars and World History', which he read as a child, as an early inspiration. In recent decades scientists have used principles similar to those first imagined by Eberty to examine, not the early history of the earth, but the early history of the outer reaches of the universe. With the launch of extremely sensitive satellite telescopes, in orbit far away from the interference of earth-based signals, scientists have been able to 'observe' the background radiation left over from just after the 'Big Bang', the mysterious expansion event that is believed to have begun the universe some 13.6 billion years ago, giving them a window into the long history of the universe itself.

29. The use of light-years as a measure of distance relies upon:

    A. rotating mirrors in order to measure distance travelled.
    B. knowing the absolute speed of light in meters per second.
    C. a theory proposed by Felix Eberty.
    D. the speed of light being countable and reasonably fixed.

30. The author would most likely agree that Eberty's theory:

    A. has been adapted by modern scientists to aid the study of the formation of the universe.
    B. inspired Foucault's mirror experiment.
    C. led to the invention of an exceptionally sensitive satellite.
    D. has been conclusively disproved.

Light travels faster than anything else in the universe, but it still has a finite, relatively constant speed: 299,792,458 meters per second, when travelling in a vacuum. This finite speed means that we can derive a unit of distance from the speed of light: a light-year is the distance that a particle of light can travel in a year. It also means that the further away a source of light is, the older the light will be when it eventually reaches an observer. Accordingly, many of the distant stars in the night sky may already have ceased to exist – what we are actually seeing is simply the light they emitted millions of years ago.

We first began to understand light in this way during the nineteenth century, when a number of different scientists undertook experiments to calculate the speed of light to a high degree of accuracy. One of the most famous of these scientists was Michel Foucault, a Frenchman who developed a system of rotating mirrors that allowed him to measure the discrepancies in time between different channelled beams of light. Foucault's system allowed him to measure the speed of light as 298,000,000 m/s, a far more accurate reading than had previously been achieved. Foucault's method was later expanded to an even larger scale in the U.S. in 1926, bringing the measurement to an unprecedented level of accuracy.

One of the first people to recognise the implications of the constant speed of light in a vacuum was a German scientist called Felix Eberty. In 1846 he published a book called 'The Stars and World History', which used the recently discovered fact of the speed of light to imagine the possibility of looking into different points in the history of the earth. This short work – perhaps one of the earliest works of science fiction – imagined what would be possible if humans were able to travel away from Earth faster than the speed of light and then look back upon it. By varying their distance, he wrote, they would be able to vary the age of the light that reached them, and therefore see events on the surface of the earth hundreds or even thousands of years ago.

It is now generally accepted that nothing can travel faster than the speed of light, so Eberty's notion that humans could 'outrun' light and then look back upon the earth remains a fiction. But his ideas were very influential in their time. Albert Einstein, the physicist who famously developed the general theory of relativity at the start of the twentieth century, later cited 'The Stars and World History', which he read as a child, as an early inspiration. In recent decades scientists have used principles similar to those first imagined by Eberty to examine, not the early history of the earth, but the early history of the outer reaches of the universe. With the launch of extremely sensitive satellite telescopes, in orbit far away from the interference of earth-based signals, scientists have been able to 'observe' the background radiation left over from just after the 'Big Bang', the mysterious expansion event that is believed to have begun the universe some 13.6 billion years ago, giving them a window into the long history of the universe itself.

31. Eberty's book theorised that events in the past could be viewed on Earth if the observer:

   A. moved away from Earth at a speed greater than 299,792,458 meters per second.
   B. travelled away from Earth at a varying speed.
   C. measured the discrepancies between
   D. travelled towards Earth at a speed greater than 299,792,458 meters per second.

32. Foucault's experiment involving rotating mirrors:

   A. suggested that past events could be observed by travelling away from objects at great speed.
   B. led to the most accurate measurement for the speed of light being recorded.
   C. inspired Albert Einstein to develop his theory of relativity.
   D. proved that nothing can travel faster than the speed of light.

New technology and an innovative approach towards data processing in sport, known as sabermetrics, have changed the role of the talent scout. Where before, talent scouts could be found at the sides of rainy football pitches, doggedly attending to youth league games, searching for a spark of talent; a sabermetrics scout is more likely to be found passionlessly crunching statistics on a computer. Information technology, some believe, has transformed the task of spotting future football talent from something of a subjective art into a mathematical science.

Sabermetrics was first developed in the U.S., in the world of baseball. Its roots lie in early American computer experiments with sports. Essential statistics about baseball had been collected on paper for most professional matches since the nineteenth century, recording each particular player's performance across five different criteria. Davey Johnson, a manager at the start of his career, began using computers in the early seventies to write programs that simulated the outcomes of different games based on such data. Johnson continued to attempt to use computers, but it was a trio of managers at the team Oakland Athletics who later used the approach to great success, by using statistics to identify undervalued players and acquiring them cheaply. This story famously featured in Michael L. Lewis's book *Moneyball*, published in 2003, and a film released in 2011 under the same name.

The moneyball method was soon utilized by professionals from other sports, including football, and today there are a range of companies that offer vital statistics on almost all football players across all leagues around the world, statistics that are readily available to football scouts as they assess who might be best for a club to acquire and nurture next. These companies can record over 1,500 separate statistical 'events' during each game, giving scouts an unprecedented well of information from which to draw when they are making their decisions. Likewise, there are many companies that sell video clips of individual players, maintaining a database of around 160,000 different players.

Despite all this information now available to football talent scouts, however, some now believe that the ideas behind *Moneyball* cannot be so readily applied to football as they can to other sports. Though sabermetrics was heavily invested in by clubs like Liverpool and Stoke City, who both employed sports statisticians from the U.S., the term has these days fallen out of favour, and critics argue that, though statistics can be useful and have revolutionised talent scouting, there is no statistical formula for the perfect team, and the acolytes of sabermetrics are expecting too much from their numbers. Sabermetrics was perhaps the best option for a baseball team like Oakland Athletics in 2002, underfunded compared to its opponents and looking for an edge, but in the Premier League, in which most teams have ample supplies of cash, its benefits are less vital, argue critics. Perhaps the subjective art of traditional talent scouting cannot yet be fully written off.

33. Most football scouts now use the moneyball method to find new players.

   A. True
   B. False
   C. Can't tell

34. Oakland Athletics received less funding than many of its competitors.

   A. True
   B. False
   C. Can't tell

New technology and an innovative approach towards data processing in sport, known as saber-metrics, have changed the role of the talent scout. Where before, talent scouts could be found at the sides of rainy football pitches, doggedly attending to youth league games, searching for a spark of talent; a sabermetrics scout is more likely to be found passionlessly crunching statistics on a computer. Information technology, some believe, has transformed the task of spotting future football talent from something of a subjective art into a mathematical science.

Sabermetrics was first developed in the U.S., in the world of baseball. Its roots lie in early American computer experiments with sports. Essential statistics about baseball had been collected on paper for most professional matches since the nineteenth century, recording each particular player's performance across five different criteria. Davey Johnson, a manager at the start of his career, began using computers in the early seventies to write programs that simulated the outcomes of different games based on such data. Johnson continued to attempt to use computers, but it was a trio of managers at the team Oakland Athletics who later used the approach to great success, by using statistics to identify undervalued players and acquiring them cheaply. This story famously featured in Michael L. Lewis's book *Moneyball*, published in 2003, and a film released in 2011 under the same name.

The moneyball method was soon utilized by professionals from other sports, including football, and today there are a range of companies that offer vital statistics on almost all football players across all leagues around the world, statistics that are readily available to football scouts as they assess who might be best for a club to acquire and nurture next. These companies can record over 1,500 separate statistical 'events' during each game, giving scouts an unprecedented well of information from which to draw when they are making their decisions. Likewise, there are many companies that sell video clips of individual players, maintaining a database of around 160,000 different players.

Despite all this information now available to football talent scouts, however, some now believe that the ideas behind *Moneyball* cannot be so readily applied to football as they can to other sports. Though sabermetrics was heavily invested in by clubs like Liverpool and Stoke City, who both employed sports statisticians from the U.S., the term has these days fallen out of favour, and critics argue that, though statistics can be useful and have revolutionised talent scouting, there is no statistical formula for the perfect team, and the acolytes of sabermetrics are expecting too much from their numbers. Sabermetrics was perhaps the best option for a baseball team like Oakland Athletics in 2002, underfunded compared to its opponents and looking for an edge, but in the Premier League, in which most teams have ample supplies of cash, its benefits are less vital, argue critics. Perhaps the subjective art of traditional talent scouting cannot yet be fully written off.

35.   Sabermetrics has been most successful in the sporting industry when applied to football teams.

    A.   True
    B.   False
    C.   Can't tell

36.   Michael L. Lewis was the first to develop the theory of sabermetrics.

    A.   True
    B.   False
    C.   Can't tell

People are often surprised to learn that the moon is not alone in its orbit of the Earth. In 1986, astronomer Duncan Waldron discovered the object 1986 TO. Waldron later named this asteroid Cruithne, which in Old Irish refers to a Scottish tribe (In English called 'the Picts') who lived during the late Iron Age and early Medieval period. Although commonly referred to at the time of its discovery as our second moon, Cruithne is more accurately described as a 'quasi-orbital satellite' of Earth, as its orbit around Earth is simply one part of its true orbit around the sun. This contrasts to the moon's orbit, which travels directly around the Earth.

Another quasi-orbital satellite, named simply 2016 HO3, was discovered yet more recently in April 2016 by the Pan STARRS 1 asteroid telescope in Haleakala, Hawaii. This satellite, thought to be 40-100 metres in diameter, has an extremely elliptical orbit, which has been described as a horseshoe orbit by astronomers, due to the uncommon loop of its route. Describing 2016 HO3's trajectory, The Center of NEO studies commented that, 'In effect, this small asteroid is caught in a game of leap frog with Earth that will last for hundreds of years.' Astronomers have calculated that, though only recently discovered, 2016 HO3 has been a stable quasi-satellite of Earth's for over a century. More than a decade ago, another asteroid followed a similar trajectory around Earth and the sun, but as the gravitational pull on this asteroid was not as strong as the Earth's pull on 2016 HO3, it has since moved outside of Earth's gravitational pull and disappeared from view outside of our solar system.

For many, the thought that we could have an object with such a large mass so close to Earth for the past 100 years and fail to notice it is a terrifying example of our global lack of preparation in the event of an asteroid collision. Thankfully, neither Cruithne nor 2016 HO3 are expected to collide with Earth, although the possibility of an asteroid collision is not as unlikely as many believe. Numerous other asteroids passing close to Earth have been deemed 'near misses' by scientists. In 2014, asteroid 2014 DX110 passed less than one lunar distance (a measurement from the centre of the Earth to the centre of the moon) to Earth. Before it passed safely by, it was predicted to have a one in ten chance of a collision with Earth.

We know how dangerous a collision could be from the effects of the asteroid collision in the prehistoric period—it took only one collision to destroy an entire species of animal. Thankfully, for the past 65.5 million years, all asteroid collisions have been considerably smaller than the meteoroid that killed the dinosaurs, and yet these asteroids still pose a significant threat. In 1908, a meteoroid hit Tunguska, Russia with an estimated 15 megatons of TNT a force 1,000 times greater than the impact of the atomic bomb dropped on Hiroshima. Though Cruithne and 2016 HO3 will remain our peaceful companions for years to come, the risk of asteroid collision remains significant. Worldwide, we have no clear strategy in place to combat the effects of an unexpected collision with Earth, and yet, as the discovery of 2016 HO3 makes evident; even very large asteroids are capable of taking us by surprise.

37. In 2014, an asteroid passing within a lunar distance of Earth had a 10% chance of collision.

  A. True
  B. False
  C. Can't tell

38. The name Cruithne refers to both a quasi-orbital satellite and an Old Irish tribe from the late Iron Age.

  A. True
  B. False
  C. Can't tell

People are often surprised to learn that the moon is not alone in its orbit of the Earth. In 1986, astronomer Duncan Waldron discovered the object 1986 TO. Waldron later named this asteroid Cruithne, which in Old Irish refers to a Scottish tribe (In English called 'the Picts') who lived during the late Iron Age and early Medieval period. Although commonly referred to at the time of its discovery as our second moon, Cruithne is more accurately described as a 'quasi-orbital satellite' of Earth, as its orbit around Earth is simply one part of its true orbit around the sun. This contrasts to the moon's orbit, which travels directly around the Earth.

Another quasi-orbital satellite, named simply 2016 HO3, was discovered yet more recently in April 2016 by the Pan STARRS 1 asteroid telescope in Haleakala, Hawaii. This satellite, thought to be 40-100 metres in diameter, has an extremely elliptical orbit, which has been described as a horseshoe orbit by astronomers, due to the uncommon loop of its route. Describing 2016 HO3's trajectory, The Center of NEO studies commented that, 'In effect, this small asteroid is caught in a game of leap frog with Earth that will last for hundreds of years.' Astronomers have calculated that, though only recently discovered, 2016 HO3 has been a stable quasi-satellite of Earth's for over a century. More than a decade ago, another asteroid followed a similar trajectory around Earth and the sun, but as the gravitational pull on this asteroid was not as strong as the Earth's pull on 2016 HO3, it has since moved outside of Earth's gravitational pull and disappeared from view outside of our solar system.

For many, the thought that we could have an object with such a large mass so close to Earth for the past 100 years and fail to notice it is a terrifying example of our global lack of preparation in the event of an asteroid collision. Thankfully, neither Cruithne nor 2016 HO3 are expected to collide with Earth, although the possibility of an asteroid collision is not as unlikely as many believe. Numerous other asteroids passing close to Earth have been deemed 'near misses' by scientists. In 2014, asteroid 2014 DX110 passed less than one lunar distance (a measurement from the centre of the Earth to the centre of the moon) to Earth. Before it passed safely by, it was predicted to have a one in ten chance of a collision with Earth.

We know how dangerous a collision could be from the effects of the asteroid collision in the prehistoric period—it took only one collision to destroy an entire species of animal. Thankfully, for the past 65.5 million years, all asteroid collisions have been considerably smaller than the meteoroid that killed the dinosaurs, and yet these asteroids still pose a significant threat. In 1908, a meteoroid hit Tunguska, Russia with an estimated 15 megatons of TNT a force 1,000 times greater than the impact of the atomic bomb dropped on Hiroshima. Though Cruithne and 2016 HO3 will remain our peaceful companions for years to come, the risk of asteroid collision remains significant. Worldwide, we have no clear strategy in place to combat the effects of an unexpected collision with Earth, and yet, as the discovery of 2016 HO3 makes evident; even very large asteroids are capable of taking us by surprise.

39. 2016 HO3 orbits the Earth as part of its true orbit of the sun.

    A. True
    B. False
    C. Can't tell

40. The last significant asteroid collision was in 1908.

    A. True
    B. False
    C. Can't tell

Historically, three criteria have been considered necessary and sufficient for knowledge; a claim must be justified, it must be true, and it must be believed. This justified, true, belief account (JTB) of knowledge has its origins in Ancient Greece, where Plato first described the theory in his Socratic dialogue, *Meno*. Socrates, in discussion with the eponymous Thessalian, distinguishes between true belief and knowledge, using the route from Athens to the nearby town of Larissa as an example. Whether one has a true belief or knowledge about the road to Larissa, the result is the same: a successful journey to Larissa. Puzzled, Meno asks Socrates why knowledge is prized over true belief if their outcomes are the same. Socrates explains that although true beliefs are as useful as knowledge, they often fail to stay in their place or remain tied down. Knowledge, on the other hand, remains fixed, it is tethered by an account of the reasons why the claim is the case. Thus, knowledge is a true belief that is justified.

For over two millennia, a justified true belief was considered equivalent to knowledge. It was not until the early 20th century that philosophers such as Bertrand Russell and Ludwig Wittgenstein began to question the criteria. Yet, it is Edmund Gettier that is credited with the refutation of the long-held standard. By the time Gettier has secured his first teaching position at Michigan's Wayne State University, he had hardly any publications. Pressured by the institution's administration to publish, Gettier unenthusiastically wrote a three-page paper in 1963, entitled "Is Justified True Belief Knowledge?" The essay set out two counterexamples to the JTB theory. These Gettier cases, as they later became known, depicted individuals who possessed a justified true belief over a claim, but who failed to know it. With a curt and unenthusiastic paper, Gettier demonstrated that the JTB account was inadequate, as it could not account of all instances of knowledge. Gettier, who is now retired, never published another paper.

In his 1963 paper, Gettier gave birth a whole new area of study, spawning countless arguments in attempt to respond to what became known as the Gettier problem. Three approaches have been used by theorists to respond to the Gettier problem. The first involves the rejection of the Gettier cases and affirmation of the JTB account of knowledge, commonly done by arguing that individuals in Gettier cases have insufficient levels of justification. Knowledge, for these responders, demands stronger justifications than the Gettier cases exhibit. The second approach is to accept the Gettier cases, stating that they exposed a problem in the JTB theory. While JTB is necessary, it is not sufficient for knowledge, and that a complete account of knowledge will contain a fourth criterion. For these responders, knowledge is justified, true, belief, and some additional condition. Epistemologists pursuing the final approach generally accept the problem raised by Gettier cases, yet they reject the JTB account. Rather than a fourth condition, these theorists seek to replace the justification criterion with some other qualification. Despite the best efforts of modern theorists to salvage the JTB account, it might never return to its former status as a dominant theory.

41. Gettier cases challenge the justified, true, belief account of knowledge because they:

   A. demonstrate that beliefs can be fallible.
   B. detail instances in which individuals have a justified, true, belief, but are not aware that they have it.
   C. indicate that truth is not necessary for knowledge.
   D. depict individuals with insufficient justification for their beliefs.

42. Which of these conclusions must be false?

   A. The JTB account was first expounded by Plato.
   B. The JTB account is a tripartite definition of knowledge.
   C. Socrates prized knowledge over true beliefs.
   D. Prior to Gettier's publication, no one had ever questioned the justified, true, belief account.

Historically, three criteria have been considered necessary and sufficient for knowledge; a claim must be justified, it must be true, and it must be believed. This justified, true, belief account (JTB) of knowledge has its origins in Ancient Greece, where Plato first described the theory in his Socratic dialogue, *Meno*. Socrates, in discussion with the eponymous Thessalian, distinguishes between true belief and knowledge, using the route from Athens to the nearby town of Larissa as an example. Whether one has a true belief or knowledge about the road to Larissa, the result is the same: a successful journey to Larissa. Puzzled, Meno asks Socrates why knowledge is prized over true belief if their outcomes are the same. Socrates explains that although true beliefs are as useful as knowledge, they often fail to stay in their place or remain tied down. Knowledge, on the other hand, remains fixed, it is tethered by an account of the reasons why the claim is the case. Thus, knowledge is a true belief that is justified.

For over two millennia, a justified true belief was considered equivalent to knowledge. It was not until the early 20th century that philosophers such as Bertrand Russell and Ludwig Wittgenstein began to question the criteria. Yet, it is Edmund Gettier that is credited with the refutation of the long-held standard. By the time Gettier has secured his first teaching position at Michigan's Wayne State University, he had hardly any publications. Pressured by the institution's administration to publish, Gettier unenthusiastically wrote a three-page paper in 1963, entitled "Is Justified True Belief Knowledge?" The essay set out two counterexamples to the JTB theory. These Gettier cases, as they later became known, depicted individuals who possessed a justified true belief over a claim, but who failed to know it. With a curt and unenthusiastic paper, Gettier demonstrated that the JTB account was inadequate, as it could not account of all instances of knowledge. Gettier, who is now retired, never published another paper.

In his 1963 paper, Gettier gave birth a whole new area of study, spawning countless arguments in attempt to respond to what became known as the Gettier problem. Three approaches have been used by theorists to respond to the Gettier problem. The first involves the rejection of the Gettier cases and affirmation of the JTB account of knowledge, commonly done by arguing that individuals in Gettier cases have insufficient levels of justification. Knowledge, for these responders, demands stronger justifications than the Gettier cases exhibit. The second approach is to accept the Gettier cases, stating that they exposed a problem in the JTB theory. While JTB is necessary, it is not sufficient for knowledge, and that a complete account of knowledge will contain a fourth criterion. For these responders, knowledge is justified, true, belief, and some additional condition. Epistemologists pursuing the final approach generally accept the problem raised by Gettier cases, yet they reject the JTB account. Rather than a fourth condition, these theorists seek to replace the justification criterion with some other qualification. Despite the best efforts of modern theorists to salvage the JTB account, it might never return to its former status as a dominant theory.

43. The author of the passage would be most likely to agree with which of the following statements?

   A. The JTB account remains an inadequate theory.
   B. Gettier refuted the longstanding JTB theory with just one counterexample.
   C. Gettier is at the forefront of current epistemological discussions.
   D. The JTB account theory remains a prevailing theory.

44. One response to the Gettier problem is to:

   A. refute the belief criterion.
   B. substitute the justification condition.
   C. claim that knowledge is impossible.
   D. demonstrate that justified, true, belief cannot account for all knowledge.

STOP. IF YOU FINISH BEFORE TIME IS UP, CHECK ANY QUESTIONS YOU HAVE MARKED FOR REVIEW. YOU MAY GO BACK TO QUESTIONS IN THIS SECTION ONLY.

Section 2: Decision Making (31 Minutes)

This section contains 29 questions. Each question is a standalone item. Some questions may include information in the form of charts, graphs, tables or diagrams. Most questions will have five answer choices. Your task is to select the best option based on the data provided.

Some questions will include five parts, instead of five answer choices. You must drag and drop the correct answer (Yes or No) for each of the five parts. These questions are worth 2 marks each. You only get 2 marks if you answer all five parts correctly. If you answer mostly correctly, you will get 1 mark.

Answer all 29 questions in Section 2, selecting one of the possible answers and circling the letter corresponding to the appropriate answer in your test paper. For drag-and-drop questions, write YES or NO in the grey box beside each of the five parts.

When you are finished with this section, you may use any remaining time to review your work in this section only. Once you proceed to the next section, you may not return to this section.

You will have 31 minutes to answer the questions. It is in your best interest to select an answer for every item as there is no penalty for wrong answers.

Set your timer for 31 minutes, turn the page and begin the section.

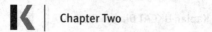

1. It is in the interest of almost all commuters to travel to work by public transport. However, no commuter should travel to work by public transport if they own a bicycle.

    Place 'Yes' if the conclusion does follow. Place 'No' if the conclusion does not follow.

It is not in the interest of some commuters to use public transport.	
Commuters who own bicycles should never use public transport.	
It is in the interest of all commuters to own bicycles.	
Most commuters should travel to work by public transport unless they own a bicycle.	
Some commuters who own bicycles should still travel to work by public transport.	

2. Of the garments in the winter collection, more than half were outdoor wear and the rest indoor wear. None of the indoor wear was made from fur, but some of it was made from suede. All items in the winter collection were hand-stitched.

Place 'Yes' if the conclusion does follow. Place 'No' if the conclusion does not follow.

Most of the items in the winter collection were made from either fur or suede.	
This garment from the winter collection is made from fur, so it must be outdoor wear.	
All outdoor wear from the winter collection is either made from fur or hand-stitched.	
This garment from the winter collection is indoor wear, so it must be made from suede.	
All indoor wear from the winter collection is either made from fur or hand-stitched.	

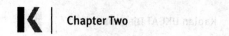

3. A farmer owns both sheep and cows. Some of the cows have horns. Apart from the horned cows, all of the animals are brown.

    Place 'Yes' if the conclusion does follow. Place 'No' if the conclusion does not follow.

All of the sheep are brown.	
An animal with horns must be a cow.	
None of the animals that are brown are cows.	
None of the sheep have horns.	
An animal that is brown and has horns must be a sheep.	

4. All of the current principals of schools in Astley were born in Brigg. Some of the previous principals of schools in Brigg were born in Astley.

    Place 'Yes' if the conclusion does follow. Place 'No' if the conclusion does not follow.

Some of the current principals of schools in Brigg were born in Astley.	
All of the previous principals of schools in Astley were born in Brigg.	
None of the current principals of schools in Astley were born in Astley.	
Some of the previous principals of schools in Brigg were not born in Astley.	
Some of the current principals of schools in Brigg were not born in Brigg.	

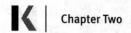

5.   A wine shop sells only red and white wines. All sparkling wines are white. Wine can be sold by the bottle or by the case (of 6 bottles), which offers a 30% discount. Sparkling wine can only be sold by the bottle.

Place 'Yes' if the conclusion does follow. Place 'No' if the conclusion does not follow.

Twelve bottles of sparkling wine can be bought for less money than ten bottles of the same wine.	
The wine shop cannot sell a case containing six bottles of sparkling wine.	
A case of six identical red wines will cost less than five bottles of the same wine.	
A bottle of wine from a case will not be white.	
Six single bottles of red wine will cost more than a case of white wine.	

Three siblings all enrolled at university when they were 19 years old. None were born in the same year and each spent a different amount of time studying: three years, four years and five years.

Lawrence and Felix both graduated in the same year.

Belinda graduated in 2016 and did not take the five-year course.

The eldest sibling enrolled at university in 2009.

Felix took the four-year course.

6.   Which of the following must be true?
   A.   Felix is at least two years younger than Lawrence.
   B.   Belinda is at least two years younger than Felix.
   C.   Felix is at least three years older than Belinda.
   D.   Lawrence is at least four years older than Belinda.

The diagram below shows a small aquarium with nine tanks, each containing one, two or three creatures. Each tank is occupied by one of three species: Nurse Sharks, Common Octopi and Green Sea Turtles. Each species occupies three tanks.

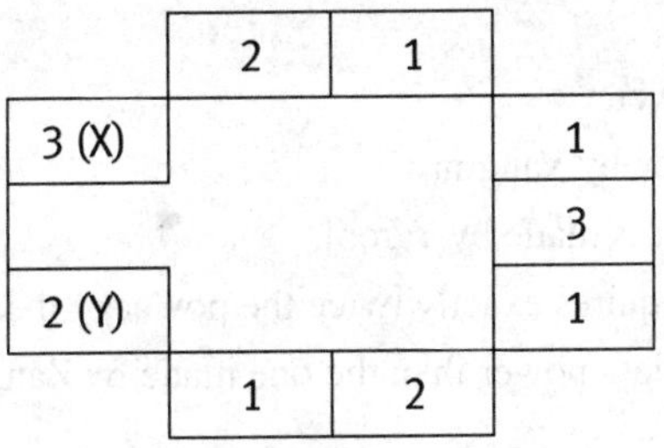

Common Octopi do not occupy the same vertical column as Nurse Sharks.

Nurse Sharks are always kept in one-creature tanks.

There are exactly five Common Octopi in the aquarium.

7.   Which species must be in the tanks labelled X and Y?
   A.   X: Green Sea Turtles, Y: Green Sea Turtles
   B.   X: Common Octopi Y: Green Sea Turtles
   C.   X: Common Octopi, Y: Common Octopi
   D.   X: Green Sea Turtles, Y: Common Octopi

A large business has split its headquarters into six sections. Each section houses one of the business's six departments.

Neither Logistics nor Customer Support are located in Epsilon-Section.

Marketing is in either Alpha-Section or Zeta-Section.

Sales is located in Delta-Section.

Human Resources is not in Epsilon-Section or Beta-Section.

Gamma-Section does not house Human Resources or Accounts.

8. In which section is Accounts located?

    A. Alpha-Section
    B. Beta-Section
    C. Epsilon-Section
    D. Zeta-Section

Five electrical appliances—a hairdryer, an ice-cream maker, a juicer, a kettle and a lamp—each require a different power supply (3V, 5V, 6V, 9V, an 12V). Each appliance also has a different manufacturer: Urbit, Vaughn, X-Tech, Yarcol and Zan.

The kettle requires the least power.

The ice-cream maker is not made by Vaughn.

Either the hairdryer or the juicer is made by Yarcol.

The appliance made by Urbit requires exactly twice the power of the ice-cream maker.

The Vaughn appliance requires less power than the one made by Zan but more than the one made by X-Tech.

9. Which pair of manufacturers made the 5V and 9V appliances (in that order)?

    A. Vaughn and Yarcol.
    B. X-Tech and Zan.
    C. Urbit and X-Tech.
    D. Vaughn and Zan.

10. Should all university students be required to do one hour per week of unpaid work, such as caring for the elderly, to improve their contribution to the community?

   Select the strongest argument from the statements below.

   A. Yes, because voluntary work has been shown to improve relationships between university students and local residents.
   B. Yes, because some university students vandalise property and are rude to members of the community.
   C. No, because some students have to spend a lot of time on their academic work.
   D. No, because some students already do voluntary work in the community.

11. Should electric cars be made available to buy at lower prices in order to cut emissions of greenhouse gases?

   Select the strongest argument from the statements below.

   A. Yes, because electric cars are good for the environment.
   B. Yes, because people are more likely to buy electric cars if they are cheaper than conventional cars.
   C. No, because electric car manufacturers might stop producing electric cars and make products with a higher profit margin instead.
   D. No, because most of the energy used to power electric cars is generated by burning fossil fuels, which releases large amounts of greenhouse gases.

12. Should the UK Government be forced to return the Elgin Marbles – carved artefacts from the Parthenon in Athens currently held at the British Museum – to Greece?

   Select the strongest argument from the statements below.

   A. Yes, because the Marbles might be damaged if somebody attempts to steal them from the British Museum.
   B. Yes, because the majority of independent polls show that both Greek and UK citizens want the Marbles to be returned to Greece.
   C. No, because then all foreign artefacts in UK museums would have to be returned.
   D. No, because the British Museum might make less money without the Elgin Marbles as an exhibit.

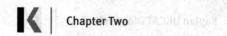

13. Would allowing employers to pay less than the minimum wage enable more disabled people to enter the workforce?

    Select the strongest argument from the statements below.

    A. Yes, because if employers are able to pay lower wages, they might be able to take on more staff.
    B. Yes, because being able to enter the workforce will allow disabled people to play a bigger role in society.
    C. No, because employers should not be able to discriminate against disabled people by paying them less.
    D. No, because even if employers could pay less than the minimum wage, disabled people still might not get hired.

14. Should all prisoners have televisions installed in their cells in order to prevent rioting?

    Select the strongest argument from the statements below.

    A. Yes, criminals are more likely to reform if they are treated well while in prison.
    B. Yes, prison riots can quickly escalate and put both guards and prisoners lives in danger.
    C. No, a lack of televisions in cells is not the reason there are riots in prisons.
    D. No, luxuries such as televisions should only be provided to prisoners as a reward for good behaviour.

15. A mortgage broker looked at the range of mortgages taken by her customers in 2010 and 2015. The percentages of customers taking each type of mortgage are indicated in the graphs.

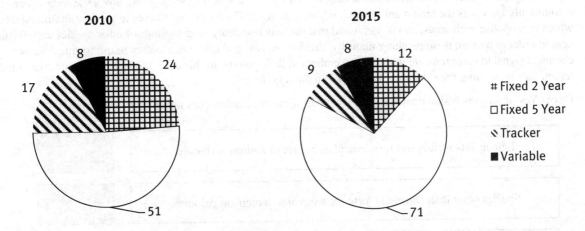

Place 'Yes' if the conclusion does follow. Place 'No' if the conclusion does not follow.

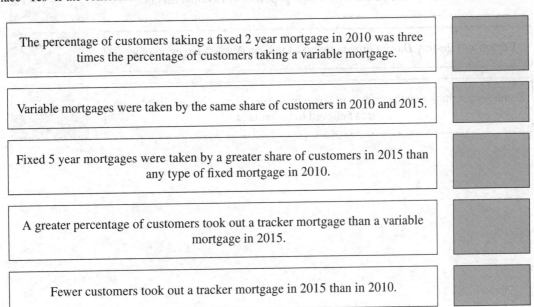

The percentage of customers taking a fixed 2 year mortgage in 2010 was three times the percentage of customers taking a variable mortgage.	
Variable mortgages were taken by the same share of customers in 2010 and 2015.	
Fixed 5 year mortgages were taken by a greater share of customers in 2015 than any type of fixed mortgage in 2010.	
A greater percentage of customers took out a tracker mortgage than a variable mortgage in 2015.	
Fewer customers took out a tracker mortgage in 2015 than in 2010.	

16. Devil's gardens are parts of the rainforest where only one species of tree appears to grow, an unusual sight in an area that is usually known for high levels of biodiversity. They are called 'devil's gardens' because the local population often considers the area to be haunted by evil spirits that prevent other flora from developing. Scientists researching the distinctive phenomena now believe that it is caused by a species of ant, *myrmelachista schumanni* – commonly known as the lemon ant – which inhabits the area. The lemon ant thrives in the *Duroia hirsuta* trees which monopolise such areas, and it was found that the ants injected young saplings of other species with formic acid in order to prevent them reaching maturity. Previously, ants had only been known to use formic acid as a chemical signal to communicate with other members of their colony. In this case, however, scientists concluded lemon ants were using the substance as a kind of natural herbicide.

Place 'Yes' if the conclusion does follow. Place 'No' if the conclusion does not follow.

Lemon ants mainly use formic acid as a form of natural herbicide.	
Species other than *Duroia hirsuta* are a threat to lemon ant colonies.	
Lemon ants flourish in areas with a high population of *Duroia hirsuta*.	
Lemon ants destroy *Duroia hirsuta* trees so they can develop larger colonies.	
Some people think that the growth of some plant species may be restricted in an area believed to be haunted.	

17. Two medications were compared in terms of how much they change the electrical activity of the heart. This is measured by recording the QTc on an electrocardiogram. A greater QTc is more dangerous. A normal QTc is less than 440 ms; anything more than this is potentially dangerous.

	Dose (mg)	Average increase in QTc (ms)
Citalopram	20	8.5
	40	12.6
	60	18.5
Escitalopram	10	4.2
	20	6.8
	30	10.7

Place 'Yes' if the conclusion does follow. Place 'No' if the conclusion does not follow.

The change in QTc at 40 mg of citalopram is double that of escitalopram at 20 mg.	
A patient with a QTc of 430 ms who starts taking a dose of 40 mg of citalopram could have potentially dangerous QTc if his QTc change matches the average for this dose of medication.	
It could be dangerous to give any of the indicated doses of either drug to a patient with a QTc of 450 ms.	
Trebling the dose of escitalopram to 30 mg trebles the QTc change.	
A patient with a QTc of 429 ms who starts taking a dose of 40 mg of escitalopram would have an average QTc increase in excess of 12 ms, which is potentially dangerous.	

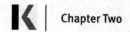

18.   A manufacturer was carrying out an assessment of three new antiseptic liquids, investigating their effectiveness against microorganisms (including both bacteria and viruses). Liquid A killed 50% more bacteria than Liquid B. However, Liquid A only killed 76% of viruses, whilst Liquid B killed 92%. Liquid C had the worst performance of all three liquids in terms of killing microorganisms, but had the best overall tolerance in those with sensitive skin, causing irritation in only 10% of all human subjects tested.

Place 'Yes' if the conclusion does follow. Place 'No' if the conclusion does not follow.

Liquid B killed 50% more bacteria than Liquid A.	
Liquid B killed 16% more bacteria than Liquid A.	
Liquid C killed 10% of viruses.	
Liquid B killed more viruses than Liquid C.	
Liquid A caused skin irritation in more than 1 in 10 human test subjects.	

Contestants in a beauty pageant were asked to name the factors that, in their view, are most important to success in pageant competition.

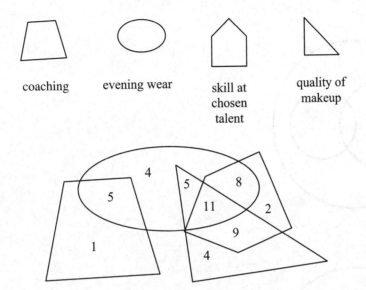

coaching   evening wear   skill at chosen talent   quality of makeup

19. Which of the following can be concluded from the diagram?

A. The number of contestants that voted for evening wear in combination with coaching is the same as the number that voted for evening wear in combination with quality of makeup.

B. Twice as many contestants selected skill at chosen talent as their sole factor as chose evening wear as their sole factor.

C. The number of contestants that selected coaching as a factor, in combination with or without any other factors, is the same as the number that selected quality of makeup in combination with or without any other factors.

D. Nine contestants selected skill at chosen talent and evening wear as their sole factors.

20. Which of the following diagrams best represents the statements 'all snakes are reptiles', 'no frogs are reptiles' and 'all frogs and reptiles are cold-blooded'?

A.

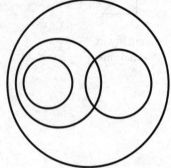

B.

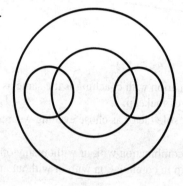

C.

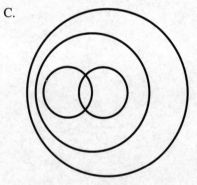

D.

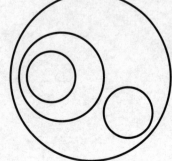

Students in their first year at university were asked which societies they belonged to.

The triangle represents the Debate Society.

The diamond represents Football Club.

The pentagon represents Boat Club.

The oval represents the Film Society.

The star represents the Dance Society.

The arch represents the Medics Society.

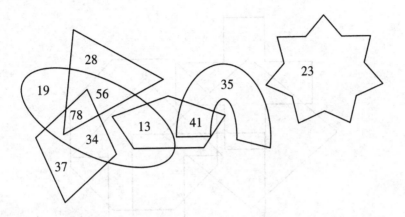

21. Which of the following must be true?

   A. Fewer than 50 students joined the Film Society in combination with the Debate Society and Football Club.
   B. More students joined the Dance Society than the Medics Society.
   C. None of the students joined Boat Club without joining at least one other society.
   D. Fewer than half the number of students that joined only Football Club joined only the Film Society.

A group of adventurous friends compare notes on their favourite mountaineering holidays. One friend makes a diagram representing the various combinations of locations that the friends have visited on mountaineering holidays.

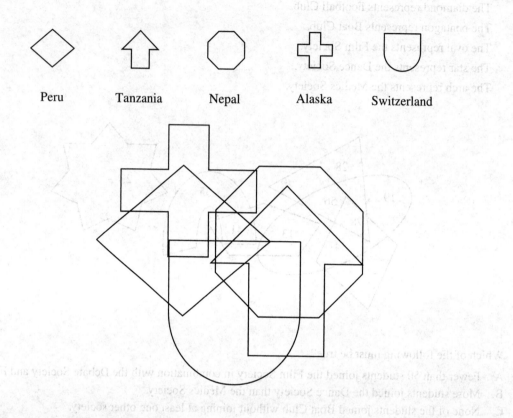

Peru   Tanzania   Nepal   Alaska   Switzerland

22.   Which of the following combinations of locations has been visited by at least one of the friends on mountaineering holidays?

A.   Alaska, Peru, Nepal and Tanzania.
B.   Nepal, Switzerland, Tanzania and Peru.
C.   Alaska, Nepal and Switzerland.
D.   Peru and Tanzania.

I like coffee and tea. Sometimes I add milk or sugar to these beverages; sometimes I add both. Sometimes I just like to drink a glass of milk. I would never drink a glass of sugar, for obvious reasons.

23.   Which of the following diagrams represents the information about my beverage preferences?

A.

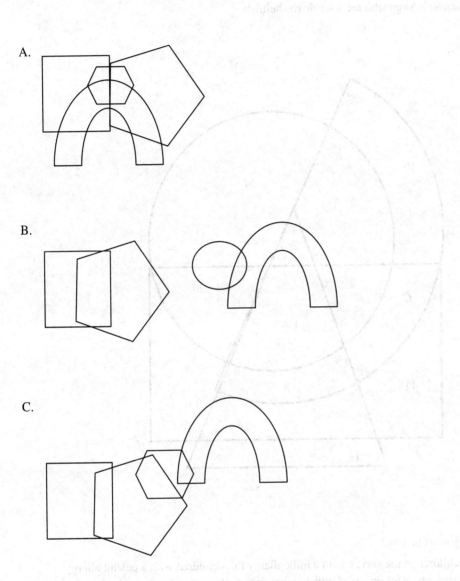

B.

C.

D.

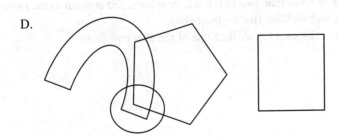

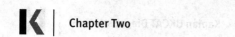
The diagram shows the results of a survey showing the food allergies of a group of children.

The semicircle represents children who are allergic to peanuts.

The rectangle represents children who are allergic to milk.

The circle represents children who are allergic to eggs.

The triangle represents children who are allergic to shellfish.

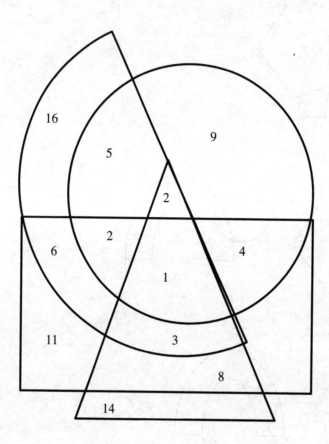

24. Which of the following must be true?

A. There were more children in the survey with a milk allergy than children with a peanut allergy.

B. Of the children in the survey allergic to shellfish, more than half were allergic to at least one other allergen.

C. The number of children who were allergic to more than two of the allergens surveyed is equal to the number of children with allergies to both milk and shellfish (but nothing else).

D. The majority of children in the survey were allergic to more than one of the allergens listed.

A bookshop tracks the customers who buy different types of books over the course of a week.

The rectangle represents the customers who bought crime novels.

The oval represents the customers who bought historical novels.

The triangle represents the customers who bought science fiction novels.

The hexagon represents the customers who bought poetry.

The star represents the customers who bought biographies.

The crescent represents the customers who bought cookbooks.

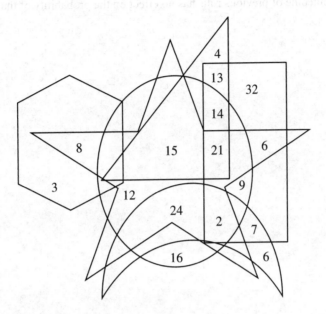

25. How many customers bought novels, but not biographies or cookbooks?

   A. 63
   B. 88
   C. 101
   D. 114

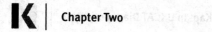

26. Amelia has a die that is rigged so that it has a 2/3 probability of landing with the 6 face showing. She rolls it three times. On the first and second rolls, the die lands with the 6 face showing.

    Amelia states that the probability that she will roll a 6 on the third attempt is 0.

    Is Amelia correct?

    A. Yes, because the chance of landing on a 6 is 2 out of 3, so on the third attempt the die must land on another face.
    B. Yes, because unfair dice never land on the same side every time.
    C. No, because the probability of rolling a 6 on the third roll is 2/3 cubed, or 8/27.
    D. No, because the outcome of previous rolls has no effect on the probability of the current roll.

27. Two new laptops are being tested at a research facility.

    Laptop Q fails the streaming test in all but 72% of trials.

    The average maximum battery life (between charges) for Laptop Q is 8.5 hours.

    Of the 200 copies of Laptop R being tested, a total of 56 fail the streaming test.

    Twenty copies of Laptop R have an average maximum battery life of 11 hours; for the rest, it's 7 hours.

    Judging **only** on the streaming test and average maximum battery life, is Laptop Q the better laptop?

    A. Yes, because its battery lasts more than an hour longer (on average) than Laptop R's battery.
    B. Yes, because it is more likely to pass the streaming test than Laptop R.
    C. No, because Laptop R has an average maximum battery life that is more than two hours longer.
    D. No, because Laptop R is 28% more likely to pass the streaming test.

28. Following an Easter egg hunt, each child selects one treat at random from a basket containing two types of treats: dark chocolate bunnies and white chocolate sheep. Each treat is contained in a box of equal size, and the basket is held above the children's eye level, so they cannot see what they are selecting.

   Three boys and three girls select bunnies; two boys and one girl select sheep; one more girl is waiting to make the final selection. There is at least one of each option remaining in the basket.

   Has the chance of a bunny being selected now increased from the start when the next girl selects a treat?

   A. Yes, if there were at least three times as many bunnies as sheep in the basket at the start.
   B. Yes, if there is exactly one sheep remaining in the basket and there were five more bunnies than sheep in the basket at the start.
   C. No, the girl is more likely to select a sheep than a bunny, compared to the first child to select a treat.
   D. No, the girl has an equal probability of selecting either treat, so a bunny is less likely to be selected than at the start.

29. The relative difficulty of two exams is compared by looking at the scores achieved by two different schools, each with the same number of students.

   Students in School A achieved an average score of 70% in Exam X, and an average score of 75% in Exam Y. Students in School B scored, on average, 28 out of 40 in Exam X, and lost 8 marks out 40 in Exam Y.

   Based **only** on the average scores for each exam, is Exam Y more difficult?

   A. Yes, the average score for Exam X is higher in both schools than the average for Exam Y.
   B. Yes, although School A scored higher on average in Exam Y than X, School B scored much more highly in Exam X than Y, which outweighs this.
   C. No, in both schools the average score for Exam Y was higher than the average score for Exam X.
   D. No, in School B the average scores for both exams were the same, but School A scored higher on average in Exam Y.

STOP. IF YOU FINISH BEFORE TIME IS CALLED, CHECK ANY QUESTIONS YOU HAVE MARKED FOR REVIEW. YOU MAY GO BACK TO QUESTIONS IN THIS SECTION ONLY.

Section 3: Quantitative Reasoning (24 Minutes)

This section contains 9 sets of data, each of which is followed by four questions. Each question will have five answer choices. Your task is to select the best option based on the data provided. Some sets may consist of four individual questions, each with its own data.

You may use a calculator to answer the questions in this section. On Test Day, you will be provided with an onscreen calculator that can perform the four basic operations (addition, subtraction, multiplication and division) along with only a few extra features (percentage, reciprocal, square root and memory buttons). You should not use any functions beyond these on the calculator used for this Mock Test.

Answer all 36 questions in Section 3, selecting one of the possible answers and circling the letter corresponding to the appropriate answer in your test paper.

When you are finished with this section, you may use any remaining time to review your work in this section only. Once you proceed to the next section, you may not return to this section.

You will have 24 minutes to answer the questions. It is in your best interest to select an answer for every item as there is no penalty for wrong answers.

Set your timer for 24 minutes, turn the page and begin the section.

The table below shows the crime rates for Lincoln, and for the UK as a whole, in 2005/2006:

Offence	Total Locally	Per 1000 Population	
		Locally	Nationally
Robbery	73	0.84	1.85
Theft of a motor vehicle	283	3.27	4.04
Theft from a motor vehicle	789	9.12	9.56
Sexual offences	186	2.15	1.17
Violence against a person	2885	33.33	19.97
Burglary	552	6.38	5.67
TOTAL	4768		

	Local	National
POPULATION	86,547	60,200,000
HOUSEHOLDS	37,000	24,900,000

1. What percentage of crimes committed locally were thefts of motor vehicles?

   A. 6%
   B. 9%
   C. 14%
   D. 17%
   E. 25%

2. What was the rate of crimes per person in Lincoln in 2005/2006?

   A. 1:22
   B. 1:21
   C. 1:20
   D. 1:19
   E. 1:18

3. Approximately how many crimes of violence against a person were committed nationally in 2005/2006?

   A. 120,000
   B. 160,000
   C. 1.2 million
   D. 1.4 million
   E. 1.6 million

4. How many burglaries were recorded in Lincoln in 2006/2007, if the total number of burglaries increased by 10% from 2005/2006?

   A. 582
   B. 607
   C. 624
   D. 648
   E. 652

Each year the University of Chalvey library keeps a record of its visitors. Below is a chart showing which subject areas the different visitors came from in 2017.

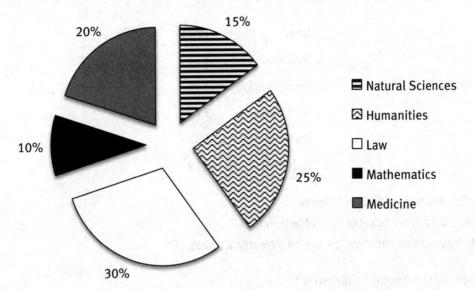

The different segments of the chart indicate the percentages of students from the different faculties.

5. Which faculty had the fewest number of student visitors to the library in 2017?
   A. Humanities
   B. Law
   C. Mathematics
   D. Medicine
   E. Natural Sciences

6. If there were 800 student visitors from the Faculty of Medicine, how many students in total visited the library in 2017?
   A. 3,200
   B. 4,000
   C. 5,000
   D. 6,500
   E. 8,000

7. If there were 400 student visitors in the Faculty of Mathematics and 25% of all student visitors are first year students, approximately how many first year Law student visitors were there in 2017?
   A. 300
   B. 600
   C. 900
   D. 1200
   E. 1500

8. What percentage of total student visitors were not students in the Law or Humanities faculties?
   A. 35%
   B. 45%
   C. 55%
   D. 65%
   E. 75%

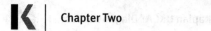

Omar is preparing for a raffle draw at a local charity event. He has made a list of prize items he purchased last week and their costs, which are the only prizes in the raffle:

Item	Price
Mountain Bike	£185
Tennis Racket	£45
MP3 Player	£75
Picnic hamper	£32
Hair dryer	£19

- Raffle tickets are priced at £1.50 each.
- Omar has set a sales target of 300 raffle tickets.
- The MP3 player and hair dryer are the only electrical prizes.

9. How much did Omar spend on the prizes?

  A. £85
  B. £115
  C. £140
  D. £356
  E. £435

10. If Omar meets the sales target exactly, how much profit will Omar make on the raffle?

  A. £77
  B. £94
  C. £114
  D. £122
  E. £144

11. This week, electrical products are on sale for 50% off. How much could Omar have saved if he bought the electrical prizes this week?

  A. £9
  B. £27
  C. £47
  D. £126
  E. £309

12. How many raffle tickets must Omar sell to make a profit of £300?

  A. 372
  B. 437
  C. 438
  D. 512
  E. 513

Russell and his friend Pauline decide to buy the total unshaded piece of land at £70 per square metre to use it as a shared vegetable patch. The unshaded piece of land has a total area of 18 m². They plan to split the land into symmetrical vegetable patches of equal area.

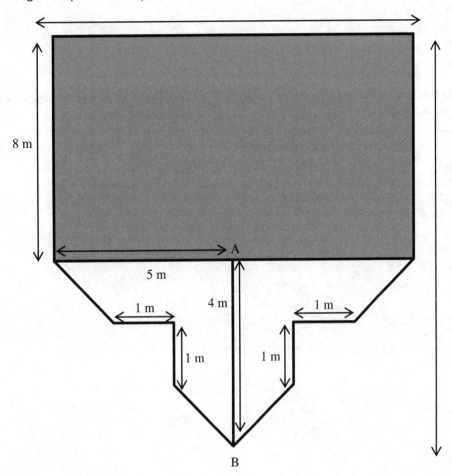

13. What is the total price that Russell and Pauline must pay for the unshaded land?

   A. £1040
   B. £1180
   C. £1260
   D. £1300
   E. £1420

14. After buying the land, they split the area equally with a 4 m fence (along line *AB*) to mark the borders of their respective vegetable patches. What is the area of Russell's vegetable patch, in cm²?

   A. 900 cm²
   B. 9,000 cm²
   C. 18,000 cm²
   D. 90,000 cm²
   E. 180,000 cm²

15. After a few months, Pauline decides to buy 30% of the shaded area to expand her vegetable patch, but the price of land has increased to £114 per square metre. How much will it cost her to buy the extra land?

    A. £2394
    B. £2736
    C. £3468
    D. £5700
    E. £6114

16. What is the total area of Pauline's vegetable patch in m², if Russell sells her half of his vegetable patch after she buys 30% of the shaded area?

    A. 28.5 m²
    B. 33 m²
    C. 37.5 m²
    D. 42 m²
    E. 44.5m²

There are four different models that car manufacturer Royal produce. Below is a graph showing how many miles each of the cars can travel for every gallon of fuel they use.

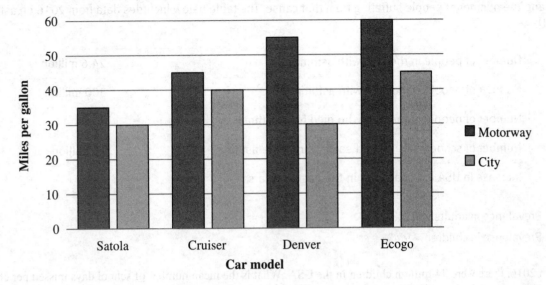

1 gallon = 4.5 litres

17. How many miles could you drive on a motorway on one gallon of fuel in the Denver car?

    A. 50
    B. 55
    C. 60
    D. 65
    E. 70

18. If fuel costs £1.10 a litre, approximately how much would a 30 mile city journey in a Satola cost?

    A. £1.10
    B. £2.20
    C. £3.65
    D. £4.50
    E. £4.95

19. Which of the models would be most economical for a journey that consists of 25 miles on the motorway and 5 miles in the city?

    A. Cruiser
    B. Denver
    C. Ecogo
    D. Satola
    E. both Cruiser and Denver

20. How many gallons of fuel do you need if you wanted to travel 405 miles on the motorway in a Cruiser?

    A. 6
    B. 7
    C. 8
    D. 9
    E. 10

Asthma is a common lung condition that causes intermittent breathing difficulties. Prevalence is the proportion of individuals within a particular group with the condition. Mortality rate is the proportion of deaths for a given cause and the number of people suffering from that cause. The table below includes data from 2016 on asthma in the USA:

Number of people in the USA with asthma	24.6 million
Number of people worldwide with asthma	300 million
Number of people in the USA who died from asthma	3,384
Number of school days missed each year due to asthma	13 million
Increase in USA asthma cases in the past 10 years	48%

- Prevalence in adults = 8.2%
- Prevalence in children = 9.4%

21. In 2016, there were 74 million children in the USA. What is the mean number of school days missed per child suffering from asthma?

    A. 1.31
    B. 1.44
    C. 1.58
    D. 1.72
    E. 1.87

22. Each year, 250,000 people die worldwide from asthma. What is the percentage difference between USA and worldwide asthma mortality rates?

    A. 172%
    B. 199%
    C. 211%
    D. 237%
    E. 251%

23. The total USA population was 323.1 million in 2016. How many asthma related deaths were there per 100,000 people in the USA that year?

    A. 1.05
    B. 1.11
    C. 1.19
    D. 1.23
    E. 1.34

24. In 2006, how many asthma sufferers were there in the USA?

    A. 14,870,000
    B. 15,020,000
    C. 15,910,000
    D. 16,620,000
    E. 17,460,000

Arabella has four horses: Dazzle, Truffles, Peppermint and Jack of Hearts.

Her brother Leander has a horse, Galaxy, with an average trotting speed of 9.2 miles per hour.

A riding trail starts at the edge of their estate, and extends a length of 11 miles through the neighbouring woodland.

25. Arabella rides Truffles at a trot for the full length of the riding trail from one end to the other, in 1 hour, 14 minutes. What is his average trotting speed on the ride, in miles per hour?

    A. 7.8
    B. 8.1
    C. 8.9
    D. 9.2
    E. 9.6

26. Arabella rides Jack of Hearts at a canter from the start of the trail to the far end, and then all the way back to the start at a trot. She notes that his speed on the ride out (which he completed in 44 minutes) was twice his speed on the ride back. What was his average speed on the total ride?

    A. 7.5 mph
    B. 10 mph
    C. 12.5 mph
    D. 15 mph
    E. 17.5 mph

27. Arabella rides Dazzle and Peppermint the full length of the trail and then all the way back to its start, both at a trot, on consecutive days. Dazzle's average trotting speed was 1.4 mph faster than Peppermint's, and Dazzle completed the ride 23 minutes faster than Peppermint's time of 2 hours, 39 minutes. What was Peppermint's average trotting speed, in miles per hour?

    A. 6.9
    B. 7.6
    C. 7.9
    D. 8.3
    E. 9.7

28. Which horse has the fastest average trotting speed?

    A. Dazzle
    B. Galaxy
    C. Jack of Hearts
    D. Peppermint
    E. Truffles

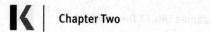

A country's prison service collects data on its prisoners. The following table contains information on prisoner's age at the end of 2017 and the age of these prisoners at admission:

Age at end of 2017	Age at Admission								Total
	≤20	21 – 30	31 – 40	41 – 50	51 – 60	61 – 70	71 – 80	> 80	
≤20	33,387	–	–	–	–	–	–	–	33,387
21 – 30	29,348	228,964	–	–	–	–	–	–	258,312
31 – 40	9,814	70,505	151,382	–	–	–	–	–	231,701
41 – 50	2,768	22,281	52,073	112,325	–	–	–	–	189,447
51 – 60	675	6,708	12,038	24,523	38,203	–	–	–	82,147
61 – 70	60	866	2,094	3,518	6,279	7,105	–	–	19,922
71 – 80	23	82	147	385	694	1,180	1,073	–	3,584
> 81	82	143	32	25	41	89	158	93	663
Total	76,157	329,549	217,766	140,776	45,217	8,374	1,231	93	819,163

29. How many per cent of prisoners were 50 or under at the end of 2017?

   A. 67%
   B. 73%
   C. 76%
   D. 82%
   E. 87%

30. What proportion of prisoners aged 71 or older at the end of 2017 were aged 30 or younger on their admission?

   A. 7.8%
   B. 8.3%
   C. 8.6%
   D. 9.1%
   E. 9.4%

There are two competing taxi companies operating at Airport X near City A. Company I charges £7.30 for the first two kilometres travelled, then charges an additional £0.90 for every additional 250 metres. Company II has a base rate of £1.50 for all journeys, followed by £0.70 per minute travelled, in addition to £1.15 per kilometer.

31. Raul takes uses Company II to travel from Airport X to his hotel. If the taxi drives at an average speed of 30 kilometres an hour, and the journey takes a total of 1 hour and 24 minutes, how much will Raul's journey cost?

   A. £58.80
   B. £96.60
   C. £108.60
   D. £125.40
   E. £156.90

32. What is the percentage increase in the cost of using Company I to travel 5 km in 10 minutes, compared to the cost of using Company II?

   A. 25%
   B. 27%
   C. 29%
   D. 31%
   E. 33%

Five weeks of single sales figures for five bands vying for the Christmas Number 1 chart position are shown below. Sales figures correspond to one single release per band. The Christmas Number 1 went to the group with the most sales in Week 3.

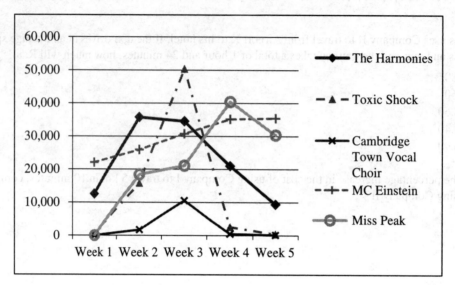

33. Which band saw the greatest percentage rise in sales from Week 2 to Week 3?

    A. Cambridge Town Vocal Choir
    B. The Harmonies
    C. MC Einstein
    D. Miss Peak
    E. Toxic Shock

34. In which week did the bands record the greatest total sales?

    A. Week 1
    B. Week 2
    C. Week 3
    D. Week 4
    E. Week 5

35. Which band saw the greatest decrease in sales from one week to the next?

    A. Cambridge Town Vocal Choir
    B. The Harmonies
    C. MC Einstein
    D. Miss Peak
    E. Toxic Shock

36. MC Einstein's Week 5 sales were what percentage of Week 5's total sales?

    A. 38%
    B. 41%
    C. 44%
    D. 47%
    E. 50%

STOP. IF YOU FINISH BEFORE TIME IS UP, CHECK ANY QUESTIONS YOU HAVE MARKED FOR REVIEW. YOU MAY GO BACK TO QUESTIONS IN THIS SECTION ONLY.

Section 4: Abstract Reasoning (13 Minutes)

This section contains 11 sets of five items each. There are four different question types:

Type 1: These items appear in sets of 5 test shapes, along with Set A and Set B. All the items in Set A are similar to each other, and all the items in Set B are similar to each other. Your task is determine in what way the shapes in each set are similar and to decide whether each test shape fits into Set A, Set B or neither set.

Type 2: These items appear as individual questions. You will see a progression of four boxes in a single row. Your task is to select the test shape that comes next in the progression.

Type 3: These items appear as individual questions. You will see a statement, with two boxes in the top row and two boxes in the bottom row. There will be some progression from the first box to the second box in the top row; the second box in the bottom row will be blank. Your task is to select the test shape that fills the blank box, so that the progression in the bottom row is the same as the progression in the top row.

Type 4: These items appear in sets of 5 questions, along with Set A and Set B. All the items in Set A are similar to each other, and all the items in Set B are similar to each other. Your task is to choose the test shape that belongs to the set mentioned in the question.

Answer all 55 questions in Section 4, selecting one of the possible answers and circling the letter corresponding to the appropriate answer in your test paper.

When you are finished with this section, you may use any remaining time to review your work in this section only. Once you proceed to the next section, you may not return to this section.

You will have 13 minutes to answer the questions. It is in your best interest to select an answer for every item as there is no penalty for wrong answers.

Set your timer for 13 minutes, turn the page and begin the section.

Set A	Set B
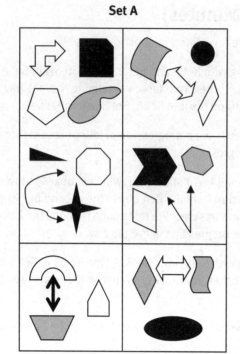	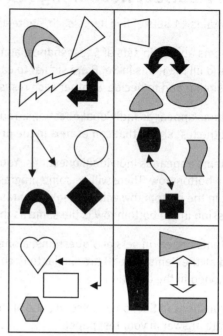

Test Shapes

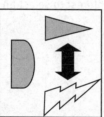

1	2	3	4	5
A. Set A	A. Set A	A. Set A	A. Set A	A. Set A
B. Set B	B. Set B	B. Set B	B. Set B	B. Set B
C. Neither	C. Neither	C. Neither	C. Neither	C. Neither

Set A   **Set B**

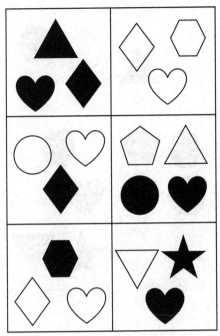 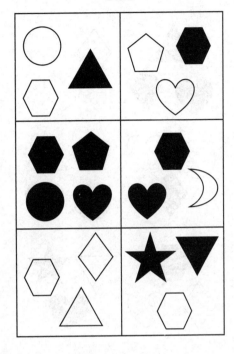

6. Which of the following test shapes belongs in Set A?

   A.   B.   C.   D.

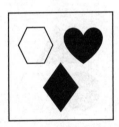 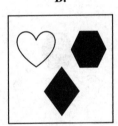 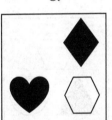 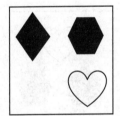

7. Which of the following test shapes belongs in Set B?

   A.   B.   C.   D.

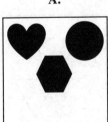 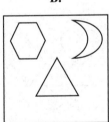 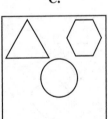 

8. Which of the following test shapes belongs in Set A?

   A.   B.   C.   D.

 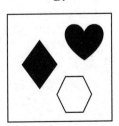 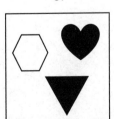 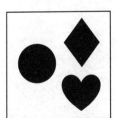

Set A   Set B

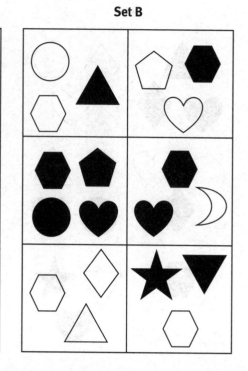

9.   Which of the following test shapes belongs in Set B?

A.   B.   C.   D.

   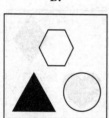   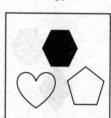   

10.   Which of the following test shapes belongs in Set A?

A.   B.   C.   D.

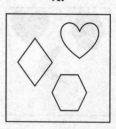   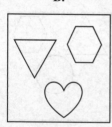      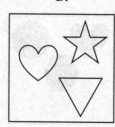

Set A

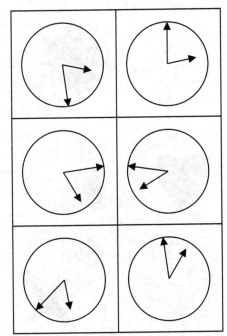

Set B

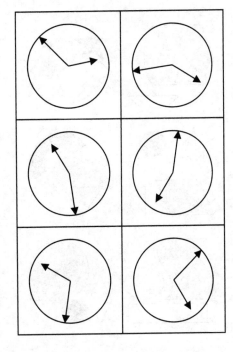

Test Shapes

11	12	13	14	15
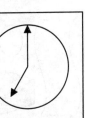	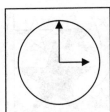	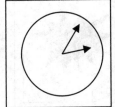	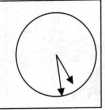	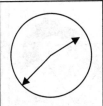

A. Set A   A. Set A   A. Set A   A. Set A   A. Set A
B. Set B   B. Set B   B. Set B   B. Set B   B. Set B
C. Neither   C. Neither   C. Neither   C. Neither   C. Neither

Set A

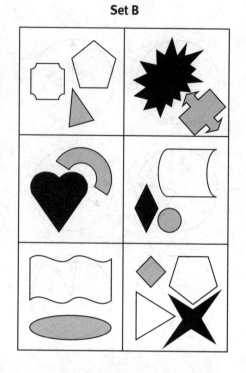

Set B

Test Shapes

16	17	18	19	20
A. Set A	A. Set A	A. Set A	A. Set A	A. Set A
B. Set B	B. Set B	B. Set B	B. Set B	B. Set B
C. Neither	C. Neither	C. Neither	C. Neither	C. Neither

Set A

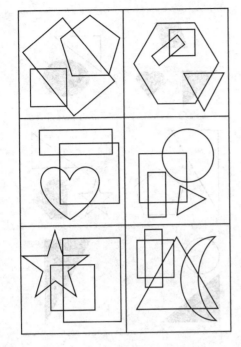

Set B

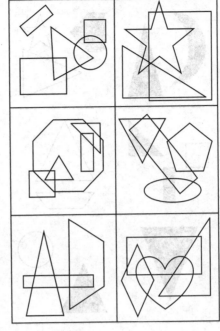

Test Shapes

| 21 | 22 | 23 | 24 | 25 |

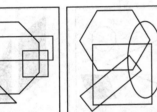 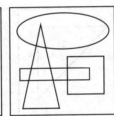 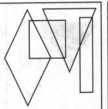

A. Set A
B. Set B
C. Neither

A. Set A
B. Set B
C. Neither

A. Set A
B. Set B
C. Neither

A. Set A
B. Set B
C. Neither

A. Set A
B. Set B
C. Neither

Set A

Set B

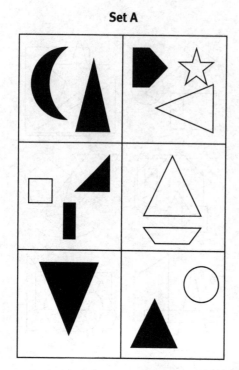

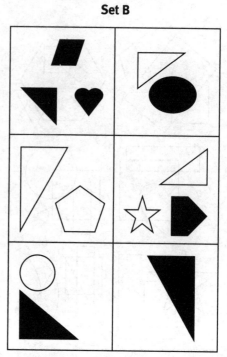

Test Shapes

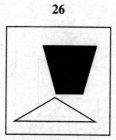

26	27	28	29	30

A. Set A
B. Set B
C. Neither

A. Set A
B. Set B
C. Neither

A. Set A
B. Set B
C. Neither

A. Set A
B. Set B
C. Neither

A. Set A
B. Set B
C. Neither

Set A

Set B

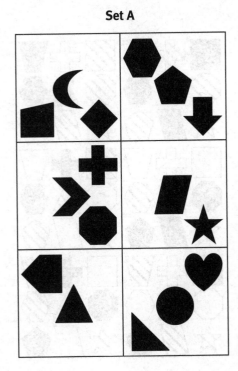
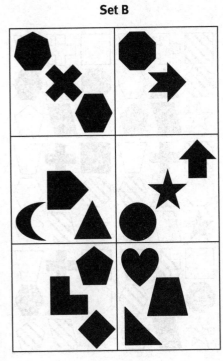

Test Shapes

31	32	33	34	35

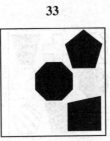

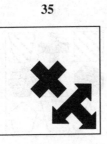

31
A. Set A
B. Set B
C. Neither

32
A. Set A
B. Set B
C. Neither

33
A. Set A
B. Set B
C. Neither

34
A. Set A
B. Set B
C. Neither

35
A. Set A
B. Set B
C. Neither

Set A   **Set B**

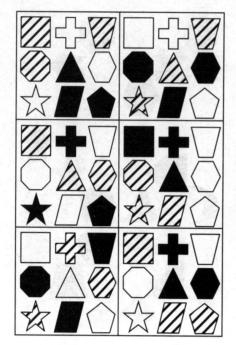 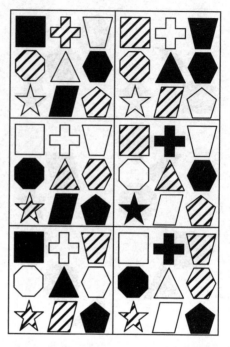

Test Shapes

36	37	38	39	40

A. Set A
B. Set B
C. Neither

A. Set A
B. Set B
C. Neither

A. Set A
B. Set B
C. Neither

A. Set A
B. Set B
C. Neither

A. Set A
B. Set B
C. Neither

Set A **Set B**

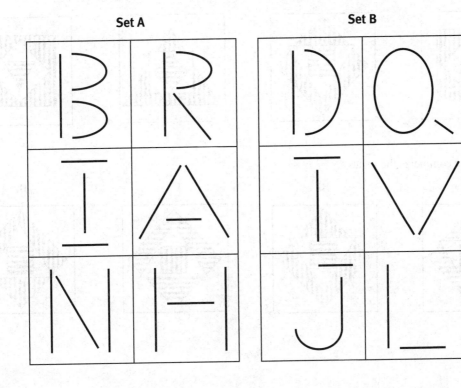

Test Shapes

41   42   43   44   45

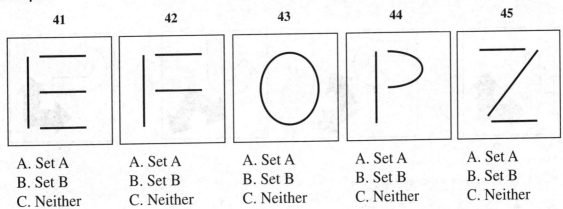

41	42	43	44	45
A. Set A	A. Set A	A. Set A	A. Set A	A. Set A
B. Set B	B. Set B	B. Set B	B. Set B	B. Set B
C. Neither	C. Neither	C. Neither	C. Neither	C. Neither

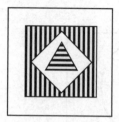 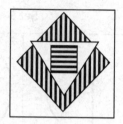 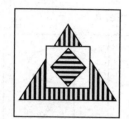 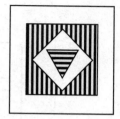

46. Which figure completes the series?

    A.   **B.**   **C.**   **D.**

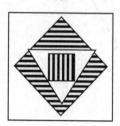   

 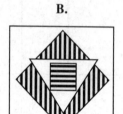 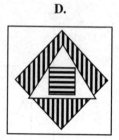

47. Which figure completes the series?

    A.   **B.**   **C.**   **D.**

  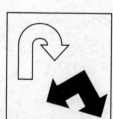 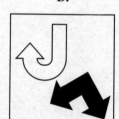

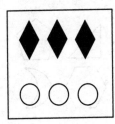

is to

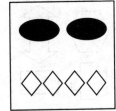

as

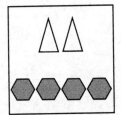

is to

48. Which figure completes the statement?

A.
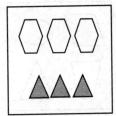

B.
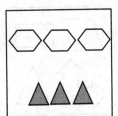

C.
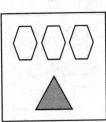

D.
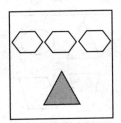

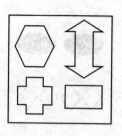

is to

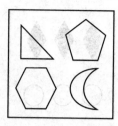

as

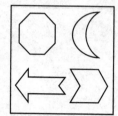

is to

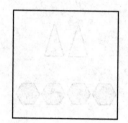

49. Which figure completes the statement?

A.   B.   C.   D.

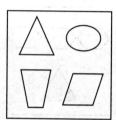 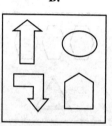 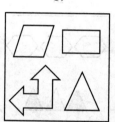 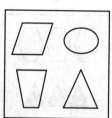

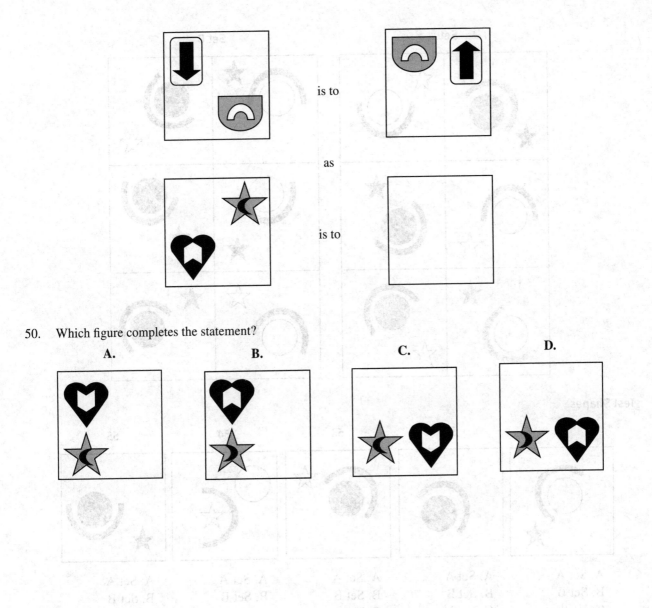

is to

as

is to

50. Which figure completes the statement?

A.   B.   C.   D.

Set A

Set B

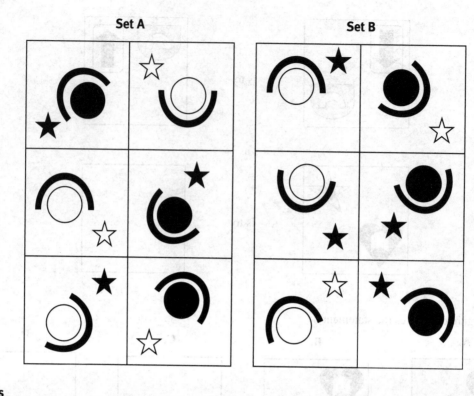

Test Shapes

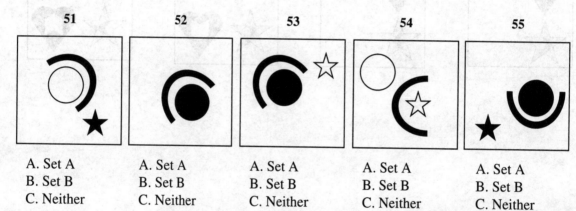

51	52	53	54	55
A. Set A	A. Set A	A. Set A	A. Set A	A. Set A
B. Set B	B. Set B	B. Set B	B. Set B	B. Set B
C. Neither	C. Neither	C. Neither	C. Neither	C. Neither

STOP. IF YOU FINISH BEFORE TIME IS UP, CHECK ANY QUESTIONS YOU HAVE MARKED FOR REVIEW. YOU MAY GO BACK TO QUESTIONS IN THIS SECTION ONLY.

Section 5: Situational Judgement (26 Minutes)

This section contains 21 theoretical scenarios, each involving a medical or dental professional, or a student preparing for a career in medicine or dentistry. Your task is to read the scenario carefully, and then make a series of judgements about possible options for responding to the situation in the scenario. There are two types of scenarios in this section:

Appropriateness: These scenarios will ask you to rate whether possible responses to the scenario are appropriate or inappropriate.

Importance: These scenarios will ask you to rate whether certain factors are important or not important to consider when responding to the scenario.

The first part of the section will contain Appropriateness scenarios; the final part of the section will contain Importance scenarios. Be sure to answer based on the appropriateness or importance of the response/factor to the person who is named in the question under the scenario. Evaluate the responses/factors independently of each other; do not assume that there will be a response/factor corresponding to each answer choice for each scenario.

Answer all 68 questions in Section 5, selecting one of the possible answers and circling the letter corresponding to the appropriate answer in your test paper.

When you are finished with this section, you may use any remaining time to review your work in this section only. Once you complete this section, you are finished with the Diagnostic Test. You may then assess your results using the scoring tables that follow.

You will have 26 minutes to answer the questions. It is in your best interest to select an answer for every item as there is no penalty for wrong answers.

Set your timer for 26 minutes, turn the page and begin the section.

Samia and Hayley are final year medical students. Their schedule includes a planned session of helping the junior doctors with work on the wards, followed by a tutorial. That morning, Samia receives a phone call from Hayley asking her to pass on the message that Hayley is unwell with diarrhoea and therefore cannot come in to the hospital today. On her way home, Samia is surprised to see Hayley working behind the counter at the local bakery.

How **appropriate** are each of the following responses by <u>Samia</u> in this situation?

1. Report Hayley to the medical school for lying about her illness

    A. A very appropriate thing to do
    B. Appropriate, but not ideal
    C. Inappropriate, but not awful
    D. A very inappropriate thing to do

2. Ask Hayley why she said she could not come to hospital if she was well enough to work in the bakery

    A. A very appropriate thing to do
    B. Appropriate, but not ideal
    C. Inappropriate, but not awful
    D. A very inappropriate thing to do

3. Ask Hayley the next day how she is feeling and whether she managed to get out and about at all the previous day

    A. A very appropriate thing to do
    B. Appropriate, but not ideal
    C. Inappropriate, but not awful
    D. A very inappropriate thing to do

Tameka is a junior doctor at a university hospital. One of the medical students whose work she supervises, Shaun, has joined her as Tameka asks a patient, Mrs Oswald, to sign the consent form for surgery to correct a bowel obstruction. Mrs Oswald is booked into theatre later in the day, and the need for the surgery is critical. Mrs Oswald says she is not sure about the surgery as she is terrified of needles, and does not think she can handle being anaesthetised. She asks if she can be hypnotised instead. Shaun sneers, and says that if Mrs Oswald is so superstitious, maybe they can hypnotise her bowel and avoid surgery altogether.

How **appropriate** are each of the following responses by **Tameka** in this situation?

4. Apologise to Mrs Oswald for the rude remark from her student

    A. A very appropriate thing to do
    B. Appropriate, but not ideal
    C. Inappropriate, but not awful
    D. A very inappropriate thing to do

5. Tell Shaun his comment is unhelpful, and ask him to apologise

    A. A very appropriate thing to do
    B. Appropriate, but not ideal
    C. Inappropriate, but not awful
    D. A very inappropriate thing to do

6. Explain to Mrs Oswald that they could hypnotise her before she is anaesthetised

    A. A very appropriate thing to do
    B. Appropriate, but not ideal
    C. Inappropriate, but not awful
    D. A very inappropriate thing to do

7. Instruct Shaun to keep his personal views to himself

    A. A very appropriate thing to do
    B. Appropriate, but not ideal
    C. Inappropriate, but not awful
    D. A very inappropriate thing to do

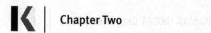

Lisa is a final year medical student and has been busy revising for her exams. She overhears several of her peers from her year group discussing a piece of coursework that is due in soon. When she questions them, it transpires the coursework was set a few weeks ago, with all the details included in an email that she did not receive.

How **appropriate** are each of the following responses by <u>**Lisa**</u> in this situation?

8.   Contact the course administrator and ask for an extension to complete the coursework

    A.   A very appropriate thing to do
    B.   Appropriate, but not ideal
    C.   Inappropriate, but not awful
    D.   A very inappropriate thing to do

9.   Concentrate on revising for exams, as she did not receive the email with the coursework assignment

    A.   A very appropriate thing to do
    B.   Appropriate, but not ideal
    C.   Inappropriate, but not awful
    D.   A very inappropriate thing to do

10.   Contact the course administrator and find out if the email should have been sent to her, and if there may have been other important emails she did not receive

    A.   A very appropriate thing to do
    B.   Appropriate, but not ideal
    C.   Inappropriate, but not awful
    D.   A very inappropriate thing to do

A consultant enters the lobby of the hospital where he works, and is approached by a patient he does not recognise. The patient starts shouting at the consultant that the hospital is worse than a zoo, and the doctors are not fit to operate on animals.

How **appropriate** are each of the following responses by **the consultant** in this situation?

11. Ask a porter to assist the patient

    A. A very appropriate thing to do
    B. Appropriate, but not ideal
    C. Inappropriate, but not awful
    D. A very inappropriate thing to do

12. Invite the patient to sit down and have a chat

    A. A very appropriate thing to do
    B. Appropriate, but not ideal
    C. Inappropriate, but not awful
    D. A very inappropriate thing to do

13. Ask the patient not to shout, and to explain his exact concerns

    A. A very appropriate thing to do
    B. Appropriate, but not ideal
    C. Inappropriate, but not awful
    D. A very inappropriate thing to do

> Haroon is a junior dentist at a large dental practice. A patient, Mrs Rahman, complains that she has had to wait 2 weeks for an appointment for a toothache. Haroon steps out to check with the receptionist, and finds the receptionist playing solitaire on her computer and typing in a chat window on a social networking site; at the same time, the phone is ringing, and a queue of patients are waiting to speak to the receptionist.

How **appropriate** are each of the following responses by **Haroon** in this situation?

14. Instruct the receptionist to answer the phone, and apologise to the patients for their wait

   A.   A very appropriate thing to do
   B.   Appropriate, but not ideal
   C.   Inappropriate, but not awful
   D.   A very inappropriate thing to do

15. Demand an immediate explanation from the receptionist for her unacceptable behaviour

   A.   A very appropriate thing to do
   B.   Appropriate, but not ideal
   C.   Inappropriate, but not awful
   D.   A very inappropriate thing to do

16. Answer the phone, asking the receptionist to speak with the patients in the queue before doing so

   A.   A very appropriate thing to do
   B.   Appropriate, but not ideal
   C.   Inappropriate, but not awful
   D.   A very inappropriate thing to do

17. Take the receptionist to a private space nearby and explain Mrs Rahman's concern about having to wait for an appointment

   A.   A very appropriate thing to do
   B.   Appropriate, but not ideal
   C.   Inappropriate, but not awful
   D.   A very inappropriate thing to do

Three medical students, James, Kyle and Avni regularly visit a patient at home as part of their first year course. The patient lives 30 minutes away so the students all meet outside the patient's house, having travelled there independently. Kyle is always at least 10 minutes late, and it is starting to annoy James. The third time it happens, Kyle calls and says he will be at least 20 minutes late. James decides he wants to go ahead and meet the patient without waiting for Kyle.

How **appropriate** are each of the following responses by **Avni** in this situation?

18. Tell James to wait for Kyle so that they can all go together
   A. A very appropriate thing to do
   B. Appropriate, but not ideal
   C. Inappropriate, but not awful
   D. A very inappropriate thing to do

19. Call Kyle and tell him that he should have tried harder to be on time
   A. A very appropriate thing to do
   B. Appropriate, but not ideal
   C. Inappropriate, but not awful
   D. A very inappropriate thing to do

20. Call the patient to apologise and explain that they will be 20 minutes late
   A. A very appropriate thing to do
   B. Appropriate, but not ideal
   C. Inappropriate, but not awful
   D. A very inappropriate thing to do

21. Explain to Kyle that they must start the visit without him, and schedule a time to meet as a group to discuss Kyle's tardiness
   A. A very appropriate thing to do
   B. Appropriate, but not ideal
   C. Inappropriate, but not awful
   D. A very inappropriate thing to do

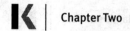

Katie is a junior doctor on a cardiology ward at a major hospital. On her day off, she plans to meet a friend for lunch; her friend works on the cardiology ward at another major hospital. On arriving in the ward, Katie sees her consultant sitting in the waiting area with the other patients, reading a newspaper. The consultant does not see her, and he is not wearing scrubs.

How **appropriate** are each of the following responses by **Katie** in this situation?

22.   Say hello to the consultant and ask why he is here

    A.   A very appropriate thing to do

    B.   Appropriate, but not ideal

    C.   Inappropriate, but not awful

    D.   A very inappropriate thing to do

23.   Pretend she didn't see the consultant, unless he brings it up later

    A.   A very appropriate thing to do

    B.   Appropriate, but not ideal

    C.   Inappropriate, but not awful

    D.   A very inappropriate thing to do

24.   Ask her friend if he knows her consultant

    A.   A very appropriate thing to do

    B.   Appropriate, but not ideal

    C.   Inappropriate, but not awful

    D.   A very inappropriate thing to do

> The infection control nurse asks Tom, a junior doctor, to remove his wristwatch because it is an infection risk. The next day, Neha, a medical student on the ward, notices that Tom is wearing his watch on his wrist again.

How **appropriate** are each of the following responses by **Neha** in this situation?

25. Report Tom to the infection control nurse

   A. A very appropriate thing to do
   B. Appropriate, but not ideal
   C. Inappropriate, but not awful
   D. A very inappropriate thing to do

26. Have a talk to Tom at the end of the week if he continues to wear the watch

   A. A very appropriate thing to do
   B. Appropriate, but not ideal
   C. Inappropriate, but not awful
   D. A very inappropriate thing to do

27. Quietly say to Tom that he should remove his watch, as it is an infection risk

   A. A very appropriate thing to do
   B. Appropriate, but not ideal
   C. Inappropriate, but not awful
   D. A very inappropriate thing to do

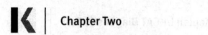

Whilst Eoghan, a medical student, is taking a history from a patient, the patient asks if the consultant will be here to see him as he has some questions to ask about his operation which is taking place tomorrow. Eoghan knows that the consultant does not get back from holiday until tomorrow.

How **appropriate** are each of the following responses by **<u>Eoghan</u>** in this situation?

28. Offer to get a doctor to come and talk to the patient

    A. A very appropriate thing to do

    B. Appropriate, but not ideal

    C. Inappropriate, but not awful

    D. A very inappropriate thing to do

29. Reassure the patient that he can answer all the patient's questions himself

    A. A very appropriate thing to do

    B. Appropriate, but not ideal

    C. Inappropriate, but not awful

    D. A very inappropriate thing to do

30. Try and answer and simple questions himself, then get a doctor to come and talk to the patient

    A. A very appropriate thing to do

    B. Appropriate, but not ideal

    C. Inappropriate, but not awful

    D. A very inappropriate thing to do

Esme is a consultant surgeon. She is on call from home but has been feeling increasingly dizzy and sick throughout the day, to the extent where is has to hold onto walls to walk along the corridor. In the middle of the night, a junior colleague calls to ask her to come in to assist with an unwell patient. Esme usually drives herself to the hospital – a journey of around 30 minutes on difficult country roads. Given how unbalanced she feels, Esme is not sure she could drive for even 5 minutes.

How **appropriate** are each of the following responses by __Esme__ in this situation?

31. Tell the junior colleague that she cannot come in, as she is unwell

   A. A very appropriate thing to do
   B. Appropriate, but not ideal
   C. Inappropriate, but not awful
   D. A very inappropriate thing to do

32. Call a taxi to take her in to the hospital to assist

   A. A very appropriate thing to do
   B. Appropriate, but not ideal
   C. Inappropriate, but not awful
   D. A very inappropriate thing to do

33. Call a different consultant who is not on call and ask them to go into hospital in her place

   A. A very appropriate thing to do
   B. Appropriate, but not ideal
   C. Inappropriate, but not awful
   D. A very inappropriate thing to do

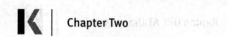

Ellen is a final year medical student, two months away from qualifying. Her friend Rupa comes to see her to ask about some symptoms she has been having for the past month. Ellen starts to become worried when Rupa describes some 'red flag symptoms' that could signify a serious disease. However, Ellen does not know very much about the disease, so she is not confident of her ability to help Rupa based on her limited knowledge at this point in her medical training.

How **appropriate** are each of the following responses by **Ellen** in this situation?

34. Tell Rupa that she is not yet experienced enough to give a diagnosis and recommend that Rupa see her GP

    A. A very appropriate thing to do
    B. Appropriate, but not ideal
    C. Inappropriate, but not awful
    D. A very inappropriate thing to do

35. Offer to examine Rupa properly, as a patient examination is often useful in making a diagnosis

    A. A very appropriate thing to do
    B. Appropriate, but not ideal
    C. Inappropriate, but not awful
    D. A very inappropriate thing to do

A patient asks Luke, a junior doctor, to explain why a new medication has been prescribed. Luke is covering on the ward for another doctor who is away on annual leave, and he has not met this patient before. Luke checks the patient's chart and sees that the doctor has prescribed a medication that Luke is entirely unfamiliar with.

How **appropriate** are each of the following responses by **Luke** in this situation?

36. Explain that the treatment is new, and that he does not know much about it

   A. A very appropriate thing to do
   B. Appropriate, but not ideal
   C. Inappropriate, but not awful
   D. A very inappropriate thing to do

37. Reassure the patient there is a good reason, and that he will follow up with more information soon

   A. A very appropriate thing to do
   B. Appropriate, but not ideal
   C. Inappropriate, but not awful
   D. A very inappropriate thing to do

38. Tell the patient he is unfamiliar with this treatment, and the doctor that prescribed it is away

   A. A very appropriate thing to do
   B. Appropriate, but not ideal
   C. Inappropriate, but not awful
   D. A very inappropriate thing to do

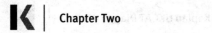

Molly is a junior doctor travelling to a training session at another hospital. Whilst on the train, Molly observes three medical students discussing the specialities they love and hate. The students voice their opinions very loudly, using profanity and crude, derogatory terms to describe the patients of certain specialities. Molly notices that several passengers appear to be offended by these comments.

How **important** to take into account are the following considerations for **Molly** when deciding how to respond to the situation?

39. The students are wearing hospital name badges that identify them as medical students, not doctors
    A. Very important
    B. Important
    C. Of minor importance
    D. Not important at all

40. The students are using offensive language to talk about patients
    A. Very important
    B. Important
    C. Of minor importance
    D. Not important at all

Jitesh is a final year medical student on geriatric wards. Every afternoon at 3:30pm the junior doctor, Rob, goes home and asks Jitesh to do his paper work, such as copying out blood results and delivering x-ray requests.

How **important** to take into account are the following considerations for **Jitesh** when deciding how to respond to the situation?

41. Rob is the sole carer for his sick father

    A. Very important
    B. Important
    C. Of minor importance
    D. Not important at all

42. The learning objectives of Jitesh's course state that he should be helping the junior doctors with their jobs to experience the real life of a junior doctor

    A. Very important
    B. Important
    C. Of minor importance
    D. Not important at all

43. 4-5pm is often the busiest time of the day on the wards

    A. Very important
    B. Important
    C. Of minor importance
    D. Not important at all

Nima, a junior doctor, enters the supply cupboard and is surprised to discover Lauren, a medical student, in the process of removing her clothes. Nima asks Lauren what she is doing, and Lauren comments that she does not like changing clothes in the presence of others.

How **important** to take into account are the following considerations for **Nima** when deciding how to respond to the situation?

44. The hospital provides a suitably private location for all staff members to change clothes

    A. Very important
    B. Important
    C. Of minor importance
    D. Not important at all

45. Nima's religious beliefs require her to wear a head scarf

    A. Very important
    B. Important
    C. Of minor importance
    D. Not important at all

46. Lauren does not have any clothes to change into – only the clothes she is removing

    A. Very important
    B. Important
    C. Of minor importance
    D. Not important at all

47. Whether someone besides Lauren was also in the supply cupboard when Nima entered

    A. Very important
    B. Important
    C. Of minor importance
    D. Not important at all

48. Whether Lauren's behaviour is heightened in other ways (slurring speech, breathing rapidly)

    A. Very important
    B. Important
    C. Of minor importance
    D. Not important at all

> Abiola is a medical student. She is in the hospital lift one day when she hears two of the junior doctors loudly discussing the sensitive details of a case that they have been involved in.

How **important** to take into account are the following considerations for **Abiola** when deciding how to respond to the situation?

49. The only other occupant of the lift is an elderly man with hearing aids

   A. Very important
   B. Important
   C. Of minor importance
   D. Not important at all

50. The junior doctors do not use the patient's name

   A. Very important
   B. Important
   C. Of minor importance
   D. Not important at all

51. The junior doctors are responsible for Abiola's report at the end of her placement

   A. Very important
   B. Important
   C. Of minor importance
   D. Not important at all

52. Abiola does not know the patient to whom they are referring

   A. Very important
   B. Important
   C. Of minor importance
   D. Not important at all

> Two medical students, Violet and Uma, are in the same tutor group, as well as being house-mates. One morning, before they have left the house for their tutor group, Violet gets a call that her grandmother is critically ill and has been rushed to hospital. Violet's grandmother is asking for her, and she must leave immediately if she is to catch the next train to her grandmother's town.

How **important** to take into account are the following considerations for <u>Violet</u> when deciding how to respond to the situation?

53. Whether she has a phone number where she can reach the tutor

    A. Very important
    B. Important
    C. Of minor importance
    D. Not important at all

54. Whether the tutor would mind if Uma explained her absence

    A. Very important
    B. Important
    C. Of minor importance
    D. Not important at all

55. Whether she will be able to email the tutor from the train before the tutor group starts

    A. Very important
    B. Important
    C. Of minor importance
    D. Not important at all

Meera is starting her first medical school placement in hospital and is paired with Adam, another student. Throughout the first week on the wards, Meera notices that Adam always looks scruffy, with his hair unbrushed, and is not dressed as smartly as she is.

How **important** to take into account are the following considerations for **Meera** when deciding how to respond to the situation?

56. The medical school has firm guidelines about how a student should dress for the wards

    A. Very important
    B. Important
    C. Of minor importance
    D. Not important at all

57. Adam has just split up with his girlfriend of 5 years

    A. Very important
    B. Important
    C. Of minor importance
    D. Not important at all

58. Meera knows that Adam has just reached his overdraft limit on his student bank account and is really short of money

    A. Very important
    B. Important
    C. Of minor importance
    D. Not important at all

59. The students have all signed an agreement declaring that they will follow the guidelines set by the medical school

    A. Very important
    B. Important
    C. Of minor importance
    D. Not important at all

Fraser is a junior doctor who has just chosen general surgery as his specialism. He is assisting the consultant who supervises his work at the hospital on a routine appendectomy when the patient suddenly arrests and dies on the operating table. The hospital opens an adverse event investigation, in which all the doctors involved must testify individually before the investigating committee. Doctors are not meant to discuss their testimony with each other until the committee's investigation is complete. Prior to the operation, Fraser had noticed in the patient's notes that she had been taking a prescription painkiller that was contraindicated for the anaesthetic used in surgery – that is, the combined effect of the anaesthetic and the painkiller caused her cardiac arrest. Fraser had mentioned the painkiller to the consultant prior to the operation. However, while Fraser is testifying to the committee, he realises that the consultant and the anaesthetist have testified that they had no prior knowledge that the patient was taking the painkiller; each blames the other for the patient's death.

How **important** to take into account are the following considerations for **Fraser** when deciding how to respond to the situation?

60. The consultant has a great deal of influence over the future of Fraser's career as a doctor

    A. Very important
    B. Important
    C. Of minor importance
    D. Not important at all

61. Fraser does not know whether the anaesthetist was aware that the patient was taking the painkiller

    A. Very important
    B. Important
    C. Of minor importance
    D. Not important at all

62. Fraser told the consultant that the patient was taking the painkiller before the operation had begun

    A. Very important
    B. Important
    C. Of minor importance
    D. Not important at all

A medical student, Sienna, is completing a placement at the university hospital. She is working closely with Lexi, a junior doctor who is only a few years older. One morning, Sienna and Lexi meet in the hospital café for a coffee before work. Lexi goes to buy another coffee and leaves her mobile on the table. Lexi's phone beeps, and a text message pops up on the screen. Sienna sees that the message is quite personal in nature, thanking Lexi for 'such a brilliant night' and signed with three kisses. The message indicates the first and last name of the sender, and Sienna recognises that he is an actor from a popular TV show who is currently on the ward, recovering from a car crash.

How **important** to take into account are the following considerations for **Sienna** when deciding how to respond to the situation?

63. Sienna cannot see whether Lexi has sent the actor any messages, or what these messages might say

   A. Very important
   B. Important
   C. Of minor importance
   D. Not important at all

64. Lexi once confided in Sienna that she had met her previous boyfriend when his mother was her patient

   A. Very important
   B. Important
   C. Of minor importance
   D. Not important at all

65. Lexi is responsible for assessing Sienna's work on the placement

   A. Very important
   B. Important
   C. Of minor importance
   D. Not important at all

> Thomas has worked at the same hospital for a few years after completing medical school. He is responsible for helping his consultant train the new junior doctors. The consultant is a man in his early 60s with an abrupt manner; he usually interrupts the junior doctors and sometimes talks over them. This year, for the first time, all the new junior doctors are women. After the first couple of weeks, Thomas notices that the consultant is particularly rude to the female junior doctors, belittling them at almost every opportunity, even in front of patients. As a result, two of the new junior doctors have confided in Thomas that they do not feel safe in saying anything in the consultant's presence, as he will just attack them. They do not know what to do if they are unsure about a patient's condition or the best course of treatment.

How **important** to take into account are the following considerations for **Thomas** when deciding how to respond to the situation?

66. Thomas has never had any complaints from male junior doctors that the consultant is intimidating them to a degree that might affect patient care

    A. Very important
    B. Important
    C. Of minor importance
    D. Not important at all

67. The consultant relies on him for support and advice whenever there is a problem with the junior doctors

    A. Very important
    B. Important
    C. Of minor importance
    D. Not important at all

68. The consultant is serving as the hospital chairman on a temporary basis; any formal complaints about the consultant would have to be submitted to the consultant

    A. Very important
    B. Important
    C. Of minor importance
    D. Not important at all

STOP. IF YOU FINISH BEFORE TIME IS CALLED, CHECK ANY QUESTIONS YOU HAVE M ARKED FOR REVIEW. YOU MAY GO BACK TO QUESTIONS IN THIS SECTION ONLY.

Kaplan UKCAT Diagnostic Test Answer Key: Sections 1–4

Verbal Reasoning

1. B
2. B
3. D
4. A
5. A
6. C
7. C
8. D
9. B
10. C
11. A
12. B
13. B
14. A
15. B
16. C
17. B
18. C
19. D
20. D
21. C
22. D
23. B
24. C
25. C
26. B
27. C
28. A
29. D
30. A
31. A
32. B
33. C
34. A
35. B
36. B
37. A
38. B
39. C
40. C
41. B
42. D
43. A
44. B

Decision Making

1. YES; NO; NO; YES; NO
2. NO; YES; NO; NO; YES
3. YES; NO; NO; NO; YES
4. NO; NO; YES; YES; NO
5. NO; YES; YES; NO; NO
6. B
7. D
8. C
9. A
10. A
11. D
12. B
13. D
14. C
15. YES; YES; NO; YES; NO
16. NO; NO; YES; NO; YES
17. NO; YES; YES; NO; NO
18. NO; NO; NO; YES; YES
19. A
20. D
21. C
22. B
23. A
24. C
25. B
26. D
27. A
28. B
29. C

Quantitative Reasoning

1. A
2. E
3. C
4. B
5. C
6. B
7. A
8. B
9. D
10. B
11. C
12. C
13. C
14. D
15. B
16. C
17. B
18. E
19. C
20. D
21. E
22. B
23. A
24. D
25. C
26. B
27. D
28. A
29. E
30. A
31. C
32. B
33. A
34. C
35. E
36. D

Abstract Reasoning

1. C
2. C
3. B
4. A
5. C
6. D
7. B
8. A
9. C
10. A
11. B
12. C
13. C
14. A
15. B
16. C
17. A
18. B
19. B
20. C
21. A
22. A
23. C
24. B
25. B
26. A
27. C
28. C
29. A
30. B
31. B
32. C
33. B
34. C
35. A
36. C
37. A
38. C
39. B
40. C
41. C
42. A
43. C
44. B
45. A
46. D
47. A
48. B
49. D
50. C
51. A
52. C
53. B
54. C
55. B

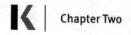

Kaplan UKCAT Diagnostic Test Scoring Table: Sections 1–4

1. Count up your number of correct answers in each scored section. For Decision Making, count multiple choice questions as 1 mark each. For each five-part question, give yourself 2 marks if you answered all five parts correctly; if you answered three or four parts correctly, give yourself 1 mark.

2. Find your approximate score for each section in the table below.

	NUMBER CORRECT	APPROXIMATE UKCAT SCORE
Verbal Reasoning	_____	_____
Decision Making	_____	_____
Quantitative Reasoning	_____	_____
Abstract Reasoning	_____	_____

3. Add your section scores to find your total score: _____

Approximate UKCAT Score	Number of Questions Answered Correctly			
	Verbal Reasoning	**Decision Making**	**Quantitative Reasoning**	**Abstract Reasoning**
300	0–5	0–4	0–3	0–6
330	6	5	4–5	7–8
350	7	6	6	9–10
370	8	7	7	11–12
400	9–10	8	8	13–14
430	11–12	9	9	15–16
450	13–14	10	10	17–18
470	15	11	11	19–20
500	16	12–13	12	21–22
530	17–18	14–15	13	23–24
550	19–20	16–17	14–15	25–26
570	21–22	18–19	16–17	27–29
600	23–24	20–21	18–19	30–32
630	25–26	22–23	20–21	33–34
650	27–28	24–25	22–23	35–36
670	29–30	26–27	24	37
700	31	28–29	25	38–39
730	32	30	26	40–41
750	33	31	27	42–43
770	34	32	28	44–45
800	35–36	33	29	46–47
830	37–38	34	30	48–49
850	39–40	35	31–32	50–51
890	41–42	36	33–34	52–53
900	43–44	37–38	35–36	54–55

N.B. These scores are for approximation purposes only. Scores on the UKCAT are given in 10-point intervals; actual scores will vary slightly from this scheme. This table is designed to err on the side of caution. In most cases, a similar performance on the UKCAT would result in a slightly higher score.

Kaplan UKCAT Diagnostic Test Answer Key: Section 5

1. D	18. D	35. D	52. D
2. B	19. C	36. D	53. A
3. A	20. D	37. A	54. C
4. A	21. A	38. C	55. A
5. A	22. D	39. D	56. A
6. A	23. A	40. A	57. D
7. B	24. D	41. D	58. D
8. B	25. D	42. D	59. A
9. D	26. D	43. B	60. D
10. A	27. A	44. B	61. C
11. C	28. A	45. D	62. A
12. A	29. D	46. A	63. A
13. A	30. D	47. A	64. B
14. A	31. B	48. B	65. D
15. D	32. D	49. D	66. C
16. C	33. A	50. C	67. A
17. A	34. A	51. D	68. C

Kaplan UKCAT Diagnostic Test Scoring Table: Section 5

1. Count up your number of correct answers in this section: _____

2. Count up your number of partially correct answers in this section: _____

   Your answers are partially correct if:

   - you chose A, but the correct answer was B.
   - you chose B, but the correct answer was A.
   - you chose C, but the correct answer was D.
   - you chose D, but the correct answer was C.

3. Multiply the number of partially correct answers by 0.5, and add to your number of correct answers for your total marks:

Partially correct answers	Correct answers	Total marks
0.5(_____) +	_____ =	_____

4. Find your approximate scoring band for this section in the table below.

Approximate UKCAT Scoring Band	Total Marks in Situational Judgement
Band 4	0–16.5
Band 3	17–33.5
Band 2	34–50.5
Band 1	51–68

Verbal Reasoning

The Task

Verbal Reasoning is the first scored subtest on the UKCAT. The Verbal section includes a total of 11 passages, each with 4 items to answer. You have 1 minute to read the instructions, and then 21 minutes to answer the items. If you divide your time equally among the 11 sets, then you will have just under 2 minutes to complete each set in the Verbal Reasoning section. As you'll see, it will be very difficult to read a full passage and answer the 4 accompanying items in 2 minutes—so you must attack the Verbal section with a strategy that will allow you to attempt all the statements within the allotted time.

The Format

Verbal passages vary in length; most passages are two to four paragraphs, and 300 to 600 words long. The passages are mostly written in a neutral and slightly engaging style, much like articles in a magazine, and can involve virtually any subject matter. Some passages will discuss topics from science or medicine, though these are likely to be a distinct minority on Test Day; most passages will focus on topics from history, the arts or everyday life.

Some Verbal Reasoning items are statements, which you must assess as True, False or Can't tell, based on the passage. Statements are fairly short—most are 10 words or fewer—and as such are relatively straightforward to compare to the passage. The answer choices for Verbal statements are always the same: True, False or Can't tell. It is essential to 'internalise' the meaning of these answers, in the context of Verbal Reasoning:

True: The passage supports the statement.

False: The statement contradicts the passage.

Can't tell: The statement is neither True nor False, or there is not enough information in the passage to evaluate the statement as True or False.

All other Verbal Reasoning items are questions. Each question will have four answer choices, and these will be particular to each question. This makes it very straightforward to distinguish questions from statements (as statements have only three answer choices, and these are always the same). Most questions will require you to select the answer that is true—the answer that is supported by the passage. A few, more difficult questions will ask you to find an answer that contradicts the passage, or is not supported by the passage. Thus, your

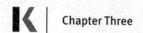

understanding of True, False and Can't tell Verbal statements will be invaluable in selecting the correct answers to Verbal questions. Each answer choice to a Verbal question is effectively a Verbal statement.

The Challenges

The most obvious challenge in Verbal Reasoning is timing: it is virtually impossible to read the passages fully and answer the questions properly in just 2 minutes per set. If you could manage to read a passage in a minute, you would have only 15 seconds to answer each of the accompanying items. That might be enough time for a simple, straightforward item—but most items will be of medium to advanced difficulty; that is, they will be very tough to assess in 15 seconds.

The other major challenge in the Verbal section is the nature of the task involved—or, to be more precise, the three different tasks. Test-takers who struggle with Verbal tend to confuse the tasks: the most common mistake is to assume that False means the statement is not True. On the UKCAT, a statement is False if it contradicts the passage. This meaning of False is very particular, and differs from the usual meaning of false ('not true'). If a Verbal statement is not True, that does not mean that it is False. A statement must contradict the passage to be False. If a statement is not True and does not contradict the passage, the answer is Can't tell. If a statement does not exactly contradict the passage, then the answer is likely to be Can't tell. Failing to distinguish between False and Can't tell is the second most common mistake in Verbal Reasoning. Thus, a confident understanding of the answer choices is key to Verbal success.

Kaplan Top Tips for Verbal Reasoning

1. Don't read the passage

This may seem counterintuitive, but there are several good reasons not to read the passage:

- *You don't have time*: With 2 minutes per set, you could allow 1 minute to read the passage and then 15 seconds per statement. However, this is not enough time to evaluate most statements. Moreover, it's not enough time to read passages that are 3 paragraphs or longer.

- *Marks come from statements*: Remember, the Verbal section does not assess your ability to read a passage, but your ability to evaluate statements based on a passage. You get a mark for each statement you correctly label as True, False or Can't tell. Reading the passage could help you earn those marks. But it's not the only way, nor is it the best way, given the time constraints of Verbal Reasoning.

- *Each question comes with four statements—the answer choices*: Verbal questions may feel like a fundamentally different format, but in fact they simply require you to apply your skill at assessing statements against the passage. The only difference is that you are given a set of four statements, and (on most questions) must select the one that is True. (A minority of 'negative' questions require you to select the answer that is False or Can't tell, and thus are more difficult.) For this reason, you must learn to assess statements with confidence, as this skill is equally essential for attacking Verbal questions.

- *Speed + accuracy = more marks*: the key to improving your Verbal score is increasing how quickly and how accurately you assess the statements. That is where you'll focus as you practise. You could try reading the passages more quickly, but that would mean reading them less accurately, and would cost you marks on the statements. So a different approach is required.

2. Scan for keywords

This approach has proven the most effective for the thousands of students we at Kaplan have prepared for the UKCAT. Instead of reading the passage:

- Read the statement/question.
- Choose a keyword (or two), and scan the passage for the keyword.
- Pick an answer (or eliminate answers) based on what you find.

A *keyword* is any word or phrase that will help you determine whether the statement is True or False. If the keywords aren't in the passage, then the answer is almost always Can't tell.

Scanning means looking very quickly through the passage for all appearances of the keyword, or related words. Scanning is not the same as reading, but it is a shortcut to save time and make the most of minimal reading: once you find the keyword, read the sentence in which it appears—and just before and after it, if necessary; in most instances, this research will be sufficient to determine that a statement is (or is not) True or False.

It is essential to scan for all appearances of the keyword. If a keyword appears twice in the passage, you may have to combine information from both of its appearances to determine the correct answer. Scanning will help you zero in on the answer to these 'pick 'n' mix' statements.

Some questions will not contain a keyword. For these questions, you must scan for a keyword from each answer choice. We will cover this approach in more detail later in the chapter.

3. If unsure, eliminate

Don't delay once you have scanned the passage and found the relevant information, even when a difficult statement makes it tough to choose an answer. Most commonly, you will be stuck choosing between Can't tell and one other answer. No matter how difficult a statement, you can always eliminate one answer choice:

- If the statement is not supported by the passage, eliminate True.
- If the statement does not contradict the passage, eliminate False.

With two remaining answers, you have a 50% chance of answering correctly. At this point, make a quick judgement call. Most of the time, you'll find yourself uncertain whether there is enough information to justify a statement as True/False. Keep it simple: if there's not enough info, then click Can't tell, flag for review and move on. There are more marks, and easier marks, ahead.

4. Skip the most difficult questions

We will spend some time considering the more challenging types of Verbal questions later in this chapter. You should practise recognising them and deciding how (or whether) to attack them. The most difficult questions can be very time-consuming, and will take more than a minute to answer. Since you have only 30 seconds per question, if you spend, say, 90 seconds on a single question, you will miss out 2 other questions later in the section—and it's likely that those 2 missed questions would be much easier than one that took 90 seconds. If a question looks very difficult or time-consuming, or you find yourself spending a minute or longer, mark an answer, flag for review and move on. Each question is worth one mark, so you will not get any extra marks for spending so much extra time on a single question. But you will run a real risk of missing out easier marks later in the section. Be quick, and be ruthless about skipping the most difficult questions. Be sure to click an answer (a random guess) as you flag for review. You might have time to come back to a few questions you skipped, but only if you are extremely rigorous about timing in this section. But you can bank a high score by picking up all the marks on the easy to medium difficulty questions, if you are not drawn in by the few questions that are especially time-consuming.

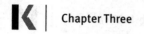

Kaplan Timed Practice Set—*Try the Kaplan Top Tips*

Set your timer for 2 minutes. Mark answers for all 4 statements before time is up!

Born in 1643 in Lincolnshire, Isaac Newton pioneered the study of optics, the properties of light detectable by the human eye, with his insight that white light is made up of the same spectrum of colour as a rainbow. Newton was also the first to demonstrate that gravity was a universal physical force, applied to everything in the universe, in his ground-breaking 1687 study, *Mathematical Principles of Natural Philosophy*. Newton furthered the study of physics in this same work by explaining the three fundamental laws of classical mechanics for the first time.

Following from insights developed by mathematicians over several centuries, Isaac Newton was the first to elucidate the fundamental theorem of calculus and the first to explore differential calculus, as well as its relation to integral calculus. Newton originally developed these concepts of calculus in a 1666 treatise that was not published in full until 1704. There are two reasons that Newton's discovery of calculus remained unknown for so long. First, publishers in the 17th century were wary of texts in the field of theoretical maths, which were so unprofitable that they drove one specialist publisher to bankruptcy. Second, Newton was very tight-lipped about his highly original work in 'the method of fluxions and fluents' (as he called calculus), not mentioning it in print until a brief reference in *Mathematical Principles of Natural Philosophy*.

After commencing study of differential calculus in the 1670s, Gottfried Leibniz, a German mathematician, developed many of the principles of calculus independently of Newton, and was initially given credit for its discovery, with a 1684 publication. However, it's not clear that Newton and Leibniz worked entirely independently, as they had many of the same friends (fellow mathematicians), and occasionally wrote to each other. Calculus as studied and applied today is more similar to the method developed by Leibniz, but this does not diminish Newton's record as an extraordinary innovator of maths as well as physics.

---

1. White light consists of a spectrum of colour.
   A. True
   B. False
   C. Can't tell

2. Newton was born in Lincoln.
   A. True
   B. False
   C. Can't tell

3. No one studied differential calculus before Leibniz.
   A. True
   B. False
   C. Can't tell

4. Newton was a leading scholar of physics.
   A. True
   B. False
   C. Can't tell

Kaplan Timed Practice Set—*Try the Kaplan Top Tips*: **Answers and Explanations**

How did you get on? Hopefully, you finished the statements in the 2 minutes, and answered them all correctly. As you practise with this book, you should **always** read through the explanations for every question, to ensure that you got the right answer for the right reasons. The explanations may also give tips that will help you on later questions with similar twists. If you didn't get them all right, don't despair – in fact, it's good to make mistakes as you practise. Each mistake you make as you practise is one you can avoid on Test Day.

1. (A)

Scan for the keywords 'white light', and you'll find them in the first sentence of the passage. This sentence states that white light is made up of the same spectrum of colour as a rainbow. The statement says the same, so it is true.

2. (C)

Scan for the keywords 'Newton' and 'Lincoln'. Newton is mentioned throughout the passage, but Lincoln is never mentioned. The first sentence states that Newton was born in Lincolnshire, but it does not specify where in Lincolnshire he was born. Thus, based on the passage, we don't know whether or not Newton was born in Lincoln. The answer is therefore **(C)**.

3. (B)

The keywords here are 'Leibniz' and 'differential calculus'. Leibniz appears in the final paragraph, which states that he developed calculus independently of Newton, and that Leibniz started to study differential calculus in the 1670s. However, differential calculus appears earlier, in the second paragraph, where it is mentioned as something that Newton was 'first to explore', and that Newton developed in 1666. Thus, we know from the passage that Newton studied differential calculus before Leibniz; this statement contradicts the passage, so it is false.

4. (A)

Scan for the keyword 'physics' in reference to Newton. The first paragraph specifies that Newton was the first to explain gravity as a universal physical force and that he was also first to explain the fundamental laws of classical mechanics, furthering the study of physics. The passage's final sentence goes even further, stating that Newton was an 'extraordinary innovator' of physics. Innovator is a synonym for leader, so the passage supports this statement. The answer is therefore **(A)**.

Now, let's move on and consider what makes a statement a valid inference.

Inferences

Many challenging Verbal Reasoning statements require you to make inferences from the passage. An inference is something that is not directly stated in the passage, but nearly so. For an inference to be True, it must stay very close to what the passage says. Here's a good rule of thumb about Verbal Reasoning inferences: If you have to work through elaborate reasoning to justify an inference, then your inference is not supported by the passage.

The following four statements involve inferences, based on the passage about Inverness and Gaelic. As you practise, try to evaluate each statement in 30 seconds before reading the answer.

In 2001, Inverness was granted city status, making it the northernmost city in the UK and also one of the smallest, with a current population of 70,000. Inverness is known as the 'capital of the Highlands', and sits amid hills at the edge of the Great Glen, where the River Ness empties into the Moray Firth. The river is nearly the shortest in Scotland, running a mere six miles from Loch Ness (*Loch Nis*, in Gaelic) to the firth. In fact, the city's Gaelic name, *Inbhir Nis*, literally means 'mouth of the river Ness'. Inverness is a popular base for tourists visiting the many historical sites in the Highlands, along with the perhaps more 'mythical' site of Loch Ness; nearly everyone takes the obligatory boat cruise.

Gaelic has always been widely spoken in the Highlands of Scotland, and Inverness is currently home to a Gaelic renaissance: the city opened a Gaelic primary school in 2007, and expanded capacity to 200 students a few years later. Many street signs in the city are bilingual, though very few adults or children in Inverness (approximately 5% of the population) speak Gaelic.

Whilst Inverness has the highest proportion of Gaelic speakers of any Scottish city, there are considerably more Gaelic speakers (as a percentage of the population) in the Outer Hebrides. Just over 52% of the population of the Outer Hebrides speak Gaelic, and the predominance of the language in this region is reflected in the name of its parliamentary constituency: not 'Outer Hebrides' but *Na h-Eileannan Siar*, which is Gaelic for Western Isles, another name for the Outer Hebrides. Thus, you are most likely to find a Gaelic speaker among the general population by visiting one of these remote, beautiful islands. The largest population of Gaelic speakers in Scotland—in terms of number of people, not as a percentage of the population—is in Glasgow, home to 10% of Scottish Gaelic speakers today.

---

5. The River Ness is Scotland's shortest river.
    A. True
    B. False
    C. Can't tell

Answer: Scan for the keywords 'shortest river', and you will find the relevant detail midway through the first paragraph. The passage explains that the River Ness is nearly the shortest river in Scotland. The statement is more extreme than the passage: the River Ness is not the shortest river in Scotland, so the statement is false.

---

6. Most children in Inverness speak Gaelic.
    A. True
    B. False
    C. Can't tell

Answer: Scan for the keywords 'children' and 'speak Gaelic'; they appear in the next-to-last sentence, which states that very few children in Inverness speak Gaelic. 'Very few' means a very small number, and 'most' means a majority. Thus, this statement contradicts the passage, and is false.

---

7.   No city is further north than Inverness.

    A.   True

    B.   False

    C.   Can't tell

Answer: 'No city is further north' is very extreme language. The keyword 'north' leads to the passage's first sentence, which says that Inverness is the northernmost city in the UK. At first glance, it may appear that the passage supports the statement. However, notice the subtle shift in terms – the statement does not say that no city in the UK is further north than Inverness. Since the passage does not mention other cities, it is impossible to say whether there are no cities anywhere that are further north than Inverness (in which case the statement would be true) or whether there is at least one such city (in which case the statement would be false). Since the statement cannot be assessed based on the passage, the answer is **(C)**.

8.   In Gaelic, *Inbhir* means 'mouth of the river'.

    A.   True

    B.   False

    C.   Can't tell

Answer: The keyword *Inbhir* is easy to scan for, since it is given in italics. The next-to-last sentence of the first paragraph says that *Inbhir Nis* is Gaelic for 'mouth of the river Ness'. The previous sentence specifies that *Loch Nis* is Gaelic for Loch Ness, so it is safe to infer that *Nis* is Gaelic for Ness. *Inbhir* must therefore mean 'mouth of the river' in Gaelic. This inference from the passage supports the statement, so the statement is true.

Difficult Statements

Some Verbal Reasoning statements will be very difficult to assess quickly. Statements can be difficult for any number of reasons:

- The statement is very long, with lots of details to compare to the passage.
- The statement combines details from the passage in an unusual way that is challenging to compare to the passage.
- The statement asserts a strong opinion that is at least somewhat supported by the passage.
- The statement mentions people, places or things that are not specifically named in the passage, but defines these people, places or things in a way that allows comparison to the passage.

Note that in these examples, it will usually be a choice between True and Can't tell, or between False and Can't tell. There should be one answer that you can eliminate fairly quickly, but it could be quite challenging to decide between the two remaining answers. Note as well that even if a statement mentions people, places or things that are not specified in the passage, it is not necessarily Can't tell; it could be True or False, if the statement defines the new information clearly enough that you can compare the rest of the statement to the passage.

There is a trend towards longer statements in recent Verbal questions—i.e., the sets that have been added to the official practice content in the last few years. You can expect to see some shorter, quicker statements on Test Day, but you should expect some long, twisty statements as well.

You will now have a chance to practise with some difficult statements. You might want to cover the answer with your hand until you have had a chance to check the statement against the passage.

All languages, and certainly widely spoken ones like English, are distillations of numerous converging linguistic influences. In particular, many languages around the world can locate their origins in linguistic exchanges brought about in the last 500 years or so by interactions of conquest, commerce and exploration between different peoples. Often, people who live their day-to-day lives between two languages will combine elements of the grammar and vocabulary of both to form a new, simplified language, known by linguists as a pidgin. Pidgins tend to be developed in the context of trade, and usually have a basic grammatical structure and limited vocabulary. If a pidgin begins to be spoken as a first language by a population of any size, it ceases to be a pidgin and is instead categorised as a creole language. Creole languages may then go on to develop rich lexicons and intricate grammatical structures of their own, and in many cases can become the sole or primary languages of large populations. For instance, Tok Pisin—once pejoratively referred to as 'Pidgin English'—is now the official language of Papua New Guinea, spoken by several million people, 100,000 of whom speak it as a first language. Tok Pisin is loosely based on English, but also includes traces of numerous other tongues, including Portuguese, German and various indigenous languages; it is often a useful *lingua franca*, given that Papua New Guinea is home to over 800 separate languages! Another case study of a vibrant creole language is that of Haitian Creole, spoken in one dialect or another by all of Haiti's 11 million residents. Haitian Creole has a vocabulary based largely on French, but its grammatical structure reflects the impact of various African and Amerindian languages.

The study of creoles often opens the door to the study of a whole broader range of considerations around the sociology of language. Given the hierarchical colonial societies in which many creole languages originated, one common area of interest for scholars is the way in which these languages register different levels of respect for authority in their day-to-day usage. Often, more 'European' inflections of a given creole language are seen as socially higher-status. For example, the Haitian Creole used in formal settings is often more similar to French than the form of the language spoken in the home. This is an incidence of what linguists call diglossia: a situation in which one language, or one variant of a given language, is commonly used in one social setting, and another, more formal and prestigious, language or variant is commonly used in another—even by one and the same language user. Diglossia seems to many at first like a strange and foreign idea, but in fact the phenomenon can probably be located in all societies to some extent; after all, most people will speak to a judge in a different way than they would speak to an old friend. And of course, many non-creole languages also embody strict traditional social hierarchies in their forms and conventions. These linguistic conventions can have a real impact on social interactions and outcomes. For instance, it's been suggested that South Korea's high rate of airplane crashes in the 1980s and 1990s may have been linked to the fact that Korean speakers use extremely deferential honorific forms of address in speaking to workplace superiors; co-pilots, whose job is to correct the principal pilots when they make mistakes, may have felt unable or unwilling to voice concerns, resulting in fatal mistakes. Many South Korean airlines now use English for all communications between employees during flights, even between South Korean crew members.

9. Korean grammar does not allow a speaker to indicate the social standing of a person to whom they are speaking.

   A. True
   B. False
   C. Can't tell

Answer: Scan for keyword Korean; you will find it near the end of the passage, in an extended example about Korean speakers using extremely deferential honorific forms of address in speaking to workplace superiors. This detail implies that Korean allows a speaker to indicate the social standing of the person to whom they are speaking. The statement says the opposite, so the statement is false.

10. Haitians are more likely to speak French in formal context than in relaxed or familiar settings.

    A. True
    B. False
    C. Can't tell

Answer: Scan for the keywords 'Haitians' and 'French'; they appear in both paragraphs, but the relevant detail is in the second paragraph. The Haitian Creole spoken in formal settings is often more similar to French than the Haitian Creole spoken in the home. Note that this does not match the statement, which is about Haitians speaking French, not Haitian Creole. The passage does not contradict the statement, since we don't know from the passage whether Haitians are more or less likely to speak French in these circumstances. The answer is **(C)**.

11. An example of diglossia is an aristocratic 19th century Russian couple speaking French at home with their children, but speaking Russian with business colleagues and staff.

    A. True
    B. False
    C. Can't tell

Answer: Scan for the keyword 'diglossia,' and you will find it defined midway through the second paragraph as occurring when a single speaker uses one language in a social setting and another, more formal and prestigious language in another setting. The example in this statement fits the definition of diglossia in the passage. The statement is therefore true.

12. English is unique among languages in its facility for incorporating linguistic influences from varied sources.

    A. True
    B. False
    C. Can't tell

Answer: The keyword English appears in the first sentence, which explains that all languages distil numerous converging linguistic influences. English is not unique in this respect, but the statement claims that it is. The statement is false.

Remember

On the most difficult statements, you may struggle to decide between two answers—usually True and Can't tell, or False and Can't tell.

Eliminate the third answer—True or False—with confidence. Then, decide whether you have enough detail in the passage for the statement to be supported or contradicted.

At this point, if you really aren't sure, it's probably best to guess Can't tell.

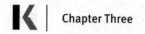

Kaplan Timed Practice Set—*Inferences and Difficult Statements*

Set your timer for 2 minutes. Mark answers for all 4 statements before time is up!

The story of Romeo and Juliet, the 'star-cross'd lovers,' is one of the most popular of all time, and has been told in several different versions. Best-known is the play *Romeo and Juliet*, which nearly everyone reads in school and which introduced such famous lines as 'What's in a name? That which we call a rose by any other name would smell as sweet.' Written and first performed in the 1590s, this highly poetical work of English theatre is set in Italy, where the legend of Romeo and Juliet and their warring families originates.

In the 18th century, the actor and producer David Garrick adapted the original play to remove material considered indecent. Among other changes, he changed references to Rosaline, Romeo's girlfriend at the start of the play, to references to Juliet, so that Romeo already knows and loves Juliet at the start of the play, and the theme is faithfulness rather than love at first sight. The original text was restored in the 19th century, with a sensational production at Sadler's Wells Theatre, London, starring the American sisters Charlotte and Susan Cushman as Romeo and Juliet. 'Gender-bending' is part of the play's tradition: in its original production, men played all the roles. Desdemona was played by a woman in a 1660 production of *Othello*, the first time a female role in a Shakespearean play was not performed by a man, some 44 years after the playwright's death; the first woman performed Juliet two years later.

By all accounts Charlotte Cushman was entirely convincing as Romeo. After seeing the Cushmans at Sadler's Wells, Queen Victoria noted in her journal that 'no one would ever have imagined she was a woman.'

In the 20th century, *Romeo and Juliet* took to the screen in a series of films, including Franco Zeffirelli's 1968 Technicolor epic, which was the first to cast unknown teenagers as the leads and to feature a controversial nude wedding scene, and Baz Luhrmann's 1996 version for the MTV generation, with a soundtrack of pop hits and gun battles instead of swordfights. The most popular film version of *Romeo and Juliet* is *West Side Story*, in which the Jets and the Sharks, rival gangs in New York City, replace the feuding Montagues and Capulets, and Romeo and Juliet become Tony and Maria. *West Side Story* also changes the ending so that one of the central couple survives, and won 10 Academy Awards in 1961, making it the most acclaimed film version of *Romeo and Juliet* to date. Who knows what twist on *Romeo and Juliet* we'll see next?

---

13. Shakespeare was the first to tell the story of Romeo and Juliet.

    A. True
    B. False
    C. Can't tell

14. Queen Victoria never went to the theatre.

    A. True
    B. False
    C. Can't tell

15. In Shakespeare's time, all the female roles in one of his plays would have been performed by male actors.

    A. True
    B. False
    C. Can't tell

16. Susan Cushman played Juliet.

    A. True
    B. False
    C. Can't tell

Kaplan Timed Practice Set—*Inferences and Difficult Statements:* Answers and Explanations

Inferences and difficult statements can be challenging to evaluate quickly. Be sure to review the worked answers in their entirety to ensure that you chose the correct answers for the correct reasons. Doing so will help to build your Verbal Reasoning skills, and help you pick up more marks within the allotted time on Test Day.

13. (C)

The keyword Shakespeare leads to the second paragraph, which implies that Shakespeare wrote *Romeo and Juliet*. The first paragraph indicates that the legend of Romeo and Juliet originates in Italy, but it is not clear from the passage whether Shakespeare was the first to tell this story or if someone else told it prior to his account in the 1590s. The correct answer is **(C)**.

14. (B)

The keyword in this statement is Queen Victoria, who appears in the third paragraph. Sadler's Wells, London, is mentioned as the home of a sensational production of *Romeo and Juliet* that featured 'gender-bending' casting, with a woman playing Romeo. Queen Victoria saw this production at Sadler's Wells Theatre, and found Charlotte Cushman entirely convincing as Romeo. Since passage states that Queen Victoria saw this performance at the theatre, we know that Queen Victoria went to the theatre at least once in her life. This statement contradicts the passage on this point, and is therefore false.

15. (A)

The keywords Shakespeare and female role lead to the second paragraph. The first woman to play a female role in a Shakespearean play did so in 1660, some 44 years after the playwright's death. Thus, it is correct to infer that all the female roles were played by men in Shakespeare's time. The statement is true.

16. (A)

Scan for the keywords Susan Cushman and Juliet. Susan Cushman appears midway through the second paragraph, which states that the sisters Charlotte and Susan Cushman played Romeo and Juliet in London sometime in the 19th century. The following paragraph specifies that Charlotte Cushman played Romeo, so it is safe to infer that Susan Cushman played Juliet. This statement is supported by the passage, so it is true.

Verbal Reasoning Questions

Most Verbal Reasoning sets will include questions instead of statements. In recent years, a slight majority of Verbal sets contained questions—most commonly, 7 out of 11 sets, as seen in the official practice tests—and it is likely that the Verbal section will be similarly balanced in future. A Verbal question has four answer choices; in most cases, the correct answer will be the one that is supported by the passage. A small number of Verbal questions will be 'negative' questions, meaning that any answers supported by the passage are incorrect. For now, let's consider how Verbal questions stand out from the Verbal statements we have practised so far:

1. They are questions, rather than statements.
2. There are four answer choices, rather than three.
3. The answer choices are not fixed-format; that is, each question will have its own four answers from which you must choose.

By far, the biggest challenge of Verbal Reasoning questions is that they require you to read a lot in order to come up with an answer. The questions and answers are usually full sentences, and will often run to more than one line of text. That is quite a lot of reading, before you have even gone to the passage! As such, Verbal questions are very challenging to answer in 30 seconds each—however, you have a good chance of answering most Verbal questions correctly, in the time allowed, if you follow the usual tips for Verbal statements, with these adjustments:

- Skip the passage—as you have even less time to read it.
- Read the question, and identify keywords that will lead to the correct answer.
- Scan the passage for the keywords. In most cases, the correct answer will paraphrase something that occurs in the passage just before or after the keywords.
- You are looking for the one answer that is supported by the passage. Even though questions may use wording such as 'best supported' or 'most likely to be true', only one answer will be supported by the passage, or true based on the passage. The other answers will either contradict the passage (just like a False statement) or will fall partially or entirely outside it (like a Can't tell statement). Thus, the skills you've practised so far are equally useful for Verbal questions.
- The exceptions to this rule are negative questions—those containing a 'negative' word, such as 'cannot', 'except' or 'least'. On a negative question, answer choices supported by the passage are incorrect. Thus, these questions are like a photographic 'negative' of most Verbal questions, in which the answer supported by the passage is correct. We'll look at these questions in more detail a bit later in the chapter.

Let's practise with the passage and questions starting on the next page. As always, try to answer each question in 30 seconds before reading the answer.

Pluto was considered the Solar System's ninth planet, and the furthest from the sun, from the time of its discovery in 1930 until 2006, when the International Astronomical Union (IAU) voted to define *planet* for the first time. According to this definition, a planet has three characteristics: it must orbit the sun, be of approximately round shape and have 'cleared its neighbourhood'—that is, it must be the only body of its size, other than its own satellites, in its region of outer space.

Because its orbit, which is eccentrically elliptical compared to those of the other planets, overlaps significantly with the orbit of Neptune—its nearest neighbouring planet in the Solar System—Pluto fails to meet the third criterion of the definition, and so it is no longer considered a planet, but instead a 'dwarf planet'. This decision by the IAU caused considerable controversy in the popular press at the time it was taken, due to the fact that generations of children had learnt in school that the Solar System includes nine planets; people often have difficulty facing reality when further scientific discovery complicates what they had previously thought to be settled, definite fact.

The IAU's decision to 'demote' Pluto from planet to dwarf planet was not taken lightly, and became necessary due to the discovery of a number of objects in the Kuiper Belt—the region of outer space that extends some 55 astronomical units beyond the orbit of Neptune. (An astro-nomical unit equals the distance from the Earth to the sun—so the Kuiper Belt extends very far out indeed!) A space object discovered in 2003 and since named Eris (after the ancient Greek goddess of discord) has a greater diameter than Pluto, with 25% more mass; both Pluto and Eris are thought to consist of the same mixture of ice and rock. Scientists could not justify calling Pluto a planet and Eris a Kuiper Belt object; since Eris was larger than Pluto, why shouldn't it also be a planet? The matter was further complicated by the fact that a second Kuiper Belt ob-ject, Makemake, discovered in 2005, is only slightly smaller than Pluto. Due to their significantly smaller mass and their resulting weaker gravitational pull, dwarf planets such as Pluto, Eris and Makemake are unable to clear other nearby space objects—either by repelling them, or by collid-ing and absorbing much of their mass, and thus growing larger and increasing their gravitational pull—and so are unlikely ever to become planets.

For these reasons, the IAU considered three options for defining planets at its meeting in 2006: the first would have increased the number of known planets to 12, keeping Pluto and adding Eris, Makemake and Ceres, long-known as the Solar System's largest asteroid; the second would have defined a planet as being one of the 9 planets discovered as of 1930; the third was the definition ultimately approved. Eris and Ceres were recognised as the first official dwarf planets a month later, with the same status extended to Makemake and Haumea in 2008. There are at least a dozen other trans-Neptunian objects that leading astronomers believe could fit the criteria for dwarf planets, though the IAU has not classified any further objects as dwarf planets since 2008.

Despite popular sentiment, scientists could not justify defining planets according to what was already known, as ongoing improvements in technology continue to allow us to observe the deepest reaches of the Solar System with increasing accuracy. The major problem with the first definition is that its broad nature could allow for an astonishing number of planets, once the expanse of the Kuiper Belt is further explored: since the Kuiper Belt is thought to contain 70,000 or more icy objects, its very possible that some of these will be as large as—or much larger than—Pluto. More than a decade on from the decision to demote Pluto, some astronomers think there could be as many as 200 dwarf planets in the Solar System. Given the extreme distance of some of these Kuiper Belt objects from the sun, they are very likely to further challenge our understanding of what is (and is not) a planet.

17. According to information in the passage, what is the primary reason that Pluto is no longer considered a planet?

    A. Pluto is not as round in shape as Eris.
    B. Astronomers voted to limit the number of planets to eight.
    C. Pluto is too far from the Sun to be considered a planet.
    D. Pluto's orbit is unusual in shape and intersects Neptune's.

Answer: The keywords in this question are Pluto and 'no longer considered a planet'—these appear near the end of the first sentence of the second paragraph. The early part of the sentence explains that Pluto is no longer considered a planet because its orbit is eccentrically elliptical, compared to the other planets' orbits, and that its orbit overlaps significantly with that of its neighbour, Neptune; for this reason, Pluto fails the third criterion of the IAU's definition of planet. Answer **(D)** is a very close paraphrase of the reason that Pluto fails to qualify as a planet under the new definition, so it must be correct. On Test Day, you'd simply click **(D)** and move on to the next question. To improve your understanding of how Verbal questions work, take a moment and try to find support for the remaining answer choices. You could take much longer than a moment, but you won't find support. In a standard Verbal question, only the correct answer is true, based on the passage.

18. The passage most strongly supports which of the following statements about Eris?

    A. Eris is smaller than Neptune.
    B. Eris is nearer to the sun than Pluto.
    C. Eris is currently classified as a dwarf planet.
    D. Eris is approximately round in shape.

Answer: The keyword in this question is Eris, which is mentioned several times in the third paragraph and once in the fourth paragraph. Since there are so many references to Eris, check a keyword from each answer choice to see if the answer is supported by the passage. The keyword in the first answer is Neptune, but Neptune is never mentioned in connection with Eris, so the comparison in **(A)** is not supported; eliminate **(A)**. The sun is never mentioned in connection with Eris, so eliminate **(B)** for the same reason. The keyword dwarf planet appears in the final sentence of the third paragraph, which states that Pluto, Eris and Makemake are dwarf planets; **(C)** is therefore correct, and there's no need to check **(D)**. For the record: If you did check **(D)**, you would see that Eris's shape never comes up in the passage.

19. The writer of the passage would most likely agree that which of the following was the ultimate cause of the public controversy that met Pluto's demotion from planet to dwarf planet?

    A. People have trouble aligning new scientific discoveries with what they know.
    B. Astronomers did not explain their decision in terms that the public could understand.
    C. Children are taught that there are nine planets.
    D. Astronomers demoted Pluto because they believed there were 200 other dwarf planets.

Answer: The keywords here are ultimate cause, public controversy and Pluto's demotion. Scanning for these leads to the final sentence of the second paragraph. Here, the writer of the passage attributes the controversy caused by the IAU's decision to define Pluto as a 'dwarf planet' rather than a 'planet' to the fact that people have trouble dealing with scientific discoveries that complicate what they had previously thought to be settled fact. Answer **(A)** paraphrases this point very concisely, and is therefore correct. For the record: **(C)** might be a tempting wrong answer, in that the author mentions that generations of children had learnt in school that there are nine planets; however, notice the subtle shift in **(C)** that makes it wrong: **(C)** instead talks about what children are taught, in the present tense, and therefore does not match the passage. **(B)** involves the terms used by astronomers and **(D)** refers to the belief that there are 200 other dwarf planets; both details are mentioned in the passage but not linked to public controversy regarding Pluto's demotion.

20. According to the passage, a common measurement used by space scientists involves:
    A. the radius of the sun.
    B. the interval between a planet and a star.
    C. the weight of ice.
    D. the distance between the sun and another star.

Answer: The keywords in this question are common measurement and space scientists. The word measurement never appears in the passage, so look for other words related to measuring or common measurement words. The answer choices give good examples to scan for: radius; length; weight; distance. The keyword distance appears in the third paragraph, in the bracketed remark that defines an astronomical unit as equal to the distance from the Earth to the sun. Answer **(B)** is a close paraphrase for this detail from the passage, so **(B)** is correct.

Negative Questions

Most students find negative questions to be the hardest questions in Verbal Reasoning. This is because the correct answer to a negative question will not be supported by the passage; on a negative question, answers that are supported by the passage will be incorrect. The nature of the correct/incorrect answers will vary, depending on the exact negative word in the question:

- If the question asks for an answer that 'cannot be true', then the correct answer must be false. That is, the correct answer will contradict the passage. Incorrect answers will be supported by the passage, or not included in the passage.

- If the question contains the word 'except', then the incorrect answers will normally be things that are supported by the passage. The correct answer could contradict the passage, or could be something not included in the passage. Answers supported by the passage will normally be incorrect. (We say 'normally' in this instance, as all the published examples of 'except' questions are framed this way, i.e. so that the correct answer is something that is not true based on the passage. But there is always the possibility, however unlikely, that the UKCAT could throw up a twist involving 'except' on Test Day—so double-check any 'except' question to make sure that it works this way.)

- If the question contains the word 'least', then the correct answer will not be supported by the passage. The incorrect answers will normally be supported by the passage. Even though the question says 'least', it is not a matter of comparing answers to see which is the 'less' appropriate—only one answer will not be supported by the passage, and will often contradict it.

Try applying these tips about negative questions that accompany the passage on the following page. As usual, try to keep yourself to no more than 30 seconds per question.

For over a hundred years, swimmers have been crossing the English Channel, the 350-mile-long stretch of water that separates Great Britain from the northern shores of France. Captain Matthew Webb made the first recorded attempt in 1875 when he swam the 21-mile distance across the Strait of Dover in 21 hours, 45 minutes. Webb's successful crossing was the beginning of a trend: 811 people have successfully swum across the Strait of Dover since Webb, a total of 1,185 times. In 1927 the Channel Swimming Association was founded as the governing authority of this relatively new sport. The association authenticates claims to channel swimming and keeps track of crossing times and provides regulations for approved swims. For example, the CSA's rules prohibit any assistance other than having nourishment handed to the swimmer (though direct contact is not allowed, even in this instance), and the CSA stipulates the acceptable swimming costumes and use of 'grease' (to protect the exposed parts of the body from the cold waters of the Channel). Each swimmer must also have a pilot in a nearby boat who ensures the swimmer's safety and provides assistance in an emergency situation, as well as feeding the swimmer by hand or feeding pole; if the swimmer leaves the water for any reason, the swim must be aborted.

To date, the record for the fastest Channel crossing by a swimmer belongs to Trent Grimsey, an Australian, who swam from Dover to Cap Gris-Nez, France, on 8 September 2012 in exactly 6 hours, 55 minutes, besting the previous record by nearly 3 minutes. Grimsey, who was aged 24 at the time of his historic Channel swim, had previously won a number of international open water swimming competitions in Argentina, Brazil, California, New Zealand, Queensland (his home state in Australia) and Italy, where he set a record of 6 hours, 29 minutes in the Maratona del Golfo Capri-Napoli. Grimsey retired from competitive swimming in August 2013.

The previous record was set by Petar Stoychev, a Bulgarian swimmer who is also the eight-time winner of the Open Water World Championship. Stoychev made his record-breaking crossing on 24 August 2007 in 6 hours, 57 minutes, 50 seconds, beating his previous time by over twenty minutes. Russian swimmer Yuri Kudinov, Stoychev's long-time rival, swam the Channel on the same day, starting just 18 minutes after Stoychev and finishing less than 30 minutes after the Bulgarian broke the world record. Stoychev's time broke a record set only two years before by Christof Wandratsch, who completed the feat in 7 hours, 3 minutes. Neither Stoychev nor Kudinov knew the other would be attempting the crossing that day until hours before they began. The two were neck and neck for most of the race, and Stoychev later confessed that he imagined he would hold the world record for only a few minutes before watching it be awarded to Kudinov. Grimsey and Stoychev are the only people to have swum across the English Channel in under 7 hours, an extraordinary feat of physical endurance.

21. Which of the following cannot be true?

A. Stoychev thought Kudinov would break his record.
B. Webb's first swim across the Channel was not regulated by the CSA.
C. Stoychev and Kudinov are Bulgarian rivals.
D. Fewer than 1,000 people have swum across the Strait of Dover.

Answer: This is a negative question, asking for something that cannot be true; the correct answer will contradict the passage. There aren't any keywords in the question, so scan for keywords from each answer and compare to the passage, until you find the one that contradicts the passage. The keywords in **(A)** are Stoychev and Kudinov, which appear in the final paragraph; the fifth sentence of this paragraph supports **(A)**, so **(A)** is incorrect. The keywords in **(B)** are Webb and CSA; these occur in the first paragraph, which states that Webb swam across the Channel in 1875 and that the CSA was founded in 1927. From this information, it is safe to infer that **(B)** is true, so **(B)** is incorrect. **(C)** contains the same keywords as **(A)**; checking the final paragraph, you will notice that Stoychev is Bulgarian but Kudinov is Russian. **(C)** contradicts the passage, and is therefore the correct answer. There is no need to check **(D)** against the passage.

22. All of the following statements about Trent Grimsey must be true EXCEPT:
    A. He swam competitively in many countries.
    B. He broke a record that had been set just over 5 years earlier.
    C. He no longer competes in open water swimming events.
    D. He is one of three swimmers to cross the English Channel in under 7 hours.

Answer: This negative question contains the word except; three of the answers will be true (supported by the passage), and therefore incorrect. The correct answer will be the one that is not supported by the passage—it could contradict the passage, or could include information that is not in the passage. The question also contains a helpful keyword, the name Trent Grimsey. Grimsey's name appears in the second paragraph, and at the very end of the passage. The second paragraph lists several countries where Grimsey swam competitively, so **(A)** is supported by the passage; thus, **(A)** is incorrect. The same paragraph mentions that Grimsey broke the record for swimming across the Channel in September 2012; the next paragraph states that the previous record was set in August 2007. Thus, **(B)** is supported by the passage and is also incorrect. Answer **(C)** is a close paraphrase of the final sentence of the second paragraph, so it is incorrect. The correct answer must be **(D)**, and the details in the final paragraph allow you to infer that only two swimmers—Grimsey and Stoychev—have swum across the English Channel in under 7 hours. **(D)** is false, and therefore correct.

23. The author would least likely agree with which of these claims about approved swims across the English Channel?
    A. They may involve direct contact between the swimmer and his pilot.
    B. Swimmers may use grease, subject to regulation.
    C. The choice of swimming costume for such swims is restricted.
    D. Swimmers may not participate without a pilot in a nearby boat.

Answer: Most passages, like this one, will not include direct statements of the author's opinion. Thus, you can infer that the author would agree with anything that is supported by the passage. The author would be least likely to agree with something that contradicts the passage, so that is what you are looking for here. The question contains the keywords 'approved swims', which appear in the first paragraph. The rest of that paragraph explains several of the rules of approved swims. Comparing these details from the passage to the answer choices, you will find that **(B)**, **(C)** and **(D)** are supported by the passage, but **(A)** contradicts it—direct contact with the swimmer is never allowed in approved swims. **(A)** is therefore correct.

24. Which of these conclusions about open water swimmers is not supported by the passage?

    A. They are capable of extreme accomplishments due to their physical prowess.
    B. They compete in many different countries.
    C. They never swim more than two hours without taking a break on a boat.
    D. They compete to break world records set by other swimmers.

Answer: This question contains a negative word, 'not', so any answers supported by the passage will be incorrect. The question also includes the keywords 'open water swimmers'; since these swimmers are discussed throughout the passage, it will be quicker and easier to scan for keywords from each answer choice. The keywords 'extreme accomplishments' and 'physical prowess' lead to the passage's final sentence, which uses similar words to describe the 'extraordinary feat' of Grimsey and Stoychev; **(A)** is supported by the passage, so it is incorrect. **(B)** mentions many different countries, and there is a list of countries where Grimsey won open water swimming competitions in the second paragraph; **(B)** is also supported, and thus also incorrect. The keywords 'two hours' never appear in the passage, and the keywords 'taking a break on a boat' contradict the rules of the CSA in the first paragraph, which does not allow for the swimmer to leave the water for any reason. **(C)** is not supported by the passage, so it is correct.

Difficult Passages

Some Verbal Reasoning passages will be difficult to work with under the time pressures of the section. Often, these passages would be no problem to read straight through, if you had two or three minutes just to read the passage. But with only 30 seconds per question—including the time to read the question and scan for support—some passages will be especially tough going.

The most difficult Verbal passages tend to feature one or more of the following characteristics:

- Long sentences, with multiple clauses strung together.
- A discursive style, meaning that the passage may take a lot of words to express an idea that might be stated more concisely and coherently.
- Technical descriptions or explanations of complex processes, with several steps or factors, which may be arranged sequentially or in some other order (e.g. the best process followed by two alternative processes that are insufficient or substandard in some way).
- Much of the passage might consist of comparison, qualification or competing opinions, which can involve quite a lot of detail, and quite a lot of references to earlier parts of the passage.

In difficult passages, ideas can be tough to follow or 'unpack' without taking time to read the passage properly. To answer some questions, you may need to compromise and read just the bit of the passage before and after the keyword. Just take care not to be drawn into the passage any more than is required to answer each question, and try to keep to no more than 30 seconds per question.

Do your best to answer the 4 questions that accompany the passage on the next page, which meets many of the criteria of a difficult passage, in 30 seconds each. If you need a bit longer, keep track of how much extra time you take. Make a note of your time per question in the margin before checking the answer for each question.

The phrase 'loudness war' is used by many professionals and enthusiasts of the music industry to denote the apparent increase in volume levels of recorded music over time. Sound engineers and record producers have, since the boom in popular recorded music in the 1940s, sought to make the default volume of records louder and louder, in the belief that louder recordings are more popular among consumers. Critics say this has led to a corresponding drop in quality, as there is only so 'loud' a recording can be made before it loses subtlety and becomes distorted.

Many believe the loudness war began with the introduction of jukeboxes in public bars and cafes. Jukeboxes would be set to a constant level of volume, either determined by the owner or manufacturer, and so record labels started to record at higher volumes in order to make their singles stand out from others. The notion of competition continued to drive records ever louder in the sixties and seventies, as vinyl compilations became popular, and artists and labels wanted their songs to stand out from others on the same disc. However, the technical qualities of vinyl recording meant that the ceiling for volume was much lower than later technologies. With the arrival of compact disc and digital recordings, the loudness war entered a new phase. The newer digital sound technologies of the eighties and nineties allowed for a much higher volume with less risk of distortion than had been previously available on vinyl.

Many reasons have been offered for the increase in the volume of recorded music over the last half-century. Often music is optimised by sound engineers for playback inside a vehicle, as this is where the vast majority of the public listen to music, where the song must compete for attention with advertisements, engine noise and the distractions of the outside world. There is also the prevalent belief among sound engineers and record labels that loud music simply sounds better to the ears of consumers. Finally, academics have also mooted the idea that the loudness war in music is part of a larger trend of our environment becoming louder in general—analogous rises in the volume of TV and film have also been noted.

However, despite this apparently ever-escalating rise in volume, today there is a prevailing view that the loudness war reached its peak almost a decade ago, and that volumes in recorded music have since levelled out. Part of this has to do with the technical limits of digital recording—as with vinyl in the seventies, labels have now maximised the possible volume on digital recording formats without straying into distortion and loss of quality. But changing fashions within the music industry are also at work. Since 2008, when a number of big pop releases were widely criticized for straying into distortion through loudness, there has been a backlash against very loud recordings, with one sound engineer even organising an annual 'Dynamic Range Day' to raise awareness of what is lost when the volume of a recording is boosted too far. Since then this backlash has gathered pace, and extremely successful albums have since been specifically engineered to avoid high volume, distorted effects. Such successes have severed the supposed link between high volume and record sales, meaning that the loudness war might finally be over.

25. Critics of increasingly loud recorded music:
    A. attack the anti-pop backlash of stunts like the Dynamic Range Day.
    B. blame musicians of the 1940s for escalating the loudness war.
    C. argue that recording quality has been lost through the increase in volume.
    D. present themselves as consumer champions.

Answer: There are many criticisms of loud music in this passage. If you scanned for the keyword critics, you may have spotted the final sentence of the first paragraph, which is paraphrased nicely in **(C)**, the correct answer. If you struggled to spot this reference, you might have gone on to check for keywords from each answer. The keyword Dynamic Range Day from **(A)** appears in the final paragraph, but this event was a backlash against loud music, not a backlash against pop; in any case, there is nothing in the passage to suggest a backlash against Dynamic Range Day. The 1940s are mentioned in the first paragraph, but there is no indication of critics blaming musicians of that decade, contrary to **(B)**. The keyword recording quality in **(C)** leads to the end of the first paragraph, confirming that **(C)** is correct. For the record: the keyword consumer champions does not appear in the passage, ruling out **(D)**.

26. The author would be most likely to agree with which statement about recordings made on vinyl?
    A. They were uniquely suited for jukeboxes in the fifties and sixties.
    B. They are more highly valued by music enthusiasts than recordings on compact disc.
    C. There was a technical limit to how loud they could be made.
    D. Their maximum volume was higher than the maximum volume of digital recordings.

Answer: The keyword vinyl appears primarily in the second paragraph; the fourth sentence there indicates that the technical qualities of vinyl recording resulted in a much lower volume ceiling than later recording technologies. To put it another way: There was a technical limit for the volume of vinyl recordings, which matches answer **(C)**. For the record: **(A)** and **(B)** include keywords from the passage (e.g. jukeboxes; fifties and sixties), but the ideas in these answers have no basis in the passage. **(D)** contradicts the passage: digital recordings can have a higher volume than vinyl recordings.

27. According to the passage, it must be false that:
    A. Most people listen to music at home.
    B. Many music professionals believe that listeners prefer loud music.
    C. Music played in cars must compete with many different diversions.
    D. Other media—not only music—has risen in volume over the years.

Answer: This is a negative question, meaning that the correct answer will contradict the passage, while the incorrect answer will be supported by the passage. As the third paragraph states, the vast majority of the public listen to music in their cars; this detail contradicts **(A)**, which is therefore correct. For the record: **(B)**, **(C)** and **(D)** are all confirmed by the same paragraph; since they are supported by the passage, they cannot be correct.

28. The passage supports the idea that, in recent years, the 'loudness war':
    A. has been superseded by structural problems in the music industry.
    B. caused intense squabbling among musicians.
    C. led to a drop in album sales worldwide.
    D. may have ended.

Answer: The keyword 'loudness war' isn't very helpful, so check the passage for keywords from each answer. Eliminate each answer as soon as you see that there is no support in the passage. The keywords in **(A)** do not lead to any information in the passage; eliminate **(A)**. **(B)** can be eliminated for the same reason. The keyword album sales worldwide leads to the final paragraph, which states that there is not necessarily a link between loudness and record sales, contradicting **(C)**. **(D)** is a paraphrase of the passage's final sentence; **(D)** is correct.

Kaplan Timed Practice Set—*Verbal Reasoning Questions*

Set your timer for 2 minutes. Attempt to answer 4 questions before time runs out. If you have trouble with a question, try to eliminate one or two answers, then make your best guess.

In 2011, a total of eight ancient boats were discovered in a quarry near the Flag Fen archaeological site, located immediately south-east of Peterborough in the Cambridgeshire fens. In 2013, carbon-dating revealed that the boats were from 1600 BC, a full two centuries earlier than the original approximation. The boats, made from lime, oak or maple, were buried extremely deep underground, and were so well built that they were virtually intact and, if allowed onto water, would still be buoyant. This unusual, historical treasure trove led the archaeologists to take the exceptional (and costly) decision to transport the boats from the quarry to their facility at Flag Fen without first cutting the boats into chunks, which required a system of pulleys and special transport equipment reinforced with scaffolding poles to ensure that the boats were not damaged.

The boats had been deliberately submerged to the bottom of what was then a creek, in what is believed to be a Bronze Age ritual of some religious significance. The area of the fens where the boats were found had been crisscrossed with creeks and rivers during the Bronze Age, and the custom of the time was to sink offerings to the gods underwater. Many daggers and jewels were found near the boats, leading archaeologists to believe that the site may have been of religious as well as commercial importance over 3,000 years ago. Some of the boats were well used by fishermen and must have been brought some distance inland in order to be sunk in the creek, and others appear to have been built only for that purpose. We know that they deliberately sank the boats because the transoms—the pieces of wood that close off the rear of the boat—had been removed.

The craftsmanship of the boats is extraordinarily practical and versatile, even by today's standards. The shipwrights used tools made of bronze to carve the tree trunks and shape the boats, some of which were hewn until only as thick as a finger, but so resiliently buoyant that they were able to float when rain filled the archaeologists' trench. The boats are now on display in a chilled container within a barn on the Flag Fen site. The technician responsible for conserving the boats had to spend eight hours a day spraying them with water and removing impurities; once the spraying was finished, the boats were injected with a special wax with preservative powers and then dried out, a process that took two years to complete. The boats are currently on display at Peterborough Museum.

Why did they sink the boats? The likeliest explanation is that an extended period of climate change led to a worrying rise in sea levels, so that the terrain of the fens became increasingly waterlogged over a very small number of years. As a consequence, the mostly agrarian society was not able to grow crops, and was at risk of starvation. The ritual sinking of the boats was thus likely intended to be a profoundly desperate offering to appease the gods and stop the seas from rising.

29. The passage suggests that the Bronze Age is most likely called 'the Bronze Age' because at that time people:

    A. used coins primarily made of bronze.

    B. constructed a series of prominent bronze statues.

    C. worked with bronze implements.

    D. first discovered bronze.

30. Which of the following conclusions cannot be true?

    A. Water once played a part in a religious custom.

    B. Climate change is only a contemporary concern.

    C. The Cambridgeshire fens were not always waterlogged.

    D. Some ancient people deliberately sank boats.

31. All of the following statements about the recently discovered boats are true except:

    A. They were carved from oak or other trees.

    B. Some of the boats are capable of floating.

    C. They were first estimated to date to 1600 BC.

    D. Some of the boats were fishing boats.

32. The author of the passage would most likely agree with which of these assertions?

    A. The Flag Fen boats could be used by fishermen today.

    B. Archaeologists were wrong to chop up the Flag Fen boats.

    C. Flag Fen was the most significant religious site in the Bronze Age.

    D. Conserving ancient boats is a slow, painstaking process.

Score Higher Online

In recent years, the Verbal section has included 7 or 8 sets with questions, with the remaining sets featuring True/False/Can't tell statements. Confirm this balance of questions and statements in your Kaplan Online Centre ahead of Test Day. We will post test updates in June, which will include a note of the expected balance of questions and statements in the Verbal section.

Kaplan Timed Practice Set—*Verbal Reasoning Questions*: Answers and Explanations

Passages with Verbal Reasoning questions are the most time-consuming and challenging on the UKCAT. Unprepared test-takers fall into the trap of reading everything, which can easily take 3 to 4 times as long as the time you actually have for the set. Despite the reading involved, you still have only 2 minutes per set. Scanning for keywords and selecting the answer choice that must be true based on the passage—a skill that you have practised on Verbal Reasoning statements—should be sufficient to get you to the correct answer for most Verbal Reasoning questions in 30 seconds. The more quickly and accurately you scan, the more marks you will earn in this section—even on the hardest questions!

29. (C)

Scan for the keywords Bronze Age, which appear twice in the second paragraph. None of the information here corresponds to the answer choices, so scan for a keyword from each answer choice. The keywords in **(A)** and **(B)**, coins and statues, do not appear in the passage; eliminate **(A)** and **(B)**. The keywords bronze implements in **(C)** lead to the third paragraph, which states that the Flag Fen shipwrights used tools made of bronze. This detail from the passage supports **(C)**, which is therefore correct. If you were not confident about this, you might also check **(D)** against the passage, but there is nothing in the passage to clarify whether bronze was first discovered in the Bronze Age.

30. (B)

There isn't a keyword in this question, and it's a negative question. The correct answer will be something that contradicts the passage; any answers that are supported by the passage are incorrect. The keywords in **(A)**, 'water' and 'religious', are found in the second paragraph, which explains that the boats were deliberately submerged underwater in a ritual of religious significance; the custom of the time was to sink offerings to the gods underwater. **(A)** is supported by the passage, so it is incorrect. The keyword in **(B)**, 'climate change', appears in the final paragraph. The Flag Fen boats date to an extended period of climate change which resulted in the fens becoming increasingly waterlogged in a very short time. Thus, **(B)** contradicts the passage, as climate change was a concern in the Bronze Age. **(B)** is correct.

31. (C)

This question contains a negative word, except. Thus, the three incorrect answers will be supported by the passage; the correct answer will contradict the passage, or will involve information that is not in the passage. The keywords oak or other trees lead to the first paragraph, which states that the Flag Fen boats were made of oak, lime or maple; **(A)** is supported by the passage, so it is incorrect. The keyword floating in **(B)** is found in the third paragraph; archaeologists found that some boats could float in rainwater. **(B)** is supported by the passage, and thus incorrect. The keyword 1600 BC occurs in the first paragraph; carbon dating revealed the boats are from 1600 BC, two centuries earlier than first thought. Thus, the boats were first estimated to date to 1400 BC. **(C)** contradicts the passage, so it is the correct answer.

32. (D)

This question asks what the author would agree with, so the answer choice that is supported by the passage will be correct. There isn't a keyword in the question, so scan for a keyword from each answer to find support in the passage. The Flag Fen boats are mentioned throughout the passage, so scan for fishermen today, the keywords in **(A)**. Fishermen in the Bronze Age are mentioned in the second paragraph, but fishermen today are not mentioned; while the boats could float, this does not mean that they are sturdy enough to be used by fishermen, so **(A)** is not supported by the passage. The keywords in **(B)**, archaeologists and chop up, lead to the end of the first paragraph. Archaeologists decided not to cut up the boats into chunks, so **(B)** contradicts the passage. The keywords in **(C)**, religious site and Bronze Age, guide you to the second paragraph, which explains that the fen was a site of some religious significance. The statement in **(C)** is much stronger, and is not supported by the passage. This means that **(D)** must be correct; indeed, the keywords conserving ancient boats lead to the third paragraph, which details the meticulous two-year process of preserving the boats.

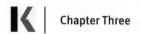

Keeping Perspective—Verbal Reasoning

You are about to complete a timed Kaplan UKCAT quiz, consisting of 6 Verbal Reasoning passage sets. If you pace yourself, and spend no more than 2 minutes per set, you should be able to attempt to answer every item. Even if you find yourself running out of time near the end, do your best to eliminate at least one answer choice and make your best guess. It is essential that you get into the mindset of marking an answer for every question, and that you practise doing so as you complete several sets under UKCAT time pressure.

As you have seen so far, Verbal statements and questions come in a range of difficulties, and all are worth one mark. If a statement or question is especially difficult, it is essential not to waste time on it. Such items are designed to draw in unprepared students, and ensure they get a poor result.

Before you begin the Kaplan UKCAT quiz, let's consider some of the key issues in Verbal Reasoning that unprepared (or underprepared) test-takers misunderstand time and again on the UKCAT:

The more elaborate your reasoning, the more likely it is to be wrong. The test-maker knows you only have 30 seconds (at most) per statement, so you are not expected to come up with an elaborate explanation to justify your answer. If you feel complicated reasoning is required, then scan the passage again for a different (or related) keyword—it is very likely that you've missed something the first time round. Or that the answer is Can't tell.

Statements can only be True or False based on what is in the passage. Support from the passage in the form of a paraphrase or an inference is required to make a statement True; similarly, a statement must contradict a detail or inference from the passage in order to be False. That is why scanning for keywords is so essential, and why you must be prepared to eliminate appropriately whenever you don't find support or contradiction (or both).

Most questions ask you to find the answer that is True (except for negative questions). Each Verbal question presents you with four statements—the answer choices—and you must normally select the one that is supported by the passage. That is, you must find the one answer that is a True statement. Negative questions are the exception to this rule, as any answers that are True will be incorrect.

Scan the entire passage for all references to your keywords, or related words. This point may seem a bit obvious, but you would be surprised how many test-takers stop scanning as soon as they find a single reference to their keyword. Sometimes, you will have to combine information from two separate references to make an inference, or to discover that the passage gives contradictory information.

Proceed carefully when the passage or the statement uses extreme language. Extreme language can be very subtle, and a shift from passage to statement could result in an unexpected answer (e.g. a statement that appears to be very similar at first glance could be False or Can't tell instead of True). Reading before and after the keyword in the passage, and checking for any other references to the keyword, will help en-sure that you pick up these marks.

Remember the many reasons why 'Can't tell' can be the correct answer. The most common reason is that the statement includes a keyword that is not mentioned in the passage. Also popular, and far more chal-lenging, is a statement that includes terms from the passage, but adds a further term that is not mentioned in (or inferable from) the passage. Another way of thinking about these statements is that they do not have adequate support from the passage to be true, but can't be false because they don't contradict the passage. Often, it is fairly straightforward to see that you can eliminate one answer straightaway on such statements (i.e. it's obviously not True, or obviously not False). Elimination is the key to saving time, and earning marks.

> # Remember
>
> It's 30 seconds per question in Verbal Reasoning.
>
> Any slower, and you will not finish the section.

Chapter 3 Kaplan UKCAT Quiz

Set your timer for 12 minutes. Try to evaluate all 24 statements and questions, and mark an answer for each before time is up. If a statement is difficult, try to eliminate one answer and then make your best guess, so you can keep to 2 minutes per set.

Because the British government has never undertaken a large-scale campaign to 'put a Briton on the moon', few people know much about the British space programme. Unlike many other national space initiatives, the British space programme's official focus was always on unmanned satellite launches, and, in fact, the UK has banned human space flight since 1986. All British astronauts who have travelled in outer space during the ban have done so with funding from non-governmental sources, either as 'space tourists' or by acquiring American citizenship and joining the NASA programme.

Interest in a British space programme, though, began much earlier. The British Interplanetary Society, founded in 1933, instigated early research in the field and developed the UK's military interest in a space programme. Throughout the 1960s and 1970s, the UK launched a number of satellites and rockets: some on the Isle of Wight, some in Woomera, Australia, where a joint Australia–UK weapons- and aerospace-testing facility was located. More than 6,000 rockets were launched from Woomera, including the hypersonic rocket Falstaff and the satellite-launching rocket Black Arrow. The Ariel programme saw the UK develop and launch six satellites from 1962 to 1979, in collaboration with NASA; the final four spacecraft in this series were designed and built in the UK. In this same era, the UK did not play a role in the 'Space Race' between the world's two military superpowers that led to the first men setting foot on the moon, in a series of American-commanded missions that captured the world's imagination from 1969 to 1972. Since the rise of manned space flight, both the USA and the Soviet Union (and, later, Russia) have included astronauts from Europe and other parts of the world on space missions.

The official programme of UK satellite launches was cancelled in the early 1980s, but in 1985 the British National Space Centre was founded to coordinate UK space activities. Today, the UK Space Agency, founded in Wiltshire in 2010, has replaced the British National Space Centre and assumed responsibility for government policy and budgets for space exploration. In the next 20 years, the agency aims to increase the size of the UK space industry from £6 billion to £40 billion, creating over 30,000 jobs. Central to this plan is the new £40 million International Space Innovation Centre in Oxfordshire, which will investigate climate change and space system security.

33. The UK did not compete in the 'Space Race'.

    A. True
    B. False
    C. Can't tell

34. No Briton has set foot on the moon.

    A. True
    B. False
    C. Can't tell

35. Most UK rockets have been launched in Australia.

    A. True
    B. False
    C. Can't tell

36. Manned space flights will now launch from Oxfordshire.

    A. True
    B. False
    C. Can't tell

City planners tend to think of 'green spaces' as something to be tightly rationed out and strictly regulated, but consider the approach being taken in Oslo, where municipal authorities are attempting to let nature run wild and free in parts of the metropolitan area. In just over a year, the city has set up 10 new public meadows. Unlike the existing public parks, these will be allowed to become overgrown with species of weeds which are known to stimulate ecological diversity, with groundskeepers ensuring that other, less beneficial weeds, are not allowed to dominate the space. The ultimate intention is to nurture the growth of wildflowers that will attract bees and other pollinators. While the meadows are far smaller than the long-standing city parks, they have an entirely distinct purpose of their own; the new meadows will be less expensive to maintain than the city's existing green spaces. Moreover, Oslo's biodiversity drive is not limited to these city-managed locations. Municipal funds are also being used to give interested members of the public crash courses on how to keep bees in their gardens, and the city government will pay for training and equipment to allow citizens to do so. Aside from the boost to national agricultural and pharmaceutical output that will result from these initiatives in years to come, the hope is that Norway can do its bit to combat the catastrophic overall decline of the global bee population, which threatens to destabilise agricultural ecosystems worldwide.

Oslo is far from the only city where plans are being made to incorporate plant life into the urban environment. New York is looking to spend some $100 million to utilise trees and other greenery to absorb solar energy and reduce the city's incidence of heatstroke, a condition that currently kills or hospitalises about 500 New Yorkers a year. A substantial amount of funding will be spent on reforestation, and a larger amount on planting more trees in public parks. The rest—some $82 million—will be spent on placing trees and plant life on the roofs of buildings, including both public property and private housing. Many other cities across the United States, which suffer from similar public health issues through the summer period, will be watching the biodiversity programme to gauge its success.

Another instance of radical applications of plant life by major cities is furnished by China, where the national government is investing millions in creating urban farming facilities in the heart of some of the world's largest metropolises. Growing food in cities is a response to a grave problem with pollution and contaminants, which have rendered some 10% of arable land in rural China unsafe. The result of using this soil for agriculture can be severe, long-term health problems for consumers eating the food in question. The pollution is even worse in the case of soil around major conurbations and industrial centres—hence the need to cultivate clean soil samples artificially for use in the new enhanced farming facilities. The results can be spectacular—the urban centres can yield up to 100 times more food per square metre than rural farming facilities. At such a rate of productivity, it may not be long before we start seeing similar techniques rolled out much more broadly around the world.

37. The author would most likely agree with which of the following statements?

    A. Oslo's new public meadows are visited far less frequently than its pre-existing parks.
    B. Oslo's new public meadows, unlike its parks, will not be tended or controlled by human staff.
    C. Oslo's meadows will require more financial support from the city government than its parks.
    D. Oslo's meadows cover less of the city than the parks that existed before the meadows.

38. The passage supports which of the following claims about beekeeping in Norway?

    A. Beekeeping has limited potential due to the northerly latitude and cold winters.
    B. Residents of Norway's cities are not expected to be interested in keeping bees.
    C. Beekeeping has the potential to increase production in more than one national industry.
    D. Local governments in Norway have not financed beekeeping to any degree.

City planners tend to think of 'green spaces' as something to be tightly rationed out and strictly regulated, but consider the approach being taken in Oslo, where municipal authorities are attempting to let nature run wild and free in parts of the metropolitan area. In just over a year, the city has set up 10 new public meadows. Unlike the existing public parks, these will be allowed to become overgrown with species of weeds which are known to stimulate ecological diversity, with groundskeepers ensuring that other, less beneficial weeds, are not allowed to dominate the space. The ultimate intention is to nurture the growth of wildflowers that will attract bees and other pollinators. While the meadows are far smaller than the long-standing city parks, they have an entirely distinct purpose of their own; the new meadows will be less expensive to maintain than the city's existing green spaces. Moreover, Oslo's biodiversity drive is not limited to these city-managed locations. Municipal funds are also being used to give interested members of the public crash courses on how to keep bees in their gardens, and the city government will pay for training and equipment to allow citizens to do so. Aside from the boost to national agricultural and pharmaceutical output that will result from these initiatives in years to come, the hope is that Norway can do its bit to combat the catastrophic overall decline of the global bee population, which threatens to destabilise agricultural ecosystems worldwide.

Oslo is far from the only city where plans are being made to incorporate plant life into the urban environment. New York is looking to spend some $100 million to utilise trees and other greenery to absorb solar energy and reduce the city's incidence of heatstroke, a condition that currently kills or hospitalises about 500 New Yorkers a year. A substantial amount of funding will be spent on reforestation, and a larger amount on planting more trees in public parks. The rest—some $82 million—will be spent on placing trees and plant life on the roofs of buildings, including both public property and private housing. Many other cities across the United States, which suffer from similar public health issues through the summer period, will be watching the biodiversity programme to gauge its success.

Another instance of radical applications of plant life by major cities is furnished by China, where the national government is investing millions in creating urban farming facilities in the heart of some of the world's largest metropolises. Growing food in cities is a response to a grave problem with pollution and contaminants, which have rendered some 10% of arable land in rural China unsafe. The result of using this soil for agriculture can be severe, long-term health problems for consumers eating the food in question. The pollution is even worse in the case of soil around major conurbations and industrial centres—hence the need to cultivate clean soil samples artificially for use in the new enhanced farming facilities. The results can be spectacular—the urban centres can yield up to 100 times more food per square metre than rural farming facilities. At such a rate of productivity, it may not be long before we start seeing similar techniques rolled out much more broadly around the world.

39. Which of these assertions about biodiversity is least likely to be true?

   A. Biodiversity schemes include efforts undertaken by governments and individuals.
   B. Cities across the USA are planting trees on rooftops to reduce hospital visits in the summer.
   C. Ecosystems in urban areas will benefit from having more wildflowers and greenery.
   D. Planting trees can reduce the heat and the summer and potentially prevent illness.

40. Which of the following cannot be true?

   A. The Chinese model of urban farming depends on soil prepared in a synthetic process.
   B. Soil in and near Chinese cities is safer for agricultural use than soil in rural China.
   C. The potential of urban farming facilities has not yet been realised on a global scale.
   D. Rural farms are less productive than the most efficient model of urban farms.

Johannes Vermeer (1632–1675) is now considered to be one of the Old Masters of Dutch painting, though only 35 of his paintings exist and very little is known about his life. Other than information in government registers and a handful of comments by other artists, Vermeer's life was so unknown (and thus inscrutably mysterious) that he was called 'the Sphinx of Delft' in the 19th century; as such, it was common to try and infer the truth about Vermeer from his paintings, as if his use of colour and light and his focus on middle-class subjects could reveal anything certain about the man who painted them. Most of what we now know about Vermeer was extensively researched in the city archives of Delft and published in the early 1980s.

Vermeer's early works were influenced by Caravaggio and Carel Fabritius, another Delft painter active in the early 1650s who was interested in the camera obscura. The Delft painters' guild made Vermeer a master in 1653, and he married in the same year. In the following two decades, Vermeer painted almost all of his extant works, which are in the mature style associated with him, such as *Girl with a Pearl Earring*, *The Music Lesson*, *The Milkmaid* and *Girl Reading a Letter at an Open Window*. This last painting was incorrectly attributed to Rembrandt for some time, until it was correctly recognised as a Vermeer in 1880. Vermeer lost everything near the end of his life and died penniless, having had to sell off the last of his paintings in his possession—though the precise reasons for his penury are lost to history.

Most of Vermeer's surviving paintings are from this mature period and feature interior scenes of tranquil domestic activity, such as reading, writing, drinking and playing musical instruments. The rooms in Vermeer's paintings are mostly dark, and he draws in the viewer's eye with his signature effect, a very distinctive 'pearly' light, achieved with miniature globules of white paint, so that the light appears to stream from a window at the left of every painting. The pearly light almost seems to gleam against the drab middle-class realities that Vermeer depicts. Objects within each painting, such as pianos and paintings, further guide the eye and define the constraints of the domestic sphere. Vermeer is also known for his use of cornflower blue and gold as common accent colours, giving his work a timeless elegance.

41. The passage suggests that the best-known feature of Vermeer's mature paintings was:

    A. his predominant use of white, gold and cornflower.
    B. an unusual, almost glowing, pearlescent light.
    C. his inclusion of musical instruments or paintings in every painting.
    D. a focus on servants and housework.

42. Which of the following was not included in any of Vermeer's paintings?

    A. windows
    B. jewellery
    C. letters
    D. seascapes

43. Based on the passage, it is correct to infer that Vermeer was called 'the Sphinx of Delft' because:

    A. he was viewed as an enigmatic artist in the 1800s.
    B. nothing was known about his life.
    C. he was the most prominent painter from Delft.
    D. his facial features resembled those of the Sphinx.

44. The author of the passage would most likely agree with which of these conclusions?

    A. You cannot determine facts about an artist from his techniques.
    B. Vermeer was uncomfortable with the everyday realities of middle-class life.
    C. The facts of an artist's life are irrelevant to an understanding of his work.
    D. Vermeer's wife was a milkmaid.

Scientists believe that the world is long overdue a serious influenza pandemic. These occur every so often when a strain of the virus possesses the correct combination of proteins to be both infectious and dangerous. These proteins are also used to describe the strain—for example, avian influenza, originating in birds, was also known as H5N1. Pandemics can be very deadly—the 'Spanish flu' pandemic in 1919 was responsible for the deaths of 20 to 40 million people, more than died in the First World War.

In 2009, a new strain of influenza, H1N1, became prominent in Mexico before spreading rapidly around the world. Known as swine flu, due to its origin in pigs, this strain of flu was highly transmissible from person to person, and fears grew that, if the virus was also dangerous, hundreds of thousands of people could die. Whilst some people seemed to suffer severely with the infection, most people seemed to have only mild symptoms lasting a few days.

Two different vaccines against this strain of flu were quickly developed and offered to those people at particular risk, such as pregnant women, health-care workers and people with certain health problems. This led to concern amongst the general population that rushing production could mean that the vaccines were not safe, and there was widespread anxiety about side effects, even though these were rare. However, many people decided that, on balance, it was a risk that they were prepared to take. Fortunately, as the winter flu season progressed, there were nowhere nearly as many serious cases of influenza as predicted, leading many people to believe that we have narrowly escaped another catastrophic pandemic.

45. Which of the following best describes the writer's view of the primary reason that the 2009 outbreak of H1N1 influenza was not as deadly as expected?

   A. Most cases were mild, and lasted for less than a week.
   B. People at high risk for H1N1 influenza were all vaccinated.
   C. The general public decided not to take the H1N1 vaccine.
   D. People who suffered most severely died quickly at the start of the outbreak.

46. The passage best supports which of the following statements about flu pandemics?

   A. They have killed more people than the World Wars.
   B. The next one will occur in the next five years.
   C. They can be averted by rushing vaccines into production.
   D. They can kill millions of people.

47. According to the information in the passage, what is it precisely that causes influenza outbreaks to develop into pandemics?

   A. An influenza strain originates in birds or swine, before passing to humans.
   B. An influenza strain develops with both dangerous and infectious proteins.
   C. An influenza strain arises on the borders of a major international conflict.
   D. An influenza strain grows stronger because the public declines an available vaccine.

48. The writer of the passage would most likely agree with which one of the following statements?

   A. The deadliest strains of flu usually emerge in Spanish-speaking countries.
   B. Avoiding contact with birds and pigs will keep you safe from deadly strains of flu.
   C. Concerns about side effects from the H1N1 vaccine were overblown.
   D. People are most vulnerable to the flu in the winter.

Drifting is a kind of automobile gymnastics, in which the driver of a car causes it to skid in a controlled manner horizontally at high speed, through judicious combination of accelerator and handbrake. For a country with seemingly strict laws and regulations, in which theft is met with capital punishment and women are restricted in public places, it is perhaps surprising that in Saudi Arabia the illegal 'sport' of drifting has become extremely popular, with the capital Riyadh proving a particular hotspot for the activity. However, there are in fact many readily understandable factors that led to the rise of drifting in Saudi Arabia.

At the start of the twentieth century, Riyadh was a small market town sandwiched between two riverbeds. Steady expansion followed by a massive boom of building in the early seventies has transformed this previously modest town into one of the region's largest cities, with a population of over five million. The key to the popularity of drifting perhaps lies in the nature of this expansion in the latter half of the twentieth century. Following a proposal drawn up by an influential urban planner in the early seventies, the Saudi government based the new city around continuous grids of large six-lane motorways, running perpendicular to each other. These grids have been extended out into the surrounding desert, awaiting the further expansion of the city, providing a perfect playground away from the city centre for errant drivers who wish to practice drifting.

Other factors, as the anthropologist Pascal Menoret argued in 2014, have led to the popularity of drifting in Saudi Arabia. Like many countries that trade heavily in oil, petrol is easily available and kept at an artificially low price by special state subsidies, meaning driving for pleasure is not a very expensive hobby for the average citizen. As the city of Riyadh, with its daunting network of motorways, is designed for cars rather than pedestrians, and (until recently) women were banned from driving, many men spent a large amount of time driving their partners or female relatives around the city, leading, Menoret argues, to a desire for rebellion that can transform the role of driver into something heroic, skilful and exhilarating, rather than quotidian and domestic. It is also posited that, in a society where politics and political activity is tightly monitored and controlled, the communities that gather around the activity of drifting form a rare site of open political dissent and rebellion against the state.

The hours around dawn, when police night patrols have returned to base, and morning patrols have yet to leave, are reported to be the most active for drifting in Riyadh. Large crowds of cars can suddenly appear in certain areas of the city, co-ordinated by mobile phone, to witness the phenomenon taking place. Sometimes the acrobatics are performed in expensive and powerful cars stolen from the super rich of Riyadh, and often there are fatal crashes in which both drivers and bystanders are killed. In 2016, in an effort to curb the high levels of accidents on Saudi roads related to drifting, the government introduced a new round of severe fines and punishments for those caught in the act, but it is unclear how far these new efforts will curb what some have called the 'national hobby' of Saudi Arabia.

49. Which of the following assertions about Saudi Arabia is supported by the passage?

A. The Saudi passion for driving increased exponentially with the hike in oil prices in the 1970s.
B. Driving is the national hobby, due to long hours spent crossing the desert in market activity.
C. The government has a history of planning for, and attempting to control, social behaviour.
D. The price of petrol was a major reason that most Saudi women did not drive until recently.

50. It must be false that:

A. Most drifting takes place in the early evening, before dinner.
B. Technology has allowed a larger population to be involved in drifting.
C. Drifting has been linked to other criminal activities.
D. Financial factors do not necessarily restrict an interest in drifting.

Drifting is a kind of automobile gymnastics, in which the driver of a car causes it to skid in a controlled manner horizontally at high speed, through judicious combination of accelerator and handbrake. For a country with seemingly strict laws and regulations, in which theft is met with capital punishment and women are restricted in public places, it is perhaps surprising that in Saudi Arabia the illegal 'sport' of drifting has become extremely popular, with the capital Riyadh proving a particular hotspot for the activity. However, there are in fact many readily understandable factors that led to the rise of drifting in Saudi Arabia.

At the start of the twentieth century, Riyadh was a small market town sandwiched between two riverbeds. Steady expansion followed by a massive boom of building in the early seventies has transformed this previously modest town into one of the region's largest cities, with a population of over five million. The key to the popularity of drifting perhaps lies in the nature of this expansion in the latter half of the twentieth century. Following a proposal drawn up by an influential urban planner in the early seventies, the Saudi government based the new city around continuous grids of large six-lane motorways, running perpendicular to each other. These grids have been extended out into the surrounding desert, awaiting the further expansion of the city, providing a perfect playground away from the city centre for errant drivers who wish to practice drifting.

Other factors, as the anthropologist Pascal Menoret argued in 2014, have led to the popularity of drifting in Saudi Arabia. Like many countries that trade heavily in oil, petrol is easily available and kept at an artificially low price by special state subsidies, meaning driving for pleasure is not a very expensive hobby for the average citizen. As the city of Riyadh, with its daunting network of motorways, is designed for cars rather than pedestrians, and (until recently) women were banned from driving, many men spent a large amount of time driving their partners or female relatives around the city, leading, Menoret argues, to a desire for rebellion that can transform the role of driver into something heroic, skilful and exhilarating, rather than quotidian and domestic. It is also posited that, in a society where politics and political activity is tightly monitored and controlled, the communities that gather around the activity of drifting form a rare site of open political dissent and rebellion against the state.

The hours around dawn, when police night patrols have returned to base, and morning patrols have yet to leave, are reported to be the most active for drifting in Riyadh. Large crowds of cars can suddenly appear in certain areas of the city, co-ordinated by mobile phone, to witness the phenomenon taking place. Sometimes the acrobatics are performed in expensive and powerful cars stolen from the super rich of Riyadh, and often there are fatal crashes in which both drivers and bystanders are killed. In 2016, in an effort to curb the high levels of accidents on Saudi roads related to drifting, the government introduced a new round of severe fines and punishments for those caught in the act, but it is unclear how far these new efforts will curb what some have called the 'national hobby' of Saudi Arabia.

51. The author of the passage would be most likely to agree that Riyadh:

A. grew more rapidly from the 1950s to the 1970s than in any earlier era.
B. is a popular location for drifting because it is less populated than the Saudi capital.
C. dwarfs the road networks of similarly sized cities in neighbouring countries.
D. is surrounded by motorways that exceed the boundaries of the city.

52. The passage suggests that one disadvantage of a living in a locality with a high rate of drifting is that:

A. petrol consumption increases, leading to a rise in the price of petrol.
B. other motorists tend to avoid the motorways at times when drifting is likely to take place.
C. the rate of drifting-related road incidents is a problem for the local authorities.
D. men who participate in drifting are more likely to hold antisocial views about women.

Cork is used in a variety of products, the most familiar of which is a wine stopper—or cork! The material's natural compressibility and near-impermeability make it ideal for this purpose, and natural cork is used for about 60% of wine stoppers today. Wine can become tainted during the process of bottling, ageing, storage and transport, and although other factors cause tainting, the stopper is usually held responsible. This association in the mind of the consumer is so strong that a bottle found on opening to have undesirable smells and tastes is usually said to have become 'corked'.

The use of alternative wine closures has grown in an attempt to prevent cork taint. For example, the synthetic cork, designed to look and function like a natural cork, avoids the risk as it is made from a resin that does not contain trichloroanisole. However, alternative closures themselves bring their own disadvantages. Wine experts have noted that a synthetic cork can impart its own slight chemical flavour to wine, replacing one type of cork taint with another. Screw-top bottles provide an alternative free of the risk of cork taint, but present an entirely new problem: consumers associate a screw-top bottle with poor quality wine, regardless of its price, vintage or reputation.

Wine experts have pointed to a larger issue facing wine lovers and casual wine drinkers, as wine sales have continued to grow over the last decade. Glass bottles are heavy and expensive, and many wines that are popular on the market do not need to be aged for more than a year. This has led some wine producers to innovate with alternative containers for wine, such as aluminium cans or polyethylene wine bottles. There is one type of alternate wine packaging that proved popular in the past: the so-called 'box of wine', a mainstay of 1980s dinner parties, which has returned more recently as an option for bulk or discounted wine purchases. A wine box most commonly contains 5 litres, compared to the standard 750 ml wine bottle. Technically of course, a 'wine box' isn't literally a 'box of wine', but rather a plastic bag of wine inside a carrier box.

53. Wine in screw-top bottles is of poor quality.

   A. True
   B. False
   C. Can't tell

54. Synthetic cork eliminates cork taint completely.

   A. True
   B. False
   C. Can't tell

55. Most wine is bottled with natural cork.

   A. True
   B. False
   C. Can't tell

56. A standard wine box would contain more than six times the amount of wine in a standard wine bottle.

   A. True
   B. False
   C. Can't tell

STOP. IF YOU FINISH BEFORE TIME IS UP, CHECK ANY QUESTIONS YOU HAVE MARKED FOR REVIEW. YOU MAY GO BACK TO QUESTIONS IN THIS QUIZ ONLY.

Chapter 3 Kaplan UKCAT Quiz: Answers and Explanations

33. (A)

Scan for the keywords Space Race, which appear in inverted commas midway through the second paragraph. The passage states here that the UK did not play a role in the Space Race; this statement paraphrases this closely, and is therefore true.

34. (C)

The keywords on the moon lead to the last sentences of the second paragraph, which say that the first men set foot on the moon in a series of US-commanded missions from 1969 to 1972, and that both the USA and the Soviet Union included European astronauts on space missions since the rise of manned space flight. Thus, the passage leaves open the possibility that a European astronaut may have been included on one of the missions to the moon; however, it is not clear whether or not a European was included, and it is also not clear whether or not any such European astronauts would have also been British. Based on the passage, then, the answer is Can't tell.

35. (C)

This statement is unusual, but scan for the keywords UK rockets and Australia. The third sentence of the second paragraph mentions that the UK launched a number of satellites and rockets in Woomera, Australia; the following sentence specifies that more than 6,000 rockets were launched from Woomera. Thus, the UK launched quite a lot of rockets in Australia; however, the passage does not mention any figures for UK rockets launched from other locations, nor does it clarify whether or not the 6,000-plus rockets launched from Woomera are a majority of UK rockets launched. The answer is therefore **(C)**.

36. (B)

Scan for the keywords manned space flight and Oxfordshire. Oxfordshire is mentioned only in the final sentence, as the location of a new space centre. This paragraph does not indicate whether manned space flights will launch from the Oxfordshire facility. Scanning the rest of the passage for manned space flight will reveal a reference to human space flight midway through the first paragraph; the UK has banned such flights since 1986. Thus, we can infer that manned space flights will not launch from Oxfordshire. This statement contradicts the passage, so the statement is false.

37. (D)

The answers all involve Oslo's new public meadows and pre-existing parks, which are discussed in the first paragraph. **(A)** mentions details about visits, which are not included in the passage. The first paragraph mentions groundskeepers in the new meadows, ruling out **(B)**. **(C)** is contradicted by the fifth sentence in the first paragraph. The same sentence matches the details in **(D)**, which is correct.

38. (C)

Beekeeping in Norway is discussed in the first paragraph. Norway's northerly latitude and cold winters are not mentioned in the passage; eliminate **(A)**. The first paragraph details a scheme to train residents of Oslo to keep bees at home, disproving the claim in **(B)**. Near the end of the first paragraph, we are told that the biodiversity schemes—including beekeeping—are expected to boost agricultural and pharmaceutical output. **(C)** paraphrases this detail from the passage; answer **(C)** is therefore correct. For the record: **(D)** contradicts the information about Oslo's local government funding beekeeping training and equipment for city residents.

39. (B)

This negative question asks for a statement that is false; the three incorrect answers will be supported by the passage, while the correct answer will contradict it. The keyword biodiversity appears in the first and second paragraphs, which detail several biodiversity schemes undertaken by governments and individuals. The second paragraph explains about New York's scheme to plant trees on rooftops to reduce the incidence of heatstroke; this scheme is being watched and considered for implementation in other US cities, which implies that New York is the only city to use this scheme so far. **(B)** contradicts the passage, so it is correct. For the record: We are told about the benefits from wildflowers and greenery expected in Oslo and New York, respectively, supporting **(C)**. **(D)** describes the goals of the tree-planting scheme in New York.

40. (B)

This negative question asks for a statement that cannot be true; the correct answer must contradict the passage, while the three incorrect answers will be supported by the passage. The Chinese model of urban farming, discussed in the final paragraph, includes clean soil that is cultivated artificially, matching the detail in **(A)**. We are told that 10% of arable land in rural China is not usable due to pollution, but the problem is much worse in major conurbations and industrial areas—that is, the soil is even more polluted in China's cities. **(B)** contradicts the passage on this point, so it must be false—and therefore correct. For the record: The details in the final sentences of the passage support the claims in **(C)** and **(D)**.

41. (B)

The keywords Vermeer's mature paintings lead to the first sentence of the final paragraph, which states that his signature effect was a distinctive pearly light that almost seems to gleam. **(B)** is a close paraphrase for this detail from the passage, so **(B)** is correct.

42. (D)

Details about Vermeer's paintings are given in the second and third paragraphs; scan these for any words that match the answer choices. Since this is a negative question, the three answers that are supported by the passage will be incorrect. Vermeer's paintings include *Girl with a Pearl Earring* and *Girl Reading a Letter by an Open Window*, so jewellery and letters were included in his paintings; eliminate **(B)** and **(C)**. The keyword window appears in the final paragraph, where it is mentioned as a common feature of Vermeer's paintings; eliminate **(A)**. Seascapes are never mentioned in the passage, so **(D)** must be correct.

43. (A)

The keywords the Sphinx of Delft appear in inverted commas in the first paragraph, so they are rather straightforward to scan for. The sentence that mentions this term also explains that it was used because Vermeer's life was so unknown and thus inscrutably mysterious in the 19th century. **(A)** is a close paraphrase for the passage, so it is correct. Beware of **(B)**, which is a classic example of a wrong answer trap that is stronger than the language in the passage. The passage says that there was some information about Vermeer's life in government registers, so the claim in **(B)** that nothing was known about his life contradicts the passage.

44. (A)

This question asks about the author's opinion, but there is no keyword in the question; you must scan for a keyword from each answer. The keywords determine facts and techniques in **(A)** lead to the first paragraph, which states that it was common to try and infer the truth about Vermeer from his use of colour and his subjects, as if these could reveal anything about the man who painted them. The 'as if' comment is a strong statement of the author's opinion, and **(A)** is a very accurate description of this same idea. **(A)** is therefore correct. If you were not sure of this, you could check the other answers; you'd find nothing in the passage to support **(B)**, **(C)** or **(D)**.

45. (A)

The keywords 2009, H1N1 influenza and not as deadly as expected lead to the second paragraph, which states that, although some people suffered severely with H1N1 infection, most people had mild symptoms lasting a few days. **(A)** paraphrases this very closely, and is therefore correct. The remaining answers are not supported by the passage.

46. (D)

Scanning for the keywords flu and pandemic is not entirely helpful, as these appear several times in the passage. Scanning for keywords from the answer choices is fairly quick in this instance, since the answers are relatively short. Answer **(A)** has the keywords World Wars, which leads to the detail in the first paragraph that the Spanish flu pandemic in 1919 killed more people than the First World War. There are no statistics about the deaths from the Second World War, so **(A)** cannot be correct. The keywords five years from **(B)** do not appear in the passage, which does not indicate precisely (or generally) when the next flu pandemic will occur, ruling out **(B)**. The keywords rushing vaccines into production do not lead to support in the passage for answer **(C)**. The only remaining answer is **(D)**; the keywords millions of people lead to the figure of deaths from the Spanish flu pandemic in the first paragraph. **(D)** is correct.

47. (B)

The keywords develop into pandemics lead to the first paragraph, which explains that flu pandemics occur when a strain of the virus has proteins that are both infectious and dangerous. Answer **(B)** matches this word for word, and is therefore correct.

48. (C)

This question is more challenging, as it does not give any keywords to scan. Instead, check for keywords from each answer choice. The keywords Spanish-speaking countries in **(A)** lead to references to Spanish flu in the first paragraph, and to Mexico, where the H1N1 strain was first prominent in the 2009 outbreak, in the second paragraph. It is not clear from these details that the writer believes that deadly flu strains originate in Spanish-speaking countries; eliminate **(A)**. The keywords birds and pigs in **(B)** lead to references to avian flu in the first paragraph and swine flu in the second; neither part of the passage indicates that you could avoid these strains of flu by avoiding birds and pigs; eliminate **(B)**. The keywords side effects and vaccine in **(C)** lead to the final paragraph, which states that there was widespread concern about side effects with the H1N1 vaccine, though these were rare. Thus, **(C)** is a safe inference based on the passage, and is correct. For the record: **(D)** has the keyword winter, which leads to the final paragraph—which does not support **(D)**.

49. (C)

The keyword Saudi appears in the second paragraph, which explains the urban planning that led to the expansion of Riyadh's motorways, and again in the third paragraph, which explains the social restrictions on women in Saudi Arabia. These details support the assertion in **(C)**, which is correct. For the record: The passage does not mention a hike in oil prices in the 1970s, nor does it refer to Saudis crossing the desert in market activity. Several phrases from **(D)** appear in the passage, but the price of petrol is not linked to restrictions on women drivers.

50. (A)

This is a negative question, meaning that the correct answer will contradict the passage, while the incorrect answers will be supported by the passage. As the first sentence of the final paragraph states, the hours around dawn are the most active for drifting in Riyadh; this contradicts **(A)**, which is therefore correct. For the record: The second sentence of the same paragraph mentions the large crowds that attend drifting events, supporting **(B)**. Likewise, **(C)** is confirmed by the next sentence, while **(D)** is supported by the final sentence.

51. (D)

The keyword Riyadh appears early in the second paragraph; later in this paragraph, we are told that Riyadh is based in a continuous grid of six-lane motorways that have been extended into the surrounding desert, awaiting the further expansion of the city. From these details, it is safe to infer that Riyadh is surrounded by motorways that exceed the boundaries of the city. **(D)** is correct. For the record: The passage does not provide details about the growth of Riyadh from the 1950s to the 1970s compared to earlier eras, ruling out **(A)**; Riyadh is the Saudi capital, contrary to **(B)**; we are not told about the road networks in other countries, eliminating **(C)**.

52. (C)

The disadvantages of drifting are mentioned in the final paragraph. The high level of accidents on Saudi roads related to drifting resulted in severe fines and punishment for drifters caught by the local authorities. This detail is a close paraphrase of **(C)**, which is therefore correct. For the record: The passage does not link an increase in petrol consumption to higher petrol prices, we are told drifting takes place when motorways are likely to be empty, and the passage does not link drifting to antisocial views about women.

53. (C)

The keywords 'screw-top bottle' appear in the final sentence of the second paragraph, which states that consumers associate such bottles with poor quality wine, regardless of the wine's price or other attributes. Thus, based on the passage, we can infer that wine in screw-top bottles may be good quality or poor quality—the quality of the wine is not necessarily connected to the screw-top bottle. Thus, on the basis of the passage, the answer is Can't tell.

54. (B)

Scanning for synthetic cork and cork taint leads to the start of the second paragraph; synthetic cork is being used in an effort to avoid cork taint. However, a few lines later, the passage states that synthetic cork can result in another type of cork taint. Thus, synthetic cork does not eliminate cork taint completely. This statement says it does, so the statement is false.

55. (A)

The keywords here are most wine and natural cork; scan for statistics, and the figure of 60% in the first paragraph will stand out. Natural cork is used for 60% of wine stoppers today. Hence, the passage supports the statement, and the statement is true.

56. (A)

The keyword wine box appears near the end of the passage. A standard wine box holds 5 litres of wine, whilst a standard bottle holds 750 ml. Six standard wine bottles would hold 4500 ml, or 4.5 litres, so a wine box holds more wine than six standard wine bottles. Answer **(A)** is correct.

Decision Making

The Task

Decision Making is the second section of the UKCAT, coming after Verbal Reasoning and before Quantitative Reasoning. This section was new to the UKCAT in 2016, becoming a scored section in 2017.

You will have 1 minute to read the directions, then you have 31 minutes to answer 29 questions. Unlike in the other sections of the UKCAT, Decision Making questions are all individual questions; they do not come in sets. If there is data in a question—such as a table or a diagram—the data applies to that question only. On average, you have a minute to answer each question, but you will want to try and answer the simpler, shorter questions more efficiently, since some questions are considerably more time-consuming—and some of these are worth two marks.

A minute per question may seem and 'feel' like a lot more time, compared to the very fast pace of other questions in other sections. However, you will find that Decision Making question require varying amounts of work. Some questions are relatively simple and can be answered briskly, in well under a minute. Other questions are terribly elaborate, and would take a good 2 or 3 minutes (or more) to work through.

As a result, you will find yourself making judgements about which questions to skip (i.e. the most time-consuming ones) and come back to, if there is any time remaining. As always, if you skip a question without working on it fully, you should mark an answer and flag it for review (with the exception of Five-Part Questions, which we will discuss below).

The Format

This section includes six different question types. Note that in the official practice tests, the questions always appear in this order:

Syllogisms: A series of initial statements are followed by five 'conclusions' in boxes, each with a grey box to its right. You must drag the word 'Yes' or 'No' into the grey box beside each conclusion, depending whether it follows from the initial statements ('Yes') or does not follow from the initial statements ('No'). The initial statements are usually relative short—just a sentence or two—though some syllogisms will have longer initial text. Syllogisms are about applying rules and categories (in the initial statements) to new information (the statements in the five parts).

Logic Puzzles: These questions will include rules that will allow you to arrange or match various elements. For example, you might have to sequence seven friends in a row of seats, or match four different cars with the colour of each car and the number of its parking space.

Strongest Argument Questions: You must select the answer that addresses the terms of the original question most strongly. In most cases, two answers will start with 'Yes' and two with 'No'; the strongest argument will have the most direct impact on the terms of the original question, either strengthening it (a 'Yes' answer) or attacking it (a 'No' answer). Wrong answers will have little or no impact on the original question.

Inference Questions: You must select the answer that is a valid inference from the data (textual, visual or both) provided. These questions are also in a five-part format; drag 'Yes' to the grey box if the inference is valid; drag 'No' if it is not. In general, there will be much more initial text with Inference Questions than with Syllogisms; Inference Questions may also include visual data, such as charts, graphs or tables.

Venn Diagram Questions: These questions will normally feature a Venn diagram; you must make a calculation or an inference based on the figures or groups in the diagram. In some cases, there will only be textual information provided, and each answer choice will be a possible Venn diagram.

Maths Questions: These questions involve probability or percentages. You may have to do a few calculations, but in most cases they are relatively straightforward (e.g. coming up with one or two probability fractions based on the figures provided). Note that while the test-maker calls these 'Probabilistic Reasoning' questions, we have found that there are several examples in the official UKCAT practice tests where the questions do not really involve probability, but rather percentages, so we have opted to call them Maths Questions instead.

All Decision Making questions (other than Syllogisms and Inference Questions) have four multiple choice answers, from **(A)** to **(D)**. Normally the answers will include text or figures (or a mix), though some Venn Diagram Questions will have Venn Diagrams in the answer choices. Syllogisms and Inference Questions are known collectively as five-part questions, since each question has five parts that must be answered yes or no.

Multiple choice questions are worth one mark each; five-part questions are worth two marks each, but only if you answer all five parts correctly. You get one mark for a partially correct answer in a five-part question; the UKCAT Consortium has declined to disclose exactly what 'partially correct' means, but we at Kaplan feel it is safe to infer that 'partially correct' means 3 or 4 out of 5 correct. That's how we score these items in our practice tests, and it's a good benchmark for assessing your performance—and for deciding how to divide up your time in this section. We'll have more to say about pacing and the two mark questions later in the chapter.

Three question types—Venn Diagram Questions, Logic Puzzles and Inference Questions—may include diagrams or visual data with each question. As a result, there may be a certain amount of analysis or deduction required in order to answer. Be prepared to use your noteboard to make any necessary sketches or notations, and be sure to use the onscreen calculator for any calculations. Calculations are most likely to be required in Venn Diagram Questions, Maths Questions and any Inference Questions with charts, graphs or tables.

The Challenges

The most obvious challenge in Decision Making is timing: 29 questions in 31 minutes means that you only have about a minute to work through and answer each question. Most questions will require a fair amount of notation, calculation or other deductive work, so there will be very few questions that you can answer in much less than a minute. You will need to practise so you can attack these question types quickly and accurately. If you work too slowly, you will run out of time.

The other major challenge in Decision Making is the wide range of question types, some of which have a very particular (we might even say peculiar) logic. Some students may excel at all six question types, but we expect that most students will have at least one or two question types that they find difficult. Remember as well, some question types (or some individual questions) will be objectively difficult. We have already discussed the objective challenges of Syllogisms and Inference Questions, with five parts and two marks each. Logic Puzzles are another question type that may in some cases be quite time-consuming or difficult, due to the amount of deductions that may be required to answer the question. Since each question is worth one mark, you will want to take care not to 'over-invest' in any single question, since 3 or 4 minutes spent on a single question will make it difficult to complete the section, meaning that you may miss out several questions (likely, much more straightforward questions) later on. Even so, we at Kaplan are confident that with a bit of practice and preparation, you can be ready to give your best performance on all six Decision Making question types on Test Day.

Kaplan Top Tips for Decision Making

1. Read the scenario first

All the question types in the Decision Making section will involve an element of logical reasoning. You will be given textual and visual information and asked to make calculations and deductions. You should expect to encounter far more information than you will actually need to determine the correct answer, so a big part of the work is separating out the relevant data, then taking the necessary steps to get to the answer. In many cases, it will be as straightforward as identifying the relevant or matching terms (i.e. in many Inference and Strongest Argument Questions) or doing a few quick calculations with the correct figures (i.e. in many Venn Diagram and Maths Questions).

In those cases, you must keep a laser-like focus on the relevant details, moving forward by selecting only those bits that you need and discarding the rest. In other questions, such as many Logic Puzzles and Syllogisms, you will find that some details are less helpful than others—not necessarily unhelpful, but certainly less clear or less concrete. Thus, it is essential in all Decision Making questions that you always *drive towards the definite*—focusing on the most critical, concrete, relevant details, and using this information to make deductions or calculations.

For example, in Logic Puzzles, you might be presented with 4 to 6 rules or conditions. Some will be very concrete (i.e. 'Susan sits in the chair at the left'), while others will be less definite (i.e. 'Tom sits somewhere between Ursula and Victor'). If there are, say, seven seats in a row in this Logic Puzzle, you could immediately place Susan in the leftmost chair based on the first rule, and you should do so in a sketch on your noteboard. However, you can't add Tom, Ursula or Victor to specific seats based on the second rule. You might add a notation near the sketch on your noteboard—U . . . T . . . V or V . . . T . . . U—so you remember to add in that grouping. But note that since this is a relative rule (not a definite or concrete rule, as the rule about Susan was), it is not nearly as helpful. You would likely need to fill in most or all of the other seats in order to work out exactly where Tom, Ursula and Victor would sit.

You should also be aware that in many Logic Puzzles, you cannot actually assign all the elements to a definite place, position or matching trait. In the example above, it might well turn out that there are three seats that could be taken by U . . . T . . . V or V . . . T . . . U, in either left-to-right sequence, but you cannot actually say for sure which applies. However, in the official UKCAT practice tests, all the Logic Puzzle questions ask for something that must be true . . . so the correct answer would almost certainly have to relate to one of the other people in that instance. That's the advantage in driving to the definite: it will help you pick out the correct answers more quickly.

2. Notate/calculate and eliminate

As we have explained in the last example regarding Susan and her friends, you will have to do a certain amount of notation in order to answer the questions in the Decision Making section. You will also have to do a certain amount of maths, which should be relatively straightforward—certainly compared to the maths required in the Quantitative Reasoning section—though you must take care to avoid the wrong answer traps that will be waiting for students who rush and do the calculations incorrectly (e.g. with one or more wrong figures from the data).

In most cases, then, you will have to notate or calculate (but not both) in order to answer a Decision Making question. Some questions may require several calculations or a fairly elaborate sketch in order to make the necessary deductions, so you must *always* keep an eye on the answer choices. This way, you can eliminate any answers that are clearly too large/too small or clearly impossible, as you continue with your notations and calculations.

Since the multiple choice questions in this section have only four answer choices, you will find in many cases that you can clearly eliminate 1 or 2 answers while working through a question. Sometimes you will get to the correct answer quickly by doing the straightforward maths or deductions, but if a question is longer or trickier, it can be faster to eliminate the wrong answers as you work. This approach will also keep you from 'overworking' a question, since there may be further deductions that can be made that are unnecessary to get to the correct answer. When you get to the answer, stop working, click it and move on.

3. Play to your strengths

You may find that you excel at all six Decision Making question types. If so, that's to your advantage on Test Day. However, most students will likely find that at least one question type is more difficult than the others. In most cases, we expect that you might find Syllogisms or Strongest Argument Questions a bit more challenging. With practice, even the most difficult questions can become more accessible by the time you get to Test Day.

However, since you have only one minute per question, you will want to bear in mind your relative strengths and allocate time appropriately. If you are giving the section a full attempt, then you will want to work as efficiently as possible in the questions where you are strongest, so you have a bit more time for the more challenging or more time-consuming items. This might also mean that you skip an entire question type (such as Syllogisms) on your first pass through the section, leaving sufficient time to come back to it after you've attempted all the other questions in the other question types in your first pass.

4. Skip the most difficult questions

If you skip a question, you might decide to come back to it with any remaining time, after your first pass through the section. However, we at Kaplan recommend that you keep track (with marks on your noteboard) of the total number of questions you are skipping, as this will vary depending on the exact number of difficult/time-consuming questions, and could easily be in the range of 6 to 10 questions. You should save 1 minute for each question you skip, so you have sufficient time to come back to them at the end of the section.

In that case, you may decide to leave the questions blank, or to mark answers. If you mark answers for questions that you are skipping, be sure to do this as quickly as possible, without being drawn into reading the question or answers, since this can waste valuable time for the questions that you will be attempting.

Many students will prefer to skip all the five-part questions—Syllogisms and Inference Questions—on the first pass through the section, flagging all these items for review. If you do so, be sure to count the number of items that you will have to come back to, and try to save at least 1 minute per item. A good rule of thumb is to try to save 10–12 minutes for a second pass, since there are usually 8–9 five-part questions in a Decision Making section. If you can save 10–12 minutes to attack them, then you can prioritise the simpler, quicker five-part questions, banking all the marks on those before coming to the hardest five-part questions. Since these are the most time-consuming items in the section, it makes sense to leave them for the end. You should still try to get at least one mark on each five-part question, but it is always a judgement call whether to invest more time and try to get all five parts correct, or just be satisfied that you have got at least three correct, guess for the remaining parts, and move on. If you are extremely rigorous with pacing, you might be able to answer all five parts of all questions without having to guess, but in most cases, you will find you could have used just slightly more time— don't feel bad about a few guesses here or there if you have banked a lot of marks in the section.

Syllogisms

The first question type in the Decision Making section is Syllogisms. Each Syllogism is a five-part question, with five statements in boxes, each beside a grey box. You must drag 'Yes' or 'No' into the grey box, depending whether the statement follows ('Yes') or does not follow ('No') from the initial information provided.

Each official practice test includes 4 or 5 Syllogisms, so you should expect to find a similar number of these items at the start of the Decision Making section on Test Day. Note that for Syllogisms, you must answer all five parts correctly to get two marks. You will get one mark for a partially correct answer, which we believe means it's one mark if you get three or four parts correct. You get zero marks if you get two or fewer statements correct.

Some Syllogisms will include relatively simple statements—2 or 3 short sentences—in the initial information. Others will include longer, more complicated statements in the initial information. You must compare each statement to the initial information to determine whether or not it follows; thus, if there is quite a lot of initial information, it can be quite time-consuming (e.g. it will take more than 1 minute) to answer some Syllogisms.

If you decide to save the five-part questions for a second pass through the section, flag all Syllogisms for review without reading them. Do not bother dragging any answers on the first pass, since this would waste time. If you skip the Syllogisms on the first pass, then you will be starting with Logic Puzzles. Be sure to make a note of the number of Syllogisms on your noteboard, so you can save at least 1 minute per question for your second pass.

A few tips for attacking Syllogisms:

- Most Syllogisms will include two or three possible categories, but be careful to ensure that you understand how these do (and do not) overlap. Example: *Some of the people in this room are boys, and the rest like apples*. You could deduce that any girls in the room like apples, and that anyone in the room who likes apples isn't a boy.

- Work carefully with words such as *most* and *some*. *Most* means 'a majority'; 'some' means at least one. However, *most* could also mean 'all' (since 100% is a majority), and *some* could be anything from just 1, to a narrow majority, to 100%. Example: *Some of the people in this room are boys* does not preclude the possibility that everyone in the room is a boy.

- Watch out for ambiguities and non-overlapping sets. Example: *Some of the boys are in this room, and some of the girls are on the bus*. We don't know for sure whether all of the boys/girls are in each respective location, or that any boys/girls could be in the other location—or in some third location.

- If the initial information is more than a line of text, consider whether it is worth attempting the question before all others in the section. Some Syllogisms will have very long initial information, which would make it very easy to spend well more than a minute on those five parts. The question isn't worth so much effort, unless you have already picked up all the easier/quicker marks elsewhere in the section. Use your time and energy wisely!

Let's look at a couple of Syllogisms. When attacking each question, read the initial information, then evaluate each statement, writing YES or NO in the grey box. Work as quickly as you can, but at this point, you should strive for accuracy rather than timing. It will likely take you more like 2 minutes to evaluate all five statements; make a note of your timing before moving on to the answer, so you can have a sense of how long these questions actually take—and then work to refine this timing as you continue to practise.

1. All trees are plants. If a plant has leaves, it must be a tree.

    Place 'Yes' if the conclusion does follow. Place 'No' if the conclusion does not follow.

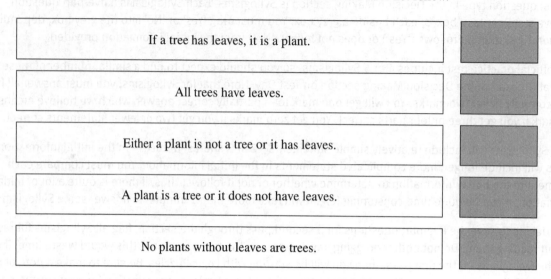

If a tree has leaves, it is a plant.	
All trees have leaves.	
Either a plant is not a tree or it has leaves.	
A plant is a tree or it does not have leaves.	
No plants without leaves are trees.	

Answer: The first conclusion follows, since we know that all trees are plants. We can also see that the second conclusion does not follow, since there could be trees without leaves. It could also be the case that all trees have leaves, but we cannot deduce this from the information provided. It is possible that there are plants that are not trees; however, we cannot say for sure that the only other option is that it is a plant with leaves, as all plants with leaves are trees. There could be trees without leaves, in which case there would be plants without leaves that are trees (since all trees are plants). For this reason, the third conclusion does not follow. The fourth conclusion follows, because plants that are not trees do not have leaves. The fifth conclusion could be true, depending whether or not there are trees without leaves. Since we don't know for sure about this possibility, this conclusion does not follow. The answers are YES; NO; NO; YES; NO.

2. All students in the society, except members of the orchestra, are required to attend society meetings on Tuesday afternoons. Only students who have missed school due to illness are excused from attending these meetings.

Place 'Yes' if the conclusion does follow. Place 'No' if the conclusion does not follow.

Members of the orchestra can attend society meetings on a Tuesday afternoon.	
Raghav missed school due to illness, so he must not have attended the society meeting on Tuesday afternoon.	
The society's monthly pizza party must take place on a Tuesday afternoon.	
Meetings of the orchestra are normally scheduled for Tuesday afternoons.	
Students in the society who are not ill or members of the orchestra cannot be excused from attending society meetings.	

Answer: Members of the orchestra are not required to attend the society's Tuesday afternoon meetings, but that does not mean they are not allowed to attend. There is no reason they could not attend if they wanted to, so the first statement follows. Students who miss school due to illness are excused from attending the Tuesday afternoon meetings, but that does not mean they are not allowed to attend; Raghav could have attended, so the second statement does not follow. It is unclear whether the society's monthly pizza party takes place at a society meeting or whether it is a separate event; the third statement does not follow. The fourth statement is possible, but there is no information about when the orchestra meets; the fourth statement does not follow. The fifth statement follows; the only excuses allowed are for members of the orchestra and students who miss school due to illness. The answers are YES; NO; NO; NO; YES.

Great work on these first two Syllogisms! Now that you have a better understanding of the question format, try to work a bit more quickly through the Syllogisms in the timed practice set. Since these questions take a bit longer than 1 minute on average, we are giving you a little extra time in the timed set. If you spot a Syllogism that looks like it will be more time-consuming, you might want to skip it and come back to it after completing the other two, so you can maximise your marks on the simpler Syllogisms first.

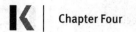
Kaplan Timed Practice Set—*Syllogisms*

Set your timer for 4 minutes. Mark answers for all 3 questions before time is up!

3. None of Yusuf's stamps are red. None of Zoe's stamps are overprints, but some are blue.

    Place 'Yes' if the conclusion does follow. Place 'No' if the conclusion does not follow.

If there's a blue stamp, it's one of Zoe's.	
There are no red stamps.	
If there's a yellow overprint stamp, it could be one of Yusuf's.	
All of Zoe's stamps are blue.	
A red overprint stamp is neither Yusuf's nor Zoe's.	

4. Three neighbouring countries—each sharing a border with both of the others—have formed the QSB zone for border controls, meaning that there are no passport controls for citizens of any of the three countries travelling between two of the countries; citizens of any country must present a valid passport (or other acceptable ID, as indicated only for citizens of the QSB zone) when they first enter the QSB zone from a country that is not in the QSB zone. Citizens of Country Q may use an identity card in place of a passport when travelling in the QSB zone. Citizens of Country S may use the same or a valid driving licence. Citizens of Country B may only use a passport when travelling to/from any other country, regardless of whether the country is in the QSB zone.

    Place 'Yes' if the conclusion does follow. Place 'No' if the conclusion does not follow.

Sage uses a passport to travel to Country S. She must be a citizen of a country that is outside the QSB zone.	
Tomasz uses his driving licence to travel to Country Q. He must be a citizen of Country S.	
Uta travels from Country S to Country B. She must use her passport to enter Country B.	
Vicki uses an identity card to travel to Country B. She must be a citizen of a country in the QSB zone.	
Wendell uses his passport to travel from Country Q to another country. He must be a citizen of Country B.	

5. Tonight's supper will be chicken nuggets or spaghetti Bolognese. We will have chips only with the former and garlic bread only with the latter. We will have a salad regardless, with tomato, carrot, and either cucumber or avocado. We will serve blackcurrant squash or apple juice, although there is only enough apple juice for three people; anyone may have tap water if they want it, in addition to, or in place of, squash or juice.

Place 'Yes' if the conclusion does follow. Place 'No' if the conclusion does not follow.

Tonight's supper will include carrot and chips or tomato and garlic bread.	
Tonight's supper will include chicken and cucumber or spaghetti and avocado.	
If there are six people at supper, exactly half of them must have apple juice.	
If tonight's salad includes carrot and avocado, it will not include cucumber.	
If there are eight people at supper, a majority of them must not have apple juice.	

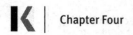

Kaplan Timed Practice Set—*Syllogisms*: Answers and Explanations

How did you get on with your first timed Decision Making set? If you worked efficiently, you should have just managed to answer all five parts of all the questions. If you struggled to finish, don't worry; you will have more opportunities to practise with five-part questions later in this chapter, and in the Kaplan UKCAT Mock Test later in the book. If you made quick work of these questions, that's great! If not, again, don't fret; most test-takers find these questions challenging to finish in a minute each, so you may decide to skip them on Test Day and come back to them on the second pass through the section. Start preparing yourself for a strategic approach to this section, which is essential if you want to earn a top score in Decision Making.

3.   NO; NO; YES; NO; YES

A blue stamp could be Zoe's, but it could also be Yusuf's; the first statement does not follow. Zoe could have red stamps, so the second statement does not follow. Either Yusuf or Zoe could have yellow stamps, but only Yusuf could have an overprint stamp; the third statement follows. It's possible that all Zoe's stamps are blue, but we don't know whether she has any stamps of other colours; the fourth statement does not follow. Yusuf cannot have red stamps, and Zoe cannot have overprint stamps; the fifth statement follows.

4.   NO; YES; NO; YES; NO

Citizens of any country must present a valid passport when entering the QSB zone, though there are exceptions (other possible documents) for citizens of QSB zone countries. However, QSB zone citizens have the option of presenting a passport; thus, if Sage uses a passport to travel to Country S, she could be a citizen of any country, inside or outside the QSB zone. The first statement does not follow. If Tomasz uses his driving licence to travel to Country Q, he must be a citizen of Country S, since those are the only people allowed to use a driving licence instead of a passport. The second statement follows. Uta could use her passport to enter Country B, but she might be able to use another option (identity card or driving licence) if she is a citizen of Country Q or Country S. The third statement does not follow. If Vicki uses an identity card to travel to Country B, she must be a citizen of Country Q or Country S; the fourth statement follows. Citizens of any country can use a passport, and we don't know which country Wendell is entering—it could be outside the QSB zone. Thus, Wendell could be a citizen of any country. The fifth statement does not follow.

5.   YES; NO; NO; YES; YES

Tonight's supper must include chips (with chicken nuggets) or garlic bread (with spag Bol); carrot and tomato will be included in the salad regardless, so the first statement follows. Tonight's supper must include chicken or spaghetti, but it could just as well include chicken and avocado (instead of cucumber) or spaghetti and cucumber (instead of avocado); the second statement does not follow. There is enough apple juice for three people, but no one is required to drink apple juice; if there are six people at supper, they could all drink squash, water or both. The third statement does not follow. The salad will always include carrot; if it includes avocado, it will not include cucumber. The fourth statement follows. Since a maximum of three people can have apple juice, there must be at least five people who do not have apple juice if there are eight people at supper; the fifth statement follows.

Logic Puzzles

Logic Puzzles usually involve one or more of the following tasks:

- Sequencing: You must arrange several people or things in a particular order. Examples: Ranking the runners who finish first to fifth place in a race; sorting items in a shop by price.

- Spatial Reasoning: You must arrange several people or things spatially, such as in a row, column, grid or circle. Examples: Arranging people in a queue; determining which flat is which in a floor plan.

- Matching: You must link people or things with one or more other categories of people or things. Examples: Matching flavours of ice cream with the amount of each flavour sold; matching vehicles to their colours and parking space numbers.

Note that there is some overlap in the tasks (e.g. spatial reasoning is often a kind of sequencing), and matching can pair easily with another task. In any case, you are likely to need to make notes on your noteboard as you work through the rules for each puzzle. Usually there will be one or more deductions—from the general set-up, an individual rule, or the rules in combination with each other or with the set-up—without which you will be unable to work out the correct answer.

If there is a sequencing or spatial element, it will often suggest an obvious sketch. For example, if arranging items or people in a row or queue, you can draw a row of blanks, then fill these in as you determine which items/people must (or mustn't) take certain positions.

If there is a matching element, it is often advisable to make a grid, so you can link the people/items to the other categories. Use the most concrete or most simple element as the basis for the grid. For example, if there are several items with different prices, then list the prices vertically (with the most expensive price at the top), since that follows the 'logic' of prices.

If you encounter a negative rule, turn it into a positive. Example: *Ava and Bob did not sit next to Charlie.* Ask yourself: *Who* did *sit next to Charlie? Who could Ava and Bob have sat next to?* Keep an eye on the number limits at the same time—most Logic Puzzles will involve four to seven people, and many will have just four or five—so knowing that two people cannot sit next to a third could be quite limiting.

Finally, you must keep an eye on the answer choices as you work. Usually you will be given just enough information to allow you to determine the correct answer. However, many times you will find that one or more wrong answers will be dismissed on the way to the correct answer—you can save time by noticing when these are no longer possible, since you may (in at least some cases) eliminate all three incorrect answers a bit more quickly than you may have otherwise realised. Do not expect that you will always be able to fill in all the information in your diagram or grid with 100% certainty. Some questions will have some uncertainty—for example, there could be two people that could occupy either of two positions—though this uncertainty will usually be reflected in the answer choices (or it will be irrelevant).

Let's look at some Logic Puzzles. When starting a question, identify the task (or tasks), then start to organise the information with some notations. For example, if you have to arrange six people in a row, you might draw six blanks, then you can start adding people (using initials, or the first two letters for names start with the same initial). If two people could go in the same spot—e.g. *Frank or Gil is immediately to the right of Helen*—notate with a slash: H F/G . Keep an eye on later rules, or deductions that arise from combining rules, that could limit the options.

Four customers buy four different items (including carrots) from a fruit and vegetable stall.

Eve does not buy raspberries.

Gus does not buy courgettes or strawberries.

Fiona does not buy berries, but Harrison does.

Neither woman (Eve or Fiona) buys carrots.

6.   Which of the following must be true?

   A.   Eve buys carrots.
   B.   Fiona buys courgettes.
   C.   Gus buys raspberries.
   D.   Harrison buys strawberries.

Answer: This Logic Puzzle contains a lot of negative rules. Since there are only four people and four items, you can turn the negatives into positives. Note the final rule—neither woman buys carrots—which will be useful to build into our notes from the start. Eve does not buy raspberries, and she can't buy carrots, so she has two options: courgettes or strawberries. Gus does not buy courgettes or strawberries, so he must buy carrots or raspberries. Fiona does not buy berries, and she can't buy carrots, so she must buy courgettes. Answer **(B)** is correct. Note the importance of keeping an eye on the answer choices as you work through a Logic Puzzle: you should do only as much work is required to identify the correct answer, or eliminate the three wrong answers. Sometimes, that will mean you will have to work through all the options and match up every person and item. In this case, you could see the correct answer before finishing work on the puzzle.

For the record: Harrison must buy raspberries or strawberries. Since Eve can't buy carrots or courgettes (as Fiona buys them), Eve must buy strawberries, so Harrison buys raspberries and Gus buys carrots.

Four teachers at an English language college—Alicia, Ben, Chloe and Dinesh—are each teaching a different afternoon lesson—reading, listening, speaking and writing—in one of four classrooms (Room 101 to Room 104) shown in the diagram.

Ben will not teach the reading lesson or the lesson in Room 101.

Chloe will teach in a room with Dinesh's room on one side and writing lesson in the room on the other side.

Alicia will teach either the listening lesson or the speaking lesson.

Alicia's room is next to the room where the reading lesson is taught.

101	102	103	104

7. Which of the following must be true?
   A. The listening lesson is taught in Room 102 or Room 104.
   B. The reading lesson is taught by Chloe in Room 103.
   C. The speaking lesson is taught in Room 101 or Room 103.
   D. The writing lesson is taught by Ben in Room 102.

Answer: This Logic Puzzle requires you to assign the teachers and lessons to rooms, to the degree necessary to work out which answer choice must be true. Thus, you should keep an eye on the answers as you work, as you may be able to eliminate some (or all) the wrong answers in the course of making deductions, before you have worked out all the exact details of the puzzle. Don't do any more work than absolutely required to get to the correct answer!

In working with the rules, start with the most definite. In this case, that's the rule about Alicia teaching listening or speaking. Make a notation of this rule: A = L/S.

The next most definite rule is the one about Alicia's room being next to reading. Again, make a notation: AR or RA (since we don't know which room is to the left/right of the other.

The next most definite rule is the one about Chloe, Dinesh and writing. Again, make a notation: DCW or WCD.

Finally, consider what we know about Ben: B ≠ 101; B ≠ R.

Now, take a moment to make some deductions. Of these notations, the most helpful is the one involving Chloe, since it assigns elements to two adjacent rooms. Since there are four rooms in a row and Chloe must have something/someone on either side of her room, we know that Chloe must be in Room 102 or Room 103, and that either Dinesh or writing must go into the other room. There are two possible groups of rooms these three could take: Rooms 101 to 103 or Rooms 102 to 104. If you put writing in 101, Chloe in 102 and Dinesh in 103, then you have a problem, since Alicia can't teach writing (she must do listening or speaking) and Ben can't teach in Room 101. If you put Dinesh in 101, Chloe in 102 and writing in 103, then it's a similar problem: Alicia can't teach writing, so she can't go in 103; if you put her in 104, then reading must go into 103, but writing is already being taught there.

Thus, Chloe, Dinesh and writing must be in Rooms 102 to 104. If writing goes into 102, then we would have Chloe in 103 and Dinesh in 104, which means that Ben must go into 102 (since he can't teach in 101), which leaves Alicia in 101. However, this would mean that Alicia teaches in the room next to the writing lesson (which must be in 102), which violates the rule that she teaches in the room next to the reading lesson.

Hence, it must be the case that the writing lesson is taught in 104, with Chloe in 103 and Dinesh in 102. Alicia can't teach writing, so Ben must teach writing in 104, putting Alicia into 101. Eliminate **(D)**, since we have now placed Ben in 104, not 102. Alicia must be next to the room where reading is taught, so Dinesh teaches reading in 102. Eliminate **(B)**, since reading is taught in 102. At this point, we can also eliminate **(A)**, since we know that reading is taught in 102 and writing in 104. Answer **(C)** must therefore be correct.

For the record: What about listening or speaking? We don't know; Alicia must teach one of these lessons, leaving Chloe to teach the other in Room 103. Note that in this instance, there is an element of uncertainty, as you cannot definitively assign all the elements. Also, in this case, the correct answer related to one of the elements (speaking) that we could not assign. Be prepared for a certain amount of uncertainty in the Logic Puzzles that you will encounter on Test Day. Some will allow you to assign all the elements to an exact position; others will have one or more elements that are uncertain, but these will not prevent you from answering the questions correctly.

Now you will complete some more Logic Puzzles in a timed set. Note that you will likely encounter a mix of different tasks on Test Day, and—as we have seen so far—some Logic Puzzles are a lot simpler than others. Normally, there are 4 or 5 Logic Puzzles, so keep an eye out for the simpler ones, and aim to complete them as quickly as possible. Most of the Logic Puzzles are likely to be relatively quick work; if you spot one that is more complicated, save it for the end of the Logic Puzzles—or even for a second pass through the section.

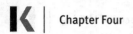

Kaplan Timed Practice Set—*Logic Puzzles*

Set your timer for 4 minutes. Mark answers for all 3 questions before time is up!

Seven students are standing in a row for the chess club photograph. Two students (Kingsley and Max) are boys; the rest are girls.

Laura is standing to the right of Nancy and immediately to the left of Priya.

Max is not standing next to Nancy.

Izzy is standing next to one boy and furthest of all the girls from the other boy.

There are exactly two people standing between Izzy and Jess.

8.   Which of the following MUST be true?

   A.   Izzy is standing between Priya and Max.
   B.   Max is standing immediately to the right of Priya.
   C.   Kingsley is standing between Izzy and Nancy.
   D.   Nancy is standing immediately to the right of Kingsley.

Four vehicles are parked along the kerb, one in front of the other. Each vehicle is a different colour. One of the vehicles is a sports car.

There are two vehicles between the blue vehicle and the van.

The white vehicle is parked directly behind the red vehicle and directly in front of the 4x4.

A single vehicle is parked between the silver vehicle and the estate car.

9.   Which of the following must be true?

   A.   The estate car is red.
   B.   The 4x4 is blue.
   C.   The sports car is silver.
   D.   The van is white.

Five stops in the nearby mountains, each with a scenic overlook, can be visited one after the other if you travel by the correct mode of transport. The modes of transport between each stop are different. The chair lift goes uphill; the other modes of transport could be uphill or downhill. All stops are uphill or downhill of all other stops; no stops are at the same elevation.

Shadow Ridge is reached by chair lift; the next stop, Tom's Peak, is reached by downhill skiing.

White Wedge is uphill of Valley Rock and downhill of Summitview, though there may be one or more intermediate stops.

You must take the cable car sometime after the cog wheel railway to visit the stops in the correct order.

You must travel uphill from the first stop to the second.

10.   Which of the following must be true?

   A.   Summitview is reached by cable car.
   B.   Shadow Ridge is the highest stop.
   C.   Summitview is the last stop.
   D.   Tom's Peak is the lowest stop.

Kaplan Timed Practice Set—*Logic Puzzles*: Answers and Explanations

These Logic Puzzles were challenging. Hopefully you were able to finish in the 4 minutes allotted. You may have noticed that some were more challenging than others; the last question was likely the most difficult, whilst the second question was relatively simple. As you continue to practise Logic Puzzles, try to hone your ability to judge whether a puzzle is relatively simple or complex at first glance. It helps to try and identify the task quickly; with more experience, you will find you become better at making snap judgements and sniffing out the puzzles that are likely to be more time-consuming. This will allow you to focus your time and energy on the puzzles (likely the majority of them) that will be simpler, faster marks.

8. (D)

The rules for this Logic Puzzle involve the relative positioning of the students in a row. Be careful not to assume too much about the exact positions based on any single rule, since there could be more than one overall arrangement that satisfies all the rules. First, we know that Laura is immediately to the left of Priya and also somewhere to the right of Nancy, so we have a partial sequence of N . . . LP. Note that it could be NLP, but use the ellipsis to indicate the uncertainty about the gap (if any) between N and L. We also know that there are exactly two people between Izzy and Jess (I __ __ J or J __ __ I), though we don't know which of this pair is further to the left. Izzy is standing next to a boy and furthest of all the girls from the other boy. This means we could have one of the boys between I and J (in the blank nearest to I), or we could have LP between I and J. If it is one of the boys, then the overall sequence must be (using b to represent a boy) IbNJLPb; since M can't be next to N, we know that K is, so the overall sequence is IKNJLPM. If LP is between I and J, then the overall sequence could be bNJLPIb; again, M can't be next to N, so the order must be KNJLPIM. In both overall sequences, we see that N is immediately to the right of K. The correct answer is **(D)**.

For the record: Note that answer **(A)** is true if the sequence is KNJLPIM, whilst **(B)** and **(C)** are true if the sequence is IKNJLPM; in each case, the answer is not true for the other sequence. If you encounter a question in which more than one answer seems to be true, consider whether there is a second sequence or arrangement that satisfies all the rules. It's likely that there is, and the correct answer will be the only one that satisfies all the rules in both sequences or arrangements.

9. (B)

This Logic Puzzle requires you to sequence four vehicles parked along a kerb. So you might start by drawing four blanks: __ __ __ __ . The first rule tells us that there are two vehicles between the blue vehicle and the van, so B and V must go at opposite ends of the sequence; it's unclear, however, which goes where. The second rule is more helpful, in combination with the first: the white vehicle is directly behind the red one and directly in front of the 4x4. If you assign 'front' to the left side of the diagram, then there are only two possibilities for this new sequence (R W 4x4): either the red vehicle is at the front, or the red vehicle is second from the front and the 4x4 is at the rear. In the first case—red vehicle at the front—we know the red vehicle must be the van, with the blue vehicle at the rear. This would make the 4x4 silver; however, this causes a problem with the final rule: a single vehicle is parked between the silver vehicle and the estate car. If the 4x4 is silver and the third vehicle from the front, then the first vehicle must be the estate car—but we have already established the front vehicle is the red van. This cannot be the sequence; we know then that the red vehicle is second from the front and the 4x4 is at the rear. Combining this detail with the first rule, we know that the van must be the front vehicle, which means that the 4x4 must be blue. Answer **(B)** is correct.

For the record: If you continue the deductions, you could assign all the vehicles and colours. We stopped once we knew that the 4x4 is blue, at which point we have the following deductions:

```
front V __ __ 4x4
        R  W   B
```

Note that the van must be silver, since that is the only remaining colour. The third rule tells us a single vehicle is parked between the silver vehicle and the estate car, so we know the estate car is white and the sports car is red. On Test Day, you must keep an eye on the answers as you make deductions, since you will often find that you will deduce the correct answer BEFORE you have worked out the complete arrangement. Don't do any more work than is required to get the correct answer. Once you have it, click it with confidence and move on.

10. (A)

In this Logic Puzzle, you must determine the order of five stops on a journey through the mountains, along with the mode of transport between stops. Shadow Ridge is reached by chair lift, which only goes uphill; the next stop, Tom's Peak, is reached by downhill skiing. Thus, we have a partial sequence:

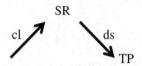

The second rule tells us that White Wedge is uphill from Valley Rock and downhill of Summitview, though there may be intermediate stops. Thus, the order must be VR ... WW ... SV. We also know that you must take the cable car (cc) sometime after the cog wheel railway (cwr) to visit the stops in the correct order, so you must take the cog wheel railway from VR to WW, and then take the cable car to SV. Hence, one possible sequence:

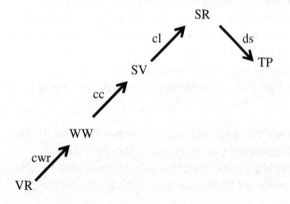

However, note carefully that while we must take the cog wheel railway between VR and WW, we only know that SV comes sometime after WW, and that SV is reached by cable car. This yields another option:

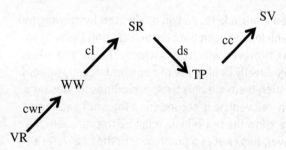

This second option meets all the original rules; in either case, we can see that Summitview must be reached by cable car. Answer **(A)** is correct.

For the record: We don't know the altitudes of the stops, so it is possible (but not assured) that Shadow Ridge is the highest stop; it must be in the first option, but in the second option, Summitview could be higher. As noted here, it would appear that Valley Rock is the lowest stop, but note that the descent from Shadow Ridge to Tom's Peak could be steeper than the initial ascent from Valley Rock—so Tom's Peak could, in fact, be the stop with the lowest elevation. We don't have enough information to know for sure.

Remember

You cannot write on the Logic Puzzles on Test Day.

Be prepared to sketch and notate on your noteboard. Use scrap paper to simulate this process as you practise.

Strongest Argument Questions

Strongest Argument Questions include four possible responses to the original question; you must select the answer that responds most directly to the terms of the original question. Note that whether the answer is a Yes or a No, or whether it is something you would actually agree with, is irrelevant. You are simply assessing based on the terms of each argument; three arguments will not impact the terms of the original question directly, while one—the correct answer—will make a direct hit.

The task is simpler than it might initially appear, since you must take a moment to read the original question and identify the key terms. Then, compare each answer choice to the original question, eliminating any that do not match the key terms exactly.

Look out for synonyms and paraphrases, as we mean 'terms' in the sense of the same logical groups or categories; the wording might be different, so long as the logical terms are the same.

Many incorrect answers will shift from the original terms. Most commonly, the terms will either be broader or narrower than the original terms, though they could also be just slightly different, e.g. not quite overlapping groups. Anything that adjusts the terms means that an answer will not make a direct hit on the original question; any such answers can be eliminated.

Since this is an elimination-based strategy, you can stop working as soon as you find the answer choice that matches the original terms exactly. Many times, that means you will stop after confirming that answer **(A)** or **(B)** is correct. If you are not 100% confident, then take a few moments to check the terms in the remaining answers, bearing in mind that most answers will not match the original terms—and only one answer in each set of 4 choices will make a direct hit.

Note that correct answers may bring in additional information or new terms, so long as they mention some (if not all) of the terms from the original question. Do not assume that an answer is incorrect simply because it includes new terms. Sometimes the original question will be faulty as it overlooks an alternative or omits some key information, which the correct answer may provide, in the context (of course) of the terms of the original question.

Let's try a few Strongest Argument Questions. With these initial questions, aim for accuracy more than timing. Identify the key terms in the original question, then eliminate any answers that do not match the key terms exactly. This approach should be sufficient to eliminate all the wrong answers on most Strongest Argument Questions. Sometimes you will need to consider the impact of an answer on the original terms, but only answers that directly affect the original terms—without shifting to slightly different categories or ideas—will be strong enough to be correct. All the wrong answers aren't 'less strong'—they are wrong.

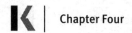

11. Should sports with a high risk of traumatic brain injury (TBI), such as boxing, be banned?

Select the strongest argument from the statements below.

A. Yes, any activity that runs a risk of damaging the brain should be prohibited in law.
B. Yes, if TBI is very likely to result when a sport, such as boxing or American football, is practised correctly.
C. No, boxers are just as likely to suffer injuries to other parts of their bodies as to their heads.
D. No, protective equipment, such as padding or mouthguards, is sufficient to protect against brain injuries in most sports.

Answer: The key terms in the original question are sports and 'high risk of traumatic brain injury'; look for the answer that matches these terms. Answer **(A)** broadens the terms considerably, shifting from sports to 'any activity' and from 'high risk of TBI' to 'runs a risk of damaging the brain'—any risk of brain damage, from any activity, is quite a wider category than the original terms. Eliminate **(A)**. Answer **(B)** addresses the condition of TBI being very likely to result from a sport being practised correctly—this matches the language of the original question ('very likely to result' = 'high risk'), so **(B)** is correct.

For the record: **(C)** makes an irrelevant comparison, comparing head injuries (which is a broader category than TBI) to injuries to other parts of the body. **(D)** suggests that protective equipment could protect against brain injuries in most sports, but this is not relevant to the question of the high risk of TBI in sports such as boxing; indeed, it's unclear how boxers would be protected from TBI by using mouthguards.

---

12. Should students aged 16 and 17 be allowed to vote in local and national elections?

Select the strongest argument from the statements below.

A. Yes, young people should have a say in deciding who represents them in councils and parliament.
B. Yes, it is important to give all citizens a voice in the future of the country.
C. No, people aged 16 and 17 have limited rights compared to older people, for example with regard to driving and buying alcohol.
D. No, it is not fair to allow students aged under 18 to vote if non-students the same age are not allowed to vote.

Answer: The key terms in the original question are 'students aged 16 and 17' and 'vote in local and national elections'. In this case, the first key term is sufficient to eliminate all the incorrect answers. Note that three answers shift from 'students aged 16 and 17' to a similar, but slightly different term: **(A)** changes from students to 'young people'; **(B)** swaps students for 'all citizens'; **(C)** is perhaps the closest, retaining the ages but switching students for 'people'. **(D)** retains students and the correct age range, so it is the only answer that could be correct.

For the record: The second key term is also useful, since **(B)** and **(C)** do not mention voting or elections. **(A)** is a classic 'strong but wrong' answer, since it matches the second key term, but it's too broad on the first—'young people' could include children aged under 16, or even people in their late teens or twenties, for example.

Note that it does not matter at all whether a 'Yes' or 'No' answer is correct—it only matters if the correct answer directly impacts the terms of the original question. Try not to be distracted by the opinions expressed in these questions, or in the answer choices. You should not assume that an answer is less likely to be correct because it expresses an extreme view, or an opinion that you find problematic or uncomfortable. Some Strongest Argument Questions in the official practice materials express views that sound like something your crotchety old uncle would say when he's in an especially foul mood. Even so, you must find the key terms in the original question, then compare the terms in the answers and eliminate all those that do not match.

The good news: Many of these questions will be relatively quick work because of this systematic approach, so you should be able to save up some extra time for five-part questions in your second pass through the section.

Kaplan Timed Practice Set—*Strongest Argument Questions*

Set your timer for 3 minutes. Mark answers for all 3 questions before time is up!

13. Should the government institute a compulsory charge per mile for every vehicle that uses the motorways, as this would have the sole effect of discouraging long journeys?

Select the strongest argument from the statements below.

A. Yes, because a motorway charge is only fair if it applies equally to everyone.
B. Yes, because reducing travel would reduce the emission of greenhouse gases, which would reduce global warming.
C. No, because most food and consumer goods are transported long distances on the motorways, so their cost would rise sharply.
D. No, because most people who use the motorways only drive short distances.

14. Should UK airports reduce the number of flights by 50%, in order to limit damage to the environment?

Select the strongest argument from the statements below.

A. Yes. Long-haul flights harm the environment more than any other activity, so airports should reduce or eliminate such flights.
B. Yes. Reducing air travel will encourage people to walk or cycle, allowing the Earth to heal.
C. No. Reducing air travel to the UK by half would severely damage the UK economy.
D. No. Restricting air travel would increase journeys by road and sea, which also damage the environment.

15. Should parents limit the amount of time each day that small children (aged 5 and under) use tablet computers?

Select the strongest argument from the statements below.

A. Yes, memory, attention span and social skills can be impaired if small children spend several hours a day on a tablet.
B. Yes, parents are best positioned to decide which devices, websites and apps their children use on a daily basis.
C. Yes, there is no good reason for babies and toddlers to use wireless devices.
D. No, long-term tablet use develops the imagination and problem solving skills of very young children.

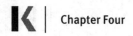

Kaplan Timed Practice Set—*Strongest Argument Questions*: Answers and Explanations

Strongest Argument Questions are a great opportunity to move a bit more quickly in the Decision Making section and bank time for the harder, longer questions. Hopefully you finished these questions with some time remaining. If you did, keep working to improve your pacing even more. If you struggled, work through the answers and see if you can improve your understanding of the question type as you continue to practise.

13. (C)

To answer a strongest argument question, you must compare each answer choice to the original question, eliminating any answers that do not have a direct impact on the terms of the original question. Here, the original question introduces the idea of a compulsory charge per mile for every vehicle on the motorways, with the sole effect of discouraging long journeys. The first answer addresses the fairness of the motorway charge, but this is not really relevant to the question of whether the charge would have the sole effect of discouraging long journeys. Similarly, the second answer raises the subject of greenhouse gas emissions; however, it is not clear that reducing journeys on the motorways would actually reduce travel (note the shift in terms from the original question to answer **(B)** on this point). For example, people might just travel by train or aeroplane instead of driving, which would also result in greenhouse gas emissions.

By contrast, the third answer has a direct impact on the original question. If it were the case that most food and consumer goods are transported long distances on motorways, then they would be subject to the compulsory charge, as it applies to every vehicle on the motorways. Since it is a charge per mile, it would be quite significant for the long journeys for these items, which would increase the price of food and consumer goods. That is quite a significant effect of the compulsory charge, beyond the stated goal of discouraging long journeys, so answer **(C)** is correct.

For the record: The compulsory charge is intended to discourage long journeys on the motorways, so people who drive short distances would presumably not be affected by it. Even if these drivers make up the majority of motorway users, as **(D)** suggests, there could still be some motorway users (as much as 49%) who drive long distances, so it is not clear that there is any real impact on the original claim if **(D)** is true.

14. (D)

The original question suggests that reducing flights by 50% would limit damage to the environment. **(A)** narrows the original term from flights to long-haul flights, which is more specific than the original question. **(B)** asserts that people would walk or cycle if not allowed to fly, but this is not logical—particularly in the context of the original question, which is about flights at UK airports; it would be impossible for visitors from overseas to walk or cycle to the UK. **(C)** mentions the UK, which is in the original question, but shifts the focus from the environment to the economy, which is not mentioned in the original question. **(D)** attacks the claim in the original question head on, pointing out that if flights were reduced, more people would travel by road and sea; these journeys would also damage the environment. **(D)** is therefore correct.

15. (A)

There are several key terms in the original question: parents; amount of time each day; small children (aged 5 and under); tablet computers. The correct answer will include most (if not all) of these terms, in some form, while not broadening or contradicting any of them. Answer **(A)** includes several additional details—memory, attention span, social skills—but it mentions small children, an amount of time each day (several hours), and tablets. Parents are not mentioned, but the answer gives a good reason that parents should restrict the daily tablet use of small children. For these reasons, **(A)** is the correct answer.

For the record: (B) mentions parents and 'daily basis', but it broadens from small children to 'children', whilst shifting from tablets to 'devices, websites and apps', which is a much wider category. **(C)** omits parents and daily use, shifting from tablets to 'wireless devices'; 'babies and toddlers' is somewhat similar to 'small children', but note that children aged 5 (included in the original question) are rather older than 'toddlers', so **(C)** is really not a good fit at all for the original terms. **(D)** is the closest of the wrong answers, since it mentions tablet use and very young children, but it shifts from daily use to long-term use, and as such, it fails to answer the original question. NB On Test Day, you must remember not only to compare key terms, but also (if an answer seems to match many of the key terms) check whether the answer makes sense as an answer to the question. Sometimes (as with **(D)** in this case) you will find answers that don't work logically. It's always best to check the key terms first, since most wrong answers can be eliminated quickly on that basis, without requiring the time and effort to consider the overall logic of each answer choice.

Inference Questions

Inference Questions come immediately after Strongest Argument Questions. They will usually include some text—often a long paragraph, sometimes two paragraphs—and may also feature visual data, such as charts, graphs or tables. You must determine whether each statement is a valid inference. Mark each valid inference 'Yes'; mark the other statements 'No.'

A valid inference (just as in Verbal Reasoning) is something that *must be true*, based on the information provided. Valid inferences may use synonyms or paraphrases, instead of the same wording from the text or visual data, but they will always match the information in the text or data.

Basic maths is always a valid inference. Be prepared to use the calculator, and be sure to make notes of any figures you calculate on the noteboard. Some questions may require quite a few calculations—in fact, you might have to do multiple calculations to evaluate a single answer choice—which is why it's important to write down the results. Otherwise, you may find yourself having to waste valuable time re-calculating the figures you thought you could hold in your head after you forget them.

Inference Questions are different from Syllogisms (the other five-part question type) in two key respects. First, Syllogisms are about applying rules and categories to new statements; Inference Questions are simply about determining whether the statements are valid inferences. Second, there will usually be quite a bit more information in Inference Questions than in Syllogisms. Visual data (such as tables) may seem quite overwhelming at first glance.

However, on the whole, most students report that they find Inference Questions a bit easier, simply because it is a case of determining whether the statements match the data. This task is actually quite similar to Verbal Reasoning. Find the keywords in the data, compare it to the statement, drag 'Yes' or 'No' to the grey box and move on to the next statement. If you work very efficiently, many of these questions can be answered in about a minute each, but note the tight timing. One minute for five parts is only 12 seconds per part, and that includes the time to drag the answer to the grey box, which usually takes several seconds.

For that reason, most students will prefer to skip Inference Questions on the first pass through the section. Make sure you note the total number of Inference Questions on your noteboard as you flag them all for review on the first pass; save at least one minute per question. Then, as you start the second pass, decide whether it will be Syllogisms or Inference Questions first. That decision depends on which you feel is your stronger question type: the one that you are more likely to finish more quickly. Then, within each question type, you can prioritise the shorter, simpler questions, saving the longer, harder ones for last.

Practise with the next few Inference Questions, focusing on accuracy more than timing. Compare each statement to the initial data. If the statement matches, it's a Yes. If it doesn't, it's a No. Mark the answers in the grey boxes as you assess each statement, then check the answer and see how you did.

16. The graph indicates, for four different age groups and years, the percentage of car owners in Country A.

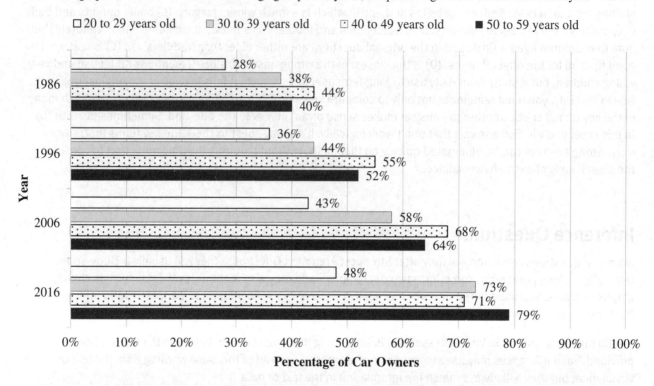

☐ 20 to 29 years old   ▨ 30 to 39 years old   ▦ 40 to 49 years old   ■ 50 to 59 years old

Place 'Yes' if the conclusion does follow. Place 'No' if the conclusion does not follow.

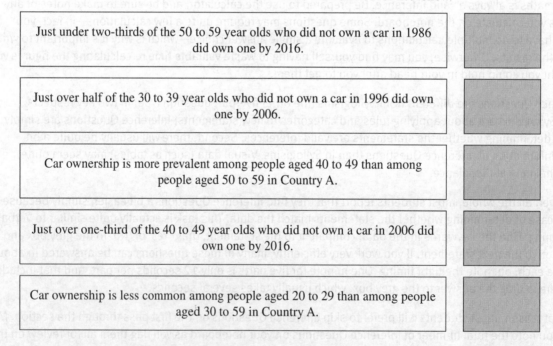

Just under two-thirds of the 50 to 59 year olds who did not own a car in 1986 did own one by 2016.	
Just over half of the 30 to 39 year olds who did not own a car in 1996 did own one by 2006.	
Car ownership is more prevalent among people aged 40 to 49 than among people aged 50 to 59 in Country A.	
Just over one-third of the 40 to 49 year olds who did not own a car in 2006 did own one by 2016.	
Car ownership is less common among people aged 20 to 29 than among people aged 30 to 59 in Country A.	

Answer: In this Inference question, it is important to note that the people from a given age cohort in one year become a different age cohort ten years later (e.g. the 30 to 39 year olds in 2006 become the 40 to 49 year olds in 2016). Thus, the first statement does not follow: the 50 to 59 year olds of 1986 would be the 80 to 89 year olds of 2016, and the percentage of car owners in that cohort is not included in the data.

In 1996, 56% (100 − 44 = 56) of 30 to 39 year olds did not own a car; half of this amount is 28% (56 ÷ 2 = 28), so the second statement suggests that 28% + 44% = 72% of 40 to 49 year olds should own a car in 2006. The actual figure is 68%; the second statement does not follow.

The third statement does not follow; 40 to 49 year olds have a higher rate of car ownership than 50 to 59 year olds in 1986, 1996 and 2006, but not in 2016.

In 2006, 32% (100 − 68 = 32) of the 40 to 49 year olds did not own a car; one-third of this amount is just under 11% (since 32 ÷ 3 = 10.67). Since 68% of 40 to 49 year olds owned cars in 2006, we can expect the percentage of 50 to 59 year olds that own cars ten years later (in 2016) to be 68% plus an additional 11%, for a total of 79%, the figure shown in the graph. The fourth statement follows.

The fifth statement also follows. The rate of car ownership among people aged 20 to 29 is the lowest of all four age groups in each of the four years; if you added the people aged 30 to 59 into a single group, they would have a higher rate of car ownership than people aged 20 to 29 in each of the four years. Thus, the answers are NO; NO; NO; YES; YES.

---

17. Scientists whose research involves highly complex calculations may require a supercomputer. Machines of this kind are designed to carry out tasks far beyond the scope of the average PC. They may, for example, be used to simulate extreme weather events or to create cellular models of organs in the human body. Supercomputers are distinguished from another type of advanced computer—the mainframe—by being adept at processing a limited set of challenging mathematical problems. Large corporations who deal with huge amounts of data, such as credit card companies or major online retailers, will typically employ a mainframe rather than a supercomputer, as they are better powered for performing great numbers of smaller and more various computations.

    Place 'Yes' if the conclusion does follow. Place 'No' if the conclusion does not follow.

The needs of big business are likely better served by a mainframe than a supercomputer.	
Supercomputers can perform calculations a normal PC cannot.	
Mainframes are not as powerful as supercomputers.	
Supercomputers usually have a more specific purpose than mainframes.	
A challenging mathematical problem is more likely to be solved by a mainframe than by a supercomputer.	

Answer: Large corporations will tend to use a mainframe rather than a supercomputer. The first statement follows.

Supercomputers are designed to carry out tasks beyond the scope of the average PC. The second statement follows.

The text states that mainframes are more powerful than supercomputers, which can process a limited amount of challenging problems by comparison. The third statement does not follow.

Supercomputers are adept at performing a limited set of challenging mathematical problems; this is a more specific purpose, so the fourth statement follows.

The text indicates that supercomputers are better for processing a limited set of challenging mathematical problems; the fifth statement does not follow. The answers are YES; YES; NO; YES; NO.

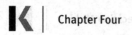

Kaplan Timed Practice Set—*Inference Questions*

Set your timer for 4 minutes. Mark answers for all 3 questions before time is up!

18. A report published in 2014 found that public funding for theatres in England has been decreasing since 2004, but this has been particularly noticeable since 2010. Arts Council England financing, funded by the government and the National Lottery, still represents almost a quarter of theatre budgets, with only a four per cent drop in actual funding in the four years prior to 2014. Alternative funding is relied upon more than ever. Although by no means consistent nationwide, it is reported that one theatre depended on philanthropic sources for 75% of its funding over the most recent financial period. Arts Council England projected that it will award £1.1 billion in government funding and £700 million in National Lottery funding between 2015 and 2018, with a renewed remit of giving more support to smaller theatres and theatres outside London.

Place 'Yes' if the conclusion does follow. Place 'No' if the conclusion does not follow.

A large theatre in London is less likely to get support from Arts Council England in 2018 than it was in 2014.	
Arts Council England will award less funding to theatres in 2018 than in 2014.	
National Lottery funding averaging £175 million per year was expected to be awarded by Arts Council England from 2015 to 2018.	
The government provided less funding for the arts in 2015 than in 2010.	
A majority of the budgets of theatres in England consists of funding from sources other than Arts Council England.	

19. Country Z includes several thousand miles of seashore and several hundred freshwater lakes; as a result, citizens of Country Z are very fond of water-based activities, and boating in particular. Sales of boats in Country Z are always the highest of any country in the region, which has more coastline than any other country in the region; most boat manufacturers spend 60% or more of their marketing and advertising budget for the region in Country Z. In 2017, a new boat manufacturer start selling the most expensive boat available for freshwater use, with all the latest high-end features, marketing the new boat exclusively in Country Z. By the end of 2017, the new boat had outsold all other boats in Country Z in that year.

Place 'Yes' if the conclusion does follow. Place 'No' if the conclusion does not follow.

More boats were sold in Country Z in 2017 than in all other countries in the region.	
Citizens of Country Z prefer a luxury boat for freshwater boating.	
People who live in a country with a lot of coastline are more likely to buy boats than people who live in a country with lesser amount of coastline.	
There are more freshwater boats in Country Z than boats for non-freshwater use.	
Citizens of Country Z will only buy boats that have been marketed in Country Z.	

20. A small zoo features four enclosures. The table below shows the number of visitors each exhibit receives at different times on a typical day in the summer months, along with the total visitors for the zoo at each time.

Exhibit	10am	1pm	4pm
Reptile House	569	960	720
Lions' Den	996	1390	1035
Avian Adventures	415	630	845
Nocturnal Wonders	220	360	480
Total Visitors (Zoo)	2200	3340	3080

Place 'Yes' if the conclusion does follow. Place 'No' if the conclusion does not follow.

There were 40% more people in the zoo at 4pm than at 10am.	
Just under half as many people visited Nocturnal Wonders as visited Avian Adventures.	
There were 25% less visitors at the Reptile House at 1pm than at 4pm.	
Ten per cent of the zoo's visitors were visiting Nocturnal Wonders at 10am.	
Attendance at the Nocturnal Wonders exhibit increased by a third between 10am and 1pm.	

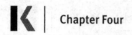

Kaplan Timed Practice Set—*Inference Questions*: Answers and Explanations

As you saw in this timed set, some Inference statements are much more straightforward than others. If a statement involves several calculations, you may have to leave it for the end of the question, or—if pressed for time—make your best guess. Remember, you get one mark if you get three or four statements correct; you only get two marks if all the statements are correct. So there may be a trade-off in deciding whether to push on and get all five statements correct, or whether to let a question go once you are sure you have answered three statements correctly. Even so, you should answer all the parts of the question, since you have fairly decent odds of guessing correctly once you have done the work for three or four of the statements.

18. YES; NO; YES; NO; YES

The final sentence suggests that large theatres and theatres in London would be less likely to get Arts Council England funding in the period from 2015 to 2018; the first statement follows.

We are not told how much funding Arts Council England awarded in 2014; the second statement does not follow.

Arts Council England was projected to award £700 million in National Lottery funding in the four years from 2015 to 2018, averaging £700 million ÷ 4 = £175 million a year. The third statement follows.

We don't know the actual amount of government arts funding in 2010 or 2015. The fourth statement does not follow.

The second sentence indicates that Arts Council England funding accounts for almost a quarter of theatre budgets, so a majority of their funding must come from other sources. The fifth statement follows.

19. NO; YES; YES; NO; NO

More boats were sold in Country Z in 2017 than any country in the region, but that does not necessarily mean that the number of boats sold in Country Z was more than all other countries in the region. The first statement does not follow.

In 2017, the new boat with all the latest high-end features, which was also the most expensive boat available for freshwater use, outsold all other boats in Country Z in that year, despite being only introduced during the year. From these details, it is correct to infer that citizens of Country Z prefer a luxury boat for freshwater boating, since they bought this high-end, most expensive boat in such vast numbers. The second statement follows.

Country Z is an example of a country that meets the criteria in the third statement, which therefore follows.

While it may sound like there are a lot of freshwater boats in Country Z, we have no idea about the relative number of non-freshwater boats; the fourth statement does not follow.

While it is true that citizens of Country Z bought one particular boat that was marketed in their country in vast numbers, it is not clear that they would (or would not) buy boats that had not been marketed in their country. The fifth statement does not follow

20. YES; NO; NO; YES; NO

There were 2200 people in the zoo at 10am and 3080 at 4pm, a difference of 3080 − 2200 = 880. This means there were 880 ÷ 2200 = 0.4, or 40% more people in the zoo at 4pm than at 10am. The first statement follows.

A total of 415 + 630 + 845 = 1,890 visited Avian Adventures, whilst a total of 220 + 360 + 480 = 1,060 visited Nocturnal Wonders. Half of 1,890 is 945; the second statement does not follow.

There were more visitors at 1pm in the Reptile House than at 4pm, not less; the third statement does not follow.

The zoo had 2200 visitors at 10am, with 220 of these visiting Nocturnal Wonders. The fourth statement follows.

The number of visitors at Nocturnal Wonders was 220 at 10am and 360 at 1pm. The increase then is (360 − 220) ÷ 220 = 140 ÷ 220 = 0.636, or 64%, which is clearly well over a third. The fifth statement does not follow.

Venn Diagram Questions

The next-to-last Decision Making question type is Venn Diagram Questions. These are quite distinctive, as they will include a range of shapes that you may not have previously seen in any Venn diagrams. As you might expect, Venn Diagram Questions are all about which categories overlap—or do not overlap.

There are four main types of Venn Diagram Questions you might encounter on Test Day:

- Questions with a Venn diagram with numbers in the diagram and the answer choices. These questions are usually fairly straightforward; you must add up all the figures from the correct overlaps in the diagram.
- Questions with a Venn diagram with numbers in the diagram but lengthy textual answer choices. These questions may involve calculations, but are more about the overlaps of the different categories.
- Questions with a Venn diagram without numbers in the diagram. These questions are about the overlaps; you may often be asked to find the answer representing groups that do *not* overlap in the diagram.
- Questions with Venn diagrams in the answer choices. These may include numbers, but sometimes you will have four diagrams without numbers. Make sure that you understand the categories in the question, and think about whether they overlap wholly, partially or not at all.

Most Venn Diagram Questions will likely be from the first two types, but you may see a few of the last two types. Do not assume that diagrams without numbers are necessarily easier or quicker than those with numbers; it can be harder to 'see' which category corresponds to each shape if there aren't numbers in the diagram.

You will generally find that you work more efficiently, and with fewer errors, if you *think in shapes instead of words*. Try to mentally translate the categories into the corresponding shapes, then check the diagram to see whether the answer is correct. This will be most helpful in the second type of Venn Diagram Question, when there are long textual answer choices. It will also be useful in the third type, as the overlaps could be quite complicated.

Another shortcut is to look for the shapes that do not overlap. This won't necessarily help, but it could be valuable information in questions that involve non-overlapping categories. For example, if the question has the word *not* in it, then that is usually a hint to look for the non-overlapping shapes.

Practise your speed and accuracy, so you can answer most Venn Diagram Questions in under a minute. In any case, you will not want to take more than a minute, as this is the most common question type. Each Decision Making section in the official practice tests includes 6 or 7 Venn Diagram Questions, while there are only 4 or 5 each of all other question types.

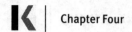

The diagram shows the duration and frequency of study sessions undertaken by members of an evening language club.

The pentagon represents the members learning French.

The oval represents the members learning Italian.

The hexagon represents members who study for at least 60 minutes in each study session.

The diamond represents members who study at least 3 days a week.

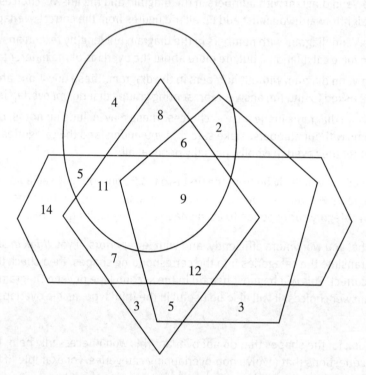

21. Which of the following statements is true?

    A. All the members learning French who study fewer than 3 days a week do it for less than an hour in each session.

    B. All the members learning Italian who study fewer than 3 days a week study for an hour or more in each session.

    C. Of all the members learning both French and Italian, less than half study for at least an hour in each session.

    D. Of all the members learning both French and Italian, more than half study for fewer than 3 days a week.

Answer: To evaluate the answer choices, compare the words to the shapes in the diagram, checking carefully to ensure that you include and exclude the correct figures. As soon as you find an answer that matches the diagram, mark it and move on—there is no need to check the remaining answers. The first answer involves members learning French (represented by the pentagon) who study fewer than 3 days a week, so look for figures that are in the pentagon but outside the diamond, which represents members who study at least 3 days a week: there are 2 members in the pentagon and oval, but not the diamond or hexagon, and another 3 members who are in the pentagon and no other shape, for a total of 5 members who are in the pentagon (studying French) and not the diamond (so they study fewer than 3 days a week). There aren't any members studying French who are in the hexagon but not the diamond, so it is true that all the members learning French who study fewer than 3 days a week do it for less than an hour in each session. Answer **(A)** is correct.

For the record, let's consider why the other answer choices are wrong:

Answer **(B)** involves the members learning Italian (the oval) who study fewer than 3 days a week, so they are in the oval but not the diamond; the statement says that all these members are also in the hexagon, as they study for an hour or more in each session. There are two figures representing members studying Italian that are outside the diamond but also outside the hexagon—there's a 4 that's only in the oval, and a 2 that's in both the oval and the pentagon, for a total of 6 members studying Italian who study for less than an hour in each session and who study fewer than 3 days a week.

Answer **(C)** involves the members learning both French and Italian, so they are inside both the pentagon and the oval. There are $9 + 6 + 2 = 17$ such members. Of these members, 9 are inside the hexagon (they study for at least 60 minutes in each session) and 8 are outside the hexagon (they study for less than 60 minutes in each session), so more than half study for an hour in each session.

Answer **(D)** involves the members learning both French and Italian, of which there are 17. Of these members, 15 are inside the diamond (they study at least 3 days a week) and 2 are outside the diamond (they study fewer than 3 days a week), so less than half study for fewer than 3 days a week.

Note how carefully you must compare the wording to the diagram. When working quickly, under the time pressures of the UKCAT, it would be very easy to invert the relationships and select a wrong answer. For example, in evaluating answer **(D)**, you might easily have thought it was correct as more than half study at least 3 days a week. Beware of wrong answer traps that are waiting for students who are rushing through the questions.

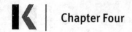

22. A garage tracks all the cars that receive one of three services over the course of a week: oil change, MOT testing and engine repair.

No car had all three services; half of the cars had an oil change with one additional service.

Five more cars had just an oil change than had just MOT testing and had just engine repair combined.

The number of cars that had MOT testing is three times the number of cars that had engine repair.

If the triangle represents cars that had an oil change, the oval represents cars that had MOT testing, and the rectangle represents cars that had engine repair, which diagram best represents the information?

A.

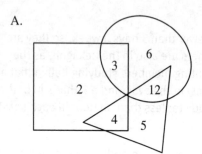

B.

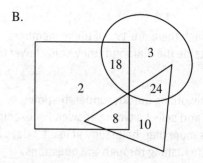

C.

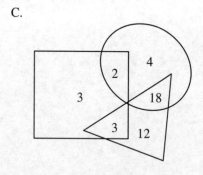

D.

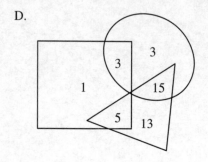

Answer: Since this question has Venn diagrams in the answers, the first step is to note which shape corresponds to which category. Note that the question does not give the categories in a helpful order; you will probably want to make a mental note (or a note on your scrap paper or noteboard) of the shapes from left to right, or clockwise from the top or left. The first rule tells us that half the cars had an oil change with one additional service; oil changes are in the triangle, so the numbers in the two overlaps with the triangle sum up to the same amount as all the other numbers in the diagram. On this basis, eliminate **(B)**, since the triangle overlaps add up to $24 + 8 = 32$, but the other numbers in the diagram add up to $10 + 18 + 2 + 3 = 33$. The second rule explains that the number of cars that had just an oil change (in the triangle only) equals five plus the number of cars that had just MOT testing (in the oval only) plus the cars that had just engine repair (in the rectangle only). Eliminate **(A)**, since 8 cars had just MOT testing or just engine repair, but only 5 cars had just oil change; eliminate **(D)** as well, since there are 9 more cars that had just an oil change (13 cars) compared to the number that had just one of the other services (4 cars). The correct answer is **(C)**.

Note the approach in the last question: We worked piece-by-piece through the initial information, comparing it to all the remaining answers and eliminating any answers that did not fit. Whilst this may seem a bit tedious, overall it is faster than the alternative approach, which would require you to attempt to construct a Venn diagram using all the rules—or combining all the rules before checking any answers. In this case, it would have been impossible to combine all the rules (or to make a Venn diagram) since we are not told the total number of cars, or any specific numbers in the categories. Be prepared to work piece-by-piece, save time through elimination, and accept that some questions will be presented in a way that is deliberately unhelpful.

With that in mind, and with practice, you can improve your pacing in Venn Diagram Questions. Most should be able to be answered in less than a minute, which is a real time-saver since there are so many of them in this section. Aim to complete the timed set in a little less than 3 minutes, and you will be off to a great start.

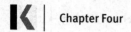

Kaplan Timed Practice Set—*Venn Diagram Questions*

Set your timer for 3 minutes. Mark answers for all 3 questions before time is up!

A restaurant tracks the desserts served over the course of a single evening.

The cross represents desserts served with ice cream.

The lightning represents desserts served with custard.

The triangle represents desserts served with chocolate sauce.

The trapezium represents cakes.

The arrow represents sundaes.

The oval represents pies.

The pentagon represents tarts.

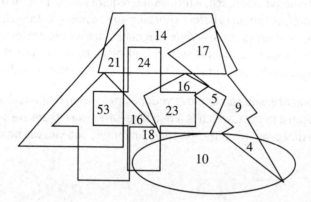

23. How many desserts were served with ice cream or custard, excluding cakes and desserts served with chocolate sauce?

    A. 66
    B. 75
    C. 92
    D. 116

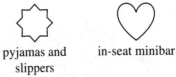

An airline offers a range of different amenities in various configurations of first class cabins on its different aircraft. The amenities available are indicated in the diagram.

USB ports

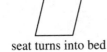

seat turns into bed

remote control

shower

pyjamas and slippers

in-seat minibar

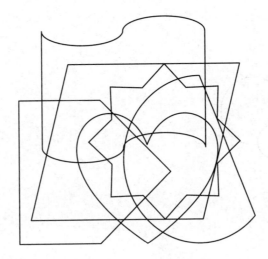

24. Which of the following combinations of first class amenities is **not** available in any aircraft on this airline?

A. Remote control and a seat that turns into a bed.

B. USB ports, in-seat minibar and a seat that turns into a bed.

C. Remote control, shower, pyjamas and slippers, in-seat minibar and a seat that turns into a bed.

D. USB ports, remote control, shower and a seat that turns into a bed.

25. Which diagram correctly depicts the relation between students, graduates, parents and babies?

A.

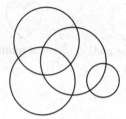

B.

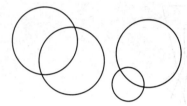

C.

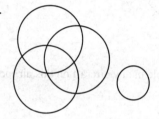

D.

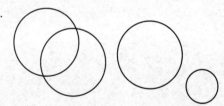

Kaplan Timed Practice Set—*Venn Diagram Questions*: Answers and Explanations

This timed set included examples of the other basic variations of Venn Diagram Questions—some without numbers, and some with just numbers in the answers. Be prepared for any variation of Venn diagrams that you may encounter on Test Day, and be ready to work through these questions as efficiently as possible. If you can answer most of them in 30 to 45 seconds—instead of a minute each—you might be able to bank a few extra minutes for the five-part questions.

23. (B)

The question asks for the total number of desserts served with ice cream (the cross) or custard (the lightning) but not chocolate sauce (triangle) or cakes (the trapezium). The figures in the cross that are not also inside the triangle or trapezium add up to $16 + 18 + 23 = 57$. The figures in the lightning that are not also inside the trapezium add up to $5 + 9 + 4 = 18$. The total desserts that meet the criteria are $57 + 18 = 75$.

24. (D)

This question asks you for to find the answer that does not represent a correct segment of overlapping shapes in the diagram. The flag (remote control) and the parallelogram (seat turns into bed) overlap without any other shapes near the top of the diagram; eliminate **(A)**. The pentagon (USB ports) and the heart (in-seat mini bar) overlap with the parallelogram, to the left of the star, below the flag; eliminate **(B)**. **(C)** includes all the shapes except the pentagon; these overlap in the narrow segment just to the left of the cleft in the heart; eliminate **(C)**. **(D)** must therefore be correct; the shapes in **(D)**—all except the heart and the star—is an impossible combination of amenities, because the pentagon (USB ports) and the half-circle (shower) only overlap inside the heart (in-seat mini bar), so you would have to have the in-seat mini bar as an amenity along with the four options listed in **(D)**.

25. (C)

Check the Venn diagrams in the answer choices against the groups in the question. Babies would not be parents, graduates or students, so there must be a separate circle that does not overlap the others. Eliminate **(A)** and **(B)**. A student could be a parent (e.g. a mature student), a graduate (e.g. a doctoral student) or both, so there must be three circles that overlap in every combination (so you could be just a student/parent/graduate, any pair of those options, or all three). The correct answer is **(C)**.

Score Higher Online

Practise using the onscreen calculator with the practice questions in your Kaplan Online Centre, so you are ready to use the calculator efficiently and accurately on Test Day.

Some Venn Diagram questions will require multiple calculations in a single answer choice; make a note of any initial or intermediate figures on your noteboard, to avoid the risk of forgetting and having to recalculate.

Maths Questions

The final Decision Making question type is identified by the test-maker as Probabilistic Reasoning. However, in reality, only some of these items will involve probability. The rest involve percentages, and you may have to do some other basic calculations before working with percentages or probability. Thus, we at Kaplan will refer to this question type as Maths Questions, since they are all about maths.

Maths Questions will generally follow one of two basic formats:

- You will have to calculate one or two probabilities, based on the information provided.
- You will have to calculate success/failure percentages for two different items/plans/devices, then compare the percentages.

In the official practice tests, all the probabilities relate to independent events, so that you would expect to multiply the probabilities if there are multiple events. For example, if you flip a fair coin three times, the probability of it landing heads up all three times is $1/2 \times 1/2 \times 1/2 = 1/8$.

Some probability questions will have a 'twist' that will often involve an incorrect deduction about the probability of an outcome. A common twist is that the text will describe several independent events, with one or more events having already happened; as a result, that event cannot be part of the probability calculation since its result is known. That might sound somewhat obvious, but it is easy to overlook if you are working quickly—and indeed, it's not the sort of detail you might have encountered on any previous schoolwork or exams involving probability.

If there are success/failure rates, be sure to keep them clear in your head. Expect to convert any failure rates to success rates, as normally the correct answers will compare success rates.

Practise attacking these questions so you can answer each in under a minute. They are generally the quickest and simplest questions in the Decision Making section, which means that they are a great opportunity to bank time that you can use for other questions. Also, because they are so quick and straightforward, it's all the more important that you get to them. Students that waste time on five-part questions before they make a first pass through the section will tend not to answer some (or all) of the Maths Questions, so they will miss out these relatively simple marks. Don't fall into that same trap on Test Day!

26. The weather forecast for a bank holiday weekend shows a 50% chance of rain for each day (Saturday, Sunday and Monday) of the three-day weekend.

    It rains all day on Saturday, so the probability that it will rain every day during the bank holiday weekend is one-half.

    A. Yes, because the probability of rain on any of the three days is 50%.
    B. Yes, because there are two days remaining, each with a 1 in 2 chance of rain.
    C. No, because there is likely to be rain on either Sunday or Monday, but not both.
    D. No, because the correct probability is one-quarter.

Answer: This question involves a three-day bank holiday weekend, Saturday to Monday, with a 50% chance of rain each day. That means there is a 1/2 chance of rain each day, or a 1/8 chance of rain every day during the bank holiday weekend; remember, you would need to multiply the probability of rain each day ($1/2 \times 1/2 \times 1/2$) to find the probability of rain on all three days, since each day is an independent event.

However, since we already know the results for Saturday (it rained), there are only two remaining days (Sunday and Monday) for which we have a remaining probability. Thus, the probability of it raining every day is $1/2 \times 1/2 = 1/4$. The correct answer is **(D)**.

With questions involving probability, you will likely find it faster (and less confusing) to simply do the maths from the initial information *before* looking at the answer choices. The wording of the wrong answers can be quite elaborate and strange, as you see with answer **(C)** here. Keep an eye on events that have already occurred (e.g. we knew it had rained on Saturday), as they will not factor into the probability of events that have not yet occurred.

27. A bowl contains twelve green sweets and nine white sweets. I select one sweet at random from the bowl; the sweet selected is white. Then I randomly select a second sweet from the bowl, without replacing the first.

Has the probability of the second sweet selected being green increased from the probability of selecting a green sweet before any sweets were selected?

A. Yes, it was 4/7 and is now 3/5.
B. Yes, it was 3/7 and is now 3/5.
C. No, it was 4/7 and is now 2/5.
D. No, it was 3/7 and is now 2/5.

Answer: Initially the bowl contains 21 sweets, of which 12 are green. Thus, at the start, the probability of selecting a green sweet at random is $12/21 = 4/7$. Eliminate **(B)** and **(C)**. The first sweet selected is white, after which there are 8 white sweets and 12 green sweets remaining in the bowl. The probability of randomly selecting a green sweet is now $12/20 = 3/5$. Answer **(A)** is correct.

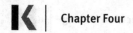

Kaplan Timed Practice Set—*Maths Questions*

Set your timer for 3 minutes. Mark answers for all 3 questions before time is up!

28. Two new vaccines for a certain disease are currently being trialled.

Vaccine P is effective at preventing the disease in 84% of patients.

Only 17% of patients experience side effects with Vaccine P.

Vaccine Q is not effective at preventing the disease in 15% of patients.

Vaccine Q does not cause any side effects in 84% of patients.

Judging **only** on side effects and effectiveness at preventing the disease, is Vaccine P the better vaccine?

A. Yes, because it has a higher rate of disease prevention, although the rate of side effects is the same.
B. Yes, because it is less likely to cause side effects than Vaccine Q.
C. No, because Vaccine Q prevents the disease in more patients, with side effects in fewer patients.
D. No, because Vaccine Q is more successful at preventing the disease, although they have the same rate of side effects.

29. A restaurant manager is keen to gather customer feedback, to understand their priorities for improving the restaurant. The manager conducts a survey by placing survey cards at the salad bar. The comment cards ask customers to rank the restaurant on a scale of 1 to 10 in five categories: seating; crockery and cutlery; ambiance; food; drink. There is also space for customers to leave comments.

80% of survey respondents included comments complaining about the salad bar. The most common complaint was that there are not enough toppings and dressings.

The manager concluded that the restaurant should expand the salad bar.

Does the survey data justify the manager's conclusion?

A. Yes, the survey was representative of the views of the restaurant's customers.
B. Yes, the restaurant's customers are more concerned with the salad bar than any other issue.
C. No, because people who eat salad are more likely to want to eat more salad.
D. No, because the survey oversampled salad bar users compared to the restaurant's other customers.

30. A bag contains six red balls, six blue balls and three black balls at the start. Balls are selected at random from the bag, one at a time, without replacing any of the balls.

The first three balls selected (in order) are blue, blue and black.

Has the chance of the fourth ball selected being blue now decreased from the chance of selecting a blue ball at the start?

A. Yes, it was 1/5 and is now 1/6.
B. Yes, it was 2/5 and is now 1/3.
C. No, it was 2/5 and is now 1/2.
D. No, it was 1/5 and is now 1/3.

Kaplan Timed Practice Set—*Maths Questions*: Answers and Explanations

Maths Questions are another question type that will hopefully be faster and more straightforward, allowing you to save time for the longer, more challenging questions. If you finished on time, that's great—but try to improve your performance in Maths Questions, so you can finish them a bit more quickly on Test Day.

28. (C)

Vaccine P prevents the disease in 84% of patients, while Vaccine Q prevents the disease in 85% of patients (100% − 15% = 85%). Vaccine P does not cause side effects in 83% of patients (100% − 17% = 83%), while Vaccine Q does not cause side effects in 84% of patients. Hence, it is clear that Vaccine Q is better than Vaccine P, in terms of preventing the disease (85% versus 84%) and also in terms of patients without side effects (84% versus 83%). Answer **(C)** is correct.

29. (D)

There is an obvious flaw in the survey, since it was conducted exclusively at the salad bar and respondents strongly favoured changes to the salad bar; this stands out even more because the salad bar was not one of the five categories being assessed. Whilst the salad bar fits into the broad category of 'food', the recommendation to expand the salad bar is based on the comments added by salad bar users, who presumably made up 100% of survey respondents. The survey did not draw from a representative sample of the restaurant's customers, oversampling salad bar users compared to other customers. The answer is **(D)**.

For the record: Note that we cannot justify the claim in **(B)** based on the data, since we only have the views of salad bar users. **(C)** does not follow from the information provided; we know that a lot of salad bar users complained about the salad bar, but this does not necessarily mean that they will eat more salad, which isn't really relevant to the issues with the survey.

30. (B)

At the start, there are a total of 6 + 6 + 3 = 15 balls in the bag. Six of these balls are blue, so the chance of selecting a blue ball at the start is 6/15 = 2/5. After the third ball is selected, the bag contains 12 balls, 4 of which are blue. At this point, the chance of selecting a blue ball is 4/12 = 1/3. The correct answer is **(B)**.

Remember

Think before you calculate.

Check you are comparing equivalent figures (e.g. success rates) and not opposites (e.g. a success rate and a failure rate).

It's easy to make an error when the question is simpler and you are working at top speed.

It's better to take an extra second to be sure you are comparing like to like and putting the right numbers into the calculator.

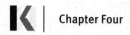

Keeping Perspective—Decision Making

You are about to complete a timed Kaplan UKCAT quiz, consisting of 15 Decision Making questions. The quiz will follow the same question type order as a full Decision Making section, with 2 or 3 questions of each type. If you pace yourself, and spend no more than 1 minute per question, you should be able to attempt and answer all of them. Even if you find yourself running out of time near the end, do your best to eliminate one or more answers before making your best guess.

Before you begin the quiz, let's consider some of the challenges in Decision Making that lead unprepared (or underprepared) test-takers to waste time and earn a lower score:

Vary your pacing, as the question types are varied—but each question is worth only one mark. Unlike other UKCAT sections, Decision Making includes much greater variety of question types and tasks. Some question types are relatively simple, with tasks that can be completed in less than a minute. Other question types (such as Syllogisms) are notably more complex, while some tasks (in some Logic Puzzles, for example) can be quite a bit more challenging. Each question is worth one mark, but the time and effort required for each mark is far from equal. Learn the question types, look out for challenges, and be prepared to vary your pacing appropriately.

Use the calculator and noteboard for maximum impact. Avoid making careless errors, such as forgetting figures you have calculated earlier in your working for a question, or miscalculating in your head. At the same time, you should aim to be efficient in calculator use, just as in the Quantitative section. The note-board will be invaluable for many Logic Puzzles, as you will need to annotate the rules and deductions more often than not.

Practise the task(s) for each question type, so they become second nature by Test Day. This is especially important for the simpler question types—Strongest Argument, Venn Diagram and Maths Questions—many of which can be answered in under a minute, if you know the task cold and can attack any such questions with brutal efficiency, without sacrificing accuracy.

Save the five-part questions for a second pass through the section. This strategic choice will ensure that you can pick up the marks on all the simpler, quicker questions before attacking the five-part questions. As a rule of thumb, there are usually 4 or 5 Syllogisms at the start of the section, with 4 to 5 Inference Questions just after the midpoint of the section. As a result, you will want to save about 10 minutes to answer these questions; you would do well to aim for 12 minutes, if you can be extremely efficient with the multiple choice questions. If you skip any other questions, then add a minute to that total. When you come to that second pass, you might want to prioritise the five-part questions that have shorter initial information, or the question type (Syllogism or Inference) that you find to be easier or more straightforward. Practise making these judgements every time you take a practice test, so you can feel confident in taking charge of the Decision Making section and maximising your marks on Test Day.

Chapter 4 Kaplan UKCAT Quiz

Set your timer for 16 minutes. Try to complete all 15 questions, and mark an answer for each before time is up. If a question is difficult, try to eliminate one answer and then make your best guess, so you can keep to 1 minute per question.

31. A volleyball team has men players and women players. Some of the women like to play hockey. The rest of the team is at the beach.

   Place 'Yes' if the conclusion does follow. Place 'No' if the conclusion does not follow.

If a volleyball player likes to play hockey, they must be a woman.	
All the men on the team are at the beach.	
Any woman on the team who is at the beach does not like to play hockey.	
None of the volleyball players at the beach like to play hockey.	
None of the women on the team are at the beach.	

32. All the black chairs have leather upholstery, but some chairs with leather upholstery are not black. Chairs with fabric upholstery are either a single colour (except brown) or patterned.

   Place 'Yes' if the conclusion does follow. Place 'No' if the conclusion does not follow.

If furniture is patterned, it must have fabric upholstery.	
If a chair is brown, it could have leather upholstery.	
None of the patterned chairs are brown.	
White chairs could have leather upholstery or fabric upholstery.	
None of the chairs with fabric upholstery are black.	

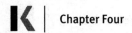

33. All of Marianna's friends have unattached earlobes, and none have an extra digit. All Katie's friends are aged 21 and over; some of Katie's friends have an extra digit, but none of Katie's friends have tattoos.

Everyone at the party is Marianna's friend or Katie's friend; at least one person at the party is both Katie's friend and Marianna's friend, but most people at the party are only Marianna's friend or only Katie's friend.

Place 'Yes' if the conclusion does follow. Place 'No' if the conclusion does not follow.

Someone at the party who is not Katie's friend has unattached earlobes.	
Someone at the party who is not Marianna's friend has an extra digit.	
At least one of Marianna's friends at the party is aged 21 and over.	
At least one of the friends at the party has an extra digit, but no tattoos.	
No one under the age of 21 at the party has tattoos.	

In the course of a morning, a charity shop is visited by four customers.

Each customer buys one item: an armchair, a record player, a wedding dress or a bowler hat.

Each item is bought at a different price: £5, £10, £20 or £25.

The articles of clothing were neither the most nor the least expensive item.

Paul's item (which wasn't the bowler hat) cost twice as much as Sally's.

Rex's item cost less than Olga's and more than the armchair.

34. Which of the following must be true?

    A. Olga's item cost £20.
    B. Paul bought the record player.
    C. Sally's item cost £10.
    D. Rex bought the bowler hat.

On a skiing holiday, five friends—Oona, Peter, Rupali, Sally and Tim—stay in the same room at the chalet.

The room has three bunk beds, each with a top and bottom bunk.

Each friend sleeps in a different bunk; one bunk is empty.

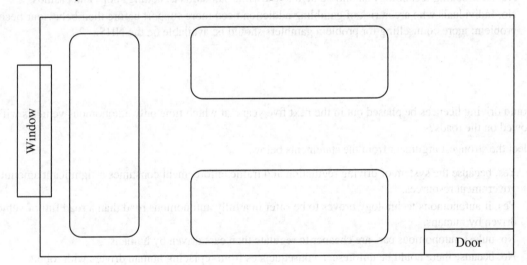

Peter sleeps nearest to the door of any of the friends.

Rupali and Tim sleep in bottom bunks.

Sally does not sleep next to the window.

Sally does not sleep above Tim.

35. Where must Oona sleep?

    A. Top bunk, furthest from the door and window.
    B. Bottom bunk, furthest from the door and window.
    C. Top bunk, nearest to the window.
    D. Bottom bunk, nearest to the door.

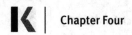

36. Should everyone be guaranteed an equal level of care in old age, regardless of their income or ability to pay?

Select the strongest argument from the statements below.

A. Yes, all citizens are entitled to food and shelter, and it is the duty of the government to ensure that this is provided.
B. Yes, otherwise some pensioners may struggle to survive without meals or nurses.
C. No, some people will require round-the-clock care in old age while others will need minimal care, and it would be an unjust expense for the government to fully take on.
D. No, older people with more resources are entitled to select a premium level of service if they desire it.

37. Should there be a strict daily limit on the amount that an individual can gamble on mobile betting apps and video betting terminals?

Select the strongest argument from the statements below.

A. Yes. Betting technology has outpaced regulation; gambling addicts are at risk of losing a fortune in under an hour with the existing very high limits (or no limits) on mobile and video bets.
B. Yes. Access to gambling technology should be prohibited unless an individual signs a legal declaration of the maximum amount they are willing to bet each day.
C. No. New betting technology should be held to the same standards as betting shops and casinos.
D. No. Individuals who are at risk of gambling addiction need more support before their behaviour becomes a problem; more counselling for problem gamblers should be available on the NHS.

38. Should driving licences be phased out in the next five years, at which time only autonomous vehicles will be allowed on the roads?

Select the strongest argument from the statements below.

A. Yes, because the system of driving regulation and traffic enforcement consumes a significant amount of government resources.
B. Yes, if autonomous technology proves to be safer in a fully autonomous road than a road full of vehicles driven by humans.
C. No, unless autonomous cars are cheaper to regulate than cars driven by humans.
D. No, because there could be unforeseen consequences from replacing human drivers with robots.

39. Archaeologists sometimes employ a technique known as magnetometry when attempting to survey an area of land for traces of historical human activity. Certain common forms of human activity, such as the construction of ditches or the burning of waste materials, permanently alter the magnetism of minute iron particles contained in the soil. By comparing the difference between the magnetic orientation of the local soil and that of the Earth's magnetic field, researchers can sometimes pinpoint the location of ancient farmland or buildings beneath the ground. These differences are usually extremely slight and so there are limits to what can be discovered with the technique. Burial sites, for instance, will often fail to show up in a survey. Nevertheless, in areas where significant changes to the soil have resulted in magnetic variation, magnetometry is an invaluable method of surveying archaeological sites of interest before committing to the laborious process of excavation.

Place 'Yes' if the conclusion does follow. Place 'No' if the conclusion does not follow.

All forms of human activity have an impact on the local soil's magnetism.	
Cemeteries tend not to result in a permanent change to the local soil's magnetism.	
Magnetometry is only possible because the Earth's magnetic field is so weak.	
Magnetometry is only used by archaeologists when excavation isn't an option.	
Archaeologists can detect human activity from an earlier era by testing small traces of a certain element in the soil.	

40. Lighting costs account for 15% of an average household's annual electricity bill, with a recent focus on both cost and energy saving measures for lighting solutions. Compulsory measures have been introduced to ban the sale of the most inefficient bulbs. In the last decade, two alternatives to the standard filament light bulb have also become popular: the light emitting diode (LED) and compact fluorescent lamp (CFL). Of the two, the former is more energy and cost efficient, but both are viable options for most existing light fittings. Per bulb, LEDs can save £3 to £6 a year, which, in a typical three-bedroom house could amount to savings of more than £200 over five years.

Place 'Yes' if the conclusion does follow. Place 'No' if the conclusion does not follow.

A typical three-bedroom house must use at least seven light bulbs.	
CFL bulbs are more energy efficient than LED bulbs.	
A new law requires old light bulbs to be replaced with a new type of bulb that is more energy efficient.	
Each year the average household spends 3 of every 20 pence of electricity costs on lighting.	
LED bulbs are more cost efficient than any other light bulbs on the market.	

All the sales and marketing jobs available on a recruitment website are indicated in the diagram.

The circle represents managerial jobs.

The triangle represents jobs in the public sector.

The pentagon represents sales jobs.

The quadrilateral represents marketing jobs.

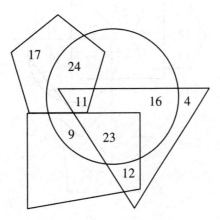

41. Which of the following must be true?

    A. None of the public sector sales jobs are managerial jobs.
    B. At least half of the marketing jobs are in the private sector.
    C. All of the private sector marketing jobs are managerial jobs.
    D. There are more managerial jobs in marketing than in sales.

The diagram below represents the books selected by undergraduate students for the final essay in a first-year module. Each student is writing the final essay about a different book.

The rectangle represents books written during the 20th century, the circle represents books written by male authors, the hexagon represents nonfiction, the triangle represents novels, and the arrow represents books written during the 19th century.

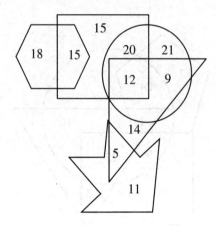

42. How many undergraduate students selected books that were written by female authors, but not during the 19th century?

    A. 48
    B. 62
    C. 78
    D. 91

A shop sells a range of perfumes containing the ingredients displayed in the diagram.

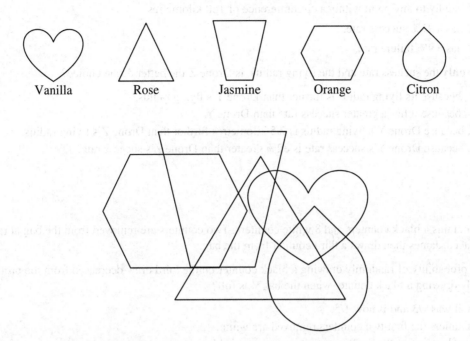

Vanilla   Rose   Jasmine   Orange   Citron

43. Which of the following combinations is **not** available in a perfume sold by the shop?

    A. A perfume with jasmine and orange.

    B. A perfume with citron and vanilla.

    C. A perfume with jasmine and rose.

    D. A perfume with orange and rose.

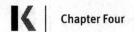

44. A researcher is testing the performance of two new drones.

    Drone Y has a flying radius of 20 kilometres.

    Drone Z can fly to any point within a circumference of 160 kilometres.

    Drone Y has a 91% success rate.

    Drone Z has a 9% failure rate.

    Judging **only** the success rate and the flying radius, is Drone Z the better drone choice?

    A. Yes, because its flying radius is further than Drone Y's flying radius.
    B. Yes, because it has a greater success rate than Drone Y.
    C. No, because Drone Y's flying radius is 2.5 kilometres further than Drone Z's flying radius.
    D. No, because Drone Y's success rate is 82% greater than Drone Z's success rate.

45. A bag contains 4 black counters and 8 white counters. Two counters are removed from the bag at random and not replaced. James then draws a third counter from the bag.

    Has the probability of randomly drawing a black counter on the third draw decreased from the probability of randomly drawing a black counter when the bag was full?

    A. Yes, it was 1/3 and is now 1/5.
    B. Yes, unless the first two counters removed are white.
    C. No, unless one of the first two counters removed is black.
    D. No, it was 1/3 and is now 2/5.

STOP. IF YOU FINISH BEFORE TIME IS UP, CHECK ANY QUESTIONS YOU HAVE MARKED FOR REVIEW. YOU MAY GO BACK TO QUESTIONS IN THIS QUIZ ONLY.

Chapter 4 Kaplan UKCAT Quiz: Answers and Explanations

31. NO; YES; YES; NO; NO

The initial information tells us about two groups of the volleyball team—some women who like to play hockey, and the rest of the team (including all the men players) who are at the beach. It is possible that the first statement is correct, but it is also possible that there are men players who like to play hockey; as there is not enough information, the first statement does not follow. The 'rest of the club' (except for the women who like to play hockey) is at the beach, so 'the rest' must include all the men players; the second statement follows. The rest of the club who are at the beach includes anyone, man or woman, who does not like to play hockey; the third statement follows. It is possible that some of the men players at the beach like to play hockey; the fourth statement does not follow. It is possible that all the women players like to play hockey, but it is also possible that some of the women players (who don't like to play hockey) are at the beach; the fifth statement does not follow.

32. NO; YES; NO; YES; YES

The initial information only covers chairs, so we don't know whether all patterned furniture must have fabric upholstery. The first statement does not follow. Some chairs with leather upholstery are not black; we are not told the colour of these chairs, so they could be brown. The second statement follows. We don't know anything about the colours in the patterned chairs; the third statement does not follow. White chairs could have leather upholstery (among the non-black leather chairs) or single-colour fabric upholstery; the fourth statement follows. All the black chairs have leather upholstery, so none of them have fabric upholstery; the final statement follows.

33. YES; NO; YES; NO; NO

Someone at the party who is not Katie's friend must be Marianna's friends, and all of her friends have unattached earlobes; the first statement follows. Someone at the party who is not Marianna's must be Katie's friend; some of these friends have an extra digit, but we don't necessarily know that any one of Katie's friends at the party would have an extra digit. The second statement does not follow. At least one of Marianna's friends at the party is also Katie's friend, and all Katie's friends are aged 21 and over; the third statement follows. We don't know that any of the friends at the party have an extra digit; this is possible, but not certain. The fourth statement does not follow. None of Katie's friends are under 21, and none have tattoos; it's possible that Marianna has a friend who is under 21 with tattoos. We can't say for sure; the fifth statement does not follow.

34. (D)

The first rule in this Logic Puzzle tells us that the wedding dress and bowler hat must cost £10 or £20; the record player and armchair must cost £5 or £25. Paul's item (not the bowler hat) cost twice as much as Sally's, which indicates two possibilities. First, it could be that Paul's item cost £20 and Sally's cost £10, in which case Paul must have bought the wedding dress and Sally the bowler hat (since the articles of clothing must cost £10 and £20, and Paul doesn't buy the bowler hat). Second, it could be that Paul's item cost £10 and Sally's cost £5, in which case Paul must buy the wedding dress (for the same reason as in the previous possibility), whilst Sally could buy the record player or the armchair. In either case, we know that Paul must buy the wedding dress. Eliminate **(B)**.

The final rule tells us that Olga's item cost more than Rex's, and that Rex's item cost more than the armchair. Since the armchair can only be £5 or £25, we know that the armchair must be the cheapest item (since there must be at least two more expensive items). This also means that Sally bought the £5 item (the armchair), since all three other customers must have bought more expensive items (since P > S and O > R > the £5 armchair). Eliminate **(C)**. That means that Paul's wedding dress cost £10 (as it must be twice the price of Sally's), so Olga's item (the record player) cost £25. Rex must have bought the bowler hat for £20. The answer is **(D)**.

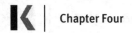

35. (C)

This Logic Puzzle requires you to allocate five friends to six possible bunks; each bed in the diagram has a top and bottom bunk, meaning that one bunk will be empty. We know from the first rule that Peter must be in the bed nearest the door, at the bottom of the diagram; we don't know if he takes the top or bottom bunk, but it doesn't matter as no one else can be in the other bunk, otherwise Peter wouldn't be nearest to the door; eliminate **(D)**. That leaves four bunks for the four remaining friends. Sally and Oona must take top bunks, since Rupali and Tim take bottom bunks; eliminate **(B)**. Sally does not sleep next to the window or above Tim, so Sally must take the top bunk at the top of the diagram, with Rupali in the bottom bunk; Tim is in the bottom bunk by the window, with Oona in the top bunk. The correct answer is **(C)**.

36. (C)

The key terms in the original question are everyone, guaranteed, equal level of care, old age, and regardless of income/ability to pay. **(A)** shifts from old age to 'all citizens', a much broader group, while also shifting from care to 'food and shelter', a narrower category; the terms are sufficiently different to rule out **(A)**. **(B)** shifts from old age to 'some pensioners', while shifting from 'care' to 'meals or nurses'; again, the terms are not quite the same. **(C)** matches the exact terms of the original question, drawing a distinction between people in old age who require 24/7 care and those who require minimal care, and pointing out it is unfair for the government to fully take on this expense. **(C)** is a direct hit, in every sense, on the original question, so it is correct.

For the record: **(D)** shifts from old age to 'older people', but note that this term is much less specific. Also, it is unclear that 'a premium level of service' relates specifically to care for people in old age.

37. (A)

The original question proposes a strict daily limit on the amount an individual can gamble on mobile betting apps and betting terminals. **(A)** responds directly to this question, acknowledging that betting technology has outpaced legislation and, as a result, gambling addicts can lose a fortune in an under an hour under current limits on mobile and video bets. **(A)** matches the key terms of the original question, so it is correct.

For the record: **(B)** suggests a way for an individual to limit their daily bet, but that is not what is being suggested in the original question. **(C)** compares new betting technology to betting shops and casinos, but this does not address the point about daily limits in mobile apps and video terminals. **(D)** shifts the focus to support for gambling addicts, specifically more NHS resources; the NHS is outside the scope of the original question.

38. (B)

The original question suggests that a shift to fully autonomous vehicles on the roads could mean an end to driving licences in the next five years. **(A)** talks instead about the cost of driving regulation and traffic enforcement, which isn't the same as driving licences and does not mention anything about autonomous vehicles, which presumably would have to be regulated by the government. **(B)** includes the key terms from the original question, suggesting that the proposal could work if the new technology is safer than a road full of cars driven by humans, i.e. humans with driving licences. The correct answer is **(B)**.

For the record: **(C)** shifts the topic to the cost of regulating autonomous cars and cars driven by humans, which is not relevant to the original question; car regulations are different from driving licences. Nothing in the original question suggests that autonomous cars would be driven by robots, contrary to **(D)**.

39. NO; YES; NO; NO; YES

Certain common forms of human activity permanently alter the magnetism of the soil, implying that not all forms of human activity impact on the magnetism of the local soil; the first statement does not follow. Burial sites often fail to show up in a magnetometric survey, and magnetometry works in areas where significant changes to the soil have resulted in permanent magnetic variation. We can therefore infer that cemeteries do not result in a permanent change to the magnetism of the local soil; the second statement follows. The text does not contain any information about the strength of the Earth's magnetic field; the third statement does not follow. The fourth statement does not follow; magnetometry is useful because it allows archaeologists to survey sites of interest before committing to excavation. The fifth statement follows; archaeologists detect human activity based on minute traces of iron particles in the soil.

40. YES; NO; NO; YES; NO

A typical three-bedroom house can save more than £200 over five years, or more than £40 per year, with LEDs, which save £3 to £6 a year per bulb. At the maximum saving per bulb, a three-bedroom house must therefore have at least £40 ÷ £6 = 6.67 LED bulbs, which means they must use at least seven light bulbs, since you can't have 0.67 of a light bulb. The first statement follows. The second statement inverts the relationship—it's LED bulbs that are more efficient—so it does not follow. The sale of the most inefficient bulbs has been banned, but that does not mean that you have to replace old light bulbs; old light bulbs are not necessarily the ones that have been banned. The third statement does not follow. The average household spends 15% of its annual electricity budget on lighting, and 3/20 = 0.15, or 15%; the fourth statement follows. LED bulbs are more cost efficient than CFL bulbs, but we are not told whether they are the most cost efficient on the market; the fifth statement does not follow.

41. (C)

There are 11 jobs in the pentagon (sales), the circle (managerial) and the triangle (public sector), so **(A)** is false. Any jobs outside the triangle are in the private sector; 9 jobs in the quadrilateral (marketing) are outside the triangle, while 23 + 12 = 35 jobs are in both shapes; 9 is less than half of 44 (9 + 35 = 44), so **(B)** is false. The marketing jobs (quadrilateral) that are outside the triangle (public sector) are all inside the circle (managerial), so all the private sector marketing jobs are managerial jobs. **(C)** is correct.

For the record: There are 23 + 9 = 32 managerial jobs in marketing (quadrilateral plus circle), whilst there are 24 + 11 = 35 managerial jobs in sales (pentagon plus circle), ruling out **(D)**.

42. (B)

Male authors are represented by the circle; all books outside the circle are written by female authors. The arrow represents books written during the 19th century. Thus, you need all the books outside the arrow and the circle. These add up to 18 + 15 + 15 + 14 = 62. The correct answer is **(B)**.

43. (D)

The hexagon (orange) and the triangle (rose) only intersect inside the trapezium (jasmine), so there isn't a perfume that includes just orange and rose—any perfumes with orange and rose would also include jasmine. Answer **(D)** is correct.

44. (A)

Drone Y has a success rate of 91%; Drone Z also has a success rate of 91% (100% − 9% = 91%). Drone Z has a flying circumference of 160 kilometres; circumference = $2\pi r = 2 \times 3.14 \times r = 160$. $r = 160 \div 6.28 = 25.48$ kilometres. Drone Y has a flying radius of 20 kilometres, so Drone Z has the further flying radius. Answer **(A)** is correct.

45. (B)

Initially the bag contains 12 counters, 4 of which are black; the probability of randomly selecting a black counter is 4/12 = 1/3. After two counters are removed, the probability of randomly selecting a black counter will depend on the colours of the counters that were removed.

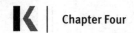

Chapter Four

If two black counters are removed: There are 2 black and 8 white counters remaining in the bag; 10 counters total. The probability of selecting a black counter is now 2/10 = 1/5.

If one black and one white counter are removed: There are 3 black and 7 white counters remaining in the bag; 10 counters total. The probability of selecting a black counter is now 3/10.

If two white counters are removed: There are 4 black and 6 white counters remaining in the bag; 10 counters total. The probability of selecting a black counter is now 4/10 = 2/5.

Note that in two of the three possibilities, the probability of selecting a black counter after removing two counters has decreased from 1/3; only if both counters removed are white would the probability increase, from 1/3 to 2/5. Answer **(B)** is correct.

Quantitative Reasoning

The Task

The Quantitative Reasoning section is the third scored section on the UKCAT. It comes straight after the Decision Making section, so it is important to have a strategy that allows you to power through the questions, despite perhaps feeling somewhat fatigued.

Again, you have 1 minute to read the directions, and then you have just 24 minutes to tackle 36 questions in sets of 4; most of these 9 sets will be accompanied by data. This section requires you to formulate and solve numerical problems by selecting relevant information—information that can be presented to you in the data in a variety of ways. On average, you must complete each question in about 30 seconds, or each set in 2 minutes.

The Format

The majority of sets in this section have data presented in charts, graphs, tables or diagrams, with varying amounts of accompanying text. Most questions come in sets of 4 items with the same data, usually a single table, chart or graph with a small amount of text. In the current Quantitative format, tables are far more common than charts or graphs. You may see one or two sets with changing data—each question in the set may have its own data, unrelated to the others, or the initial table, chart or graph may change in one or more subsequent questions. There are usually one or two sets that do not have any visual data, with only a few lines of written information. The topics covered are extremely varied, but a range of key ideas come up frequently. These will be covered later in the chapter.

Each question in the Quantitative Reasoning section has five multiple choice answers, from **(A)** to **(E)**. The format of the answer choices depends on the questions asked, but you may be required to calculate a number, or select an option (for example, a place, person or time), based on the subject matter in the question. In the most recent Quantitative sets from the UKCAT Consortium—those added to the online practice tests and sets in the past few years—virtually all the questions require two or three calculations, so you will be using the on-screen calculator quite a bit. You should have a computer with a number pad on the right side of the keyboard on Test Day, so be sure to practise using the on-screen calculator in the official practice tests with your keyboard at home. Getting to know the on-screen calculator is just as important as learning the ins and outs of the questions in this section.

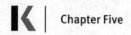

Note that (as of the time of writing) the Quantitative sections in the first two official practice tests (Test A and Test B) on the UKCAT website contain quite a few sets that were written in 2009 or earlier, when the challenges of the Quantitative section were a bit different. In these older sets, there is quite a lot of visual data. Some sets have two or three charts, graphs or tables, with nearly a full page of accompanying text, often in the form of a list of bullet points. Obviously these questions present different challenges, and they can feel quite scary when the data takes up two or more screens. But they are not representative of the current test format, so do not fret about them. The sets in Test C and the extra Quantitative practice on the UKCAT website are very representative of the current test format.

The Challenges

At Kaplan, we find that many candidates worry about the mathematics in this section, but this anxiety is misplaced. Most of the maths required in the Quantitative Reasoning section is fairly straightforward, and relatively basic—you won't see any trigonometry or calculus! The challenge in Quantitative lies in identifying exactly what each question is asking you to do, confidently manipulating formulae, accurately selecting the correct data to get to the answer, and doing it all within the time constraints of the section. Fortunately, there are a number of techniques that you can employ to enable you to answer the maximum number of questions in the time available.

Note that while you will use the same formulae over and over, you will often be asked to set up and solve for an unknown that is not the usual result of the formula. For example, if a question involves an average score on an exam, you will expect to use the average formula. But the question might tell you the average score, the number of students that took the exam, and the scores for all but one of the students—the unknown in this case would be the individual score of a single student, so you would have to manipulate the average formula to solve for the unknown. Be prepared to do a lot of mental algebra, and to apply familiar formulae and concepts in new and unexpected ways.

Kaplan Top Tips for Quantitative Reasoning

1. Don't get bogged down in the data

It can be tempting to spend time reading all of the text accompanying sets of data, getting to grips with graphs, and trying to absorb diagrams and tables. With 2 minutes to complete each set, you simply do not have time—especially as much of the data may be irrelevant to the questions. Instead, glance over pictorial data to determine key features:

- The general categories of data involved, and how they relate to each other.
- Labels and units—misreading these is a key pitfall!
- The gist of the information in any accompanying text.

2. Set up calculations to solve accurately

Several maths concepts and formulae come up time and again in the Quantitative Reasoning section. Having these at your fingertips so you can apply them quickly, confidently and accurately will help you to perform to the best of your ability on those questions. There are four basic formulae that come up very frequently on the UKCAT:

- Percentage $= \dfrac{\text{Part}}{\text{Whole}}$

- Percentage change $= \dfrac{\text{Difference}}{\text{Original}}$

- Speed $= \dfrac{\text{Distance}}{\text{Time}}$

- Mean(average) $= \dfrac{\text{Sum of the terms}}{\text{Number of terms}}$

In addition, you should know and be prepared to use any basic geometry formulae—such as those involving area, perimeter, circumference, and volume of common two- and three-dimensional shapes.

Many of the calculations you must complete in Quantitative Reasoning will require you to work quickly and comfortably with fractions and proportions; remember, a proportion is simply a fraction written side to side, so that $\dfrac{3}{4}$ has the same value as 3:4.

3. Eyeball, eliminate and estimate

The most efficient way to answer some of the questions will not be to calculate them. Eyeballing—comparing data and answers with a rough visual approximation to avoid unnecessary steps—and estimating answers based on rounded figures will help you to move quickly through the section. Eliminating answer choices that must be wrong—answers that are obviously too big, or obviously too small—is a vital skill to help you reduce the number of calculations you need to do, thus saving time.

4. Minimise the maths

Some of the questions in this section will involve no maths whatsoever. Instead, simply reading the information or eyeballing the data may find the answer. Most of the section comprises questions that involve simple calculations with one or two steps, and a few questions will be more complex, requiring several steps to get to the answer. These complex questions are often excellent targets to guess an answer choice, mark the question for review, move on, and return if there is time remaining.

Time to put Kaplan's top tips into practice! Give yourself 2 minutes to work through the Quantitative Reasoning set on the next page, and to write down answers for all 4 questions. Remember, you are allowed a calculator in Quantitative Reasoning, so be sure to use one here. Also, be sure to use scrap paper for any notations, rather than marking on the book itself, when answering practice questions: you can't write on the test itself on Test Day, as the questions appear on the computer screen; it is best to start out with good habits from now on.

Score Higher Online

Check the onscreen calculator in the official UKCAT practice questions now, so you are familiar with its functions.

Take a moment to try moving the calculator—notice that you will have to adjust it so that it does not obscure the question or the answer choices.

Be ready to adjust the calculator as needed on Test Day.

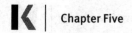

Kaplan Timed Practice Set—Try the Kaplan Top Tips

Set your timer for 2 minutes. Mark answers for all 4 questions before time is up!

The table includes the local authority areas in greater London with the greatest percentage rise in population from 2011 to 2016.

Local authority	Location	2011	2016
Barking and Dagenham	Outer	185,911	206,500
Camden	Inner	220,338	246,200
City of London	Inner	7,375	9,400
Hillingdon	Outer	273,936	302,500
Islington	Inner	206,125	232,900
Kingston upon Thames	Outer	160,060	176,100
Tower Hamlets	Inner	254,096	304,900
Westminster	Inner	219,396	247,600
Inner London (all boroughs)		3,231,901	3,515,500
Outer London (all boroughs)		4,942,040	5,258,600

- Location indicates whether the borough is located in Inner London or Outer London.
- The City of London's population grew by 2.63% from 2001 to 2011.

1. What was the mean population change in the Inner London boroughs?
   A. 21,731
   B. 23,515
   C. 26,734
   D. 28,832
   E. 31,906

2. The population of Tower Hamlets rose by what percentage?
   A. 19.99%
   B. 20.11%
   C. 20.57%
   D. 21.07%
   E. 21.33%

3. The City of London's population grew by what percentage from 2001 to 2016?
   A. 24.83%
   B. 27.46%
   C. 28.18%
   D. 29.02%
   E. 30.81%

4. The three Outer London boroughs account for how much of the population growth in Outer London?
   A. 13.17%
   B. 14.86%
   C. 18.67%
   D. 20.59%
   E. 22.99%

Kaplan Timed Practice Set—*Try the Kaplan Top Tips*: Answers and Explanations

How did you get on? Hopefully, you finished the statements in the 2 minutes, and answered them all correctly. As you practise with this book, you should **always** read through the explanations for every question, to ensure that you got the right answer for the right reasons. The explanations may also give tips that will help you on later questions with similar twists. If you didn't get them all right, don't despair—in fact, it is good to make mistakes as you practise. Each mistake you make as you practise is one you can avoid on Test Day.

1. (C)

The target here is the mean population change in the five Inner London boroughs. First, subtract the figures for each of these local authorities to find the population changes; next, add the population changes to find the total population change; finally, divide by 5 to find the mean population change for the five boroughs. You will want to make a note of the population change for each of the boroughs on scrap paper (or on your noteboard on Test Day) so you can pop them in the calculator once you are ready to find the total.

Camden: 246,200 − 220,338 = 25,862

City of London: 9,400 − 7,375 = 2,025

Islington: 232,900 − 206,125 = 26,775

Tower Hamlets: 304,900 − 254,096 = 50,804

Westminster: 247,600 − 219,396 = 28,204

Total population change: 25,862 + 2,025 + 26,775 + 50,804 + 28,204 = 133,670

Mean population change: 133,670 ÷ 5 = 26,734

The correct answer is **(C)**. Note that this question is not especially difficult to understand, but you must work very efficiently with the calculator to complete all the calculations in 30 seconds. In the Quantitative section, a question's difficulty level is often about the amount of work involved, rather than the conceptual complexity of the work involved. You can see already that it is essential to try and avoid making careless errors with the calculator, or in noting the figures from the initial calculations as you come up with them.

2. (A)

Percentage rise equals difference divided by original. The original figure is 254,096; the difference is 304,900 − 254,096 = 50,804. The percentage rise is 50,804 ÷ 254,096 = 0.19994, or 19.99%, answer **(A)**.

3. (E)

The information under the graph states that the City of London's population grew by 2.63% from 2001 to 2011. Thus, the City of London population in 2011 is 102.63% of its population in 2011; divide to find the 2001 population: 7,375 ÷ 1.0263 = 7,186. To find the percentage change from 2011 to 2016, find the difference and divide by the original (7,186). The difference is 9,400 − 7,186 = 2,214; the percentage change is 2,214 ÷ 7,186 = 0.308099, or 30.81%. Answer **(E)** is correct.

4. (D)

Outer London grew by 5,258,600 − 4,942,040 = 316,560 from 2011 to 2016. Next, find the population growth for the three Outer London boroughs in the table:

Barking and Dagenham: 206,500 − 185,911 = 20,589

Hillingdon: 302,500 − 273,936 = 28,564

Kingston upon Thames: 176,100 − 160,060 = 16,040

Total population growth: 20,589 + 28,564 + 16,040 = 65,193

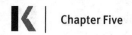

Thus, we can see that the three Outer London boroughs accounted for 65,193 ÷ 316,650 = 0.20588, or 20.59%, of the population growth in Outer London. The answer is **(D)**.

Take a moment to consider the level of maths required in this set. It is mostly just arithmetic and algebra; you had to use your knowledge of averages, percentages, and percentage change. The big challenge was working quickly, to keep to the tight timing required to finish the set in 2 minutes. You will want to practise your 'mental maths', so you can get as efficient as possible at setting up the steps BEFORE going to the calculator, and so you can make your calculations in the best order without error. This will feel quite different to any maths exam you have previously taken, but the good news is that these skills can be developed and improved.

Let's take a deeper look at a set with a table.

Working with Tables

In the current Quantitative test format, you should expect that more questions will involve tables than any other data format. There is an advantage to working with tables, since they are usually relatively straightforward, and are less vulnerable to the challenges that charts and graphs can present. For example, it is usually relatively simple to find the correct data in a table, so long as you understand the row and column labels. The UKCAT will sometimes make this more challenging by having lots of rows and columns, or subcategories of rows and columns—but the cells in the table will normally contain the actual numbers and percentages you need. So it is usually just a matter of making sure you've picked the right numbers from the right cells.

Be prepared to see some tables that are especially elaborate. Most tables will have a fair few cells that are not required for any of the questions in the set; some tables may have entire rows or columns that are irrelevant. That's why it's important that you do not spend time studying the data before attacking the first question in a set. Go straight into the first question, then take a quick look at the data (most likely a table) once you know what data you need for the first question. At that point, you will want to make sure you have a basic sense of the parameters of the table, to avoid pulling data from the wrong cell. This is usually just a matter of taking a few seconds to orient yourself to the table—it requires a certain deftness to do this quickly and accurately, and it's something to practise as you work through this chapter and your remaining Quantitative practice questions.

Let's get started with the next table and the four accompanying questions. For each question, take a moment to read the question and decide what data you need, then look at the table to pick out the data. Use the data to set up and solve—make any notations or rough workings on scrap paper, as you won't be able to write on the table or the questions and answers on Test Day. In this set, focus more on technique than timing—mastering the Quantitative technique first will help you improve speed in the long run.

A chocolate shop tests the nutritional values of its chocolates and makes the following table. All nutrition and price values are given per 100 g.

	Dark Chocolate	Milk Chocolate	White Chocolate
Energy (kcal)	598.43	563.72	560.11
Carbohydrates (g)	45.9	59.13	60.1
Fat (g)	42.63	33.6	32.9
Protein (g)	7.79	6.2	5.9
Cocoa solids	75%	35%	0%
Price	£3.20	£2.85	£2.60

- 1 kcal = 4.18 kJ
- Caloric value of carbohydrates: 4 kcal per gram
- Caloric value of fat: 9 kcal per gram

5. If one milk chocolate bar contains 320 kcal, how much would six milk chocolate bars cost?

   A. £7.24
   B. £8.86
   C. £9.71
   D. £10.90
   E. £13.56

Answer: Milk chocolate contains 563.72 kcal per 100 g. If one milk chocolate bar contains 320 kcal, then it must weigh $320 \div 563.72 \times 100 = 56.77$ g. The cost of milk chocolate is £2.85 per 100 g; six milk chocolate bars would cost $(56.77 \times 6 \div 100) \times 2.85 = £9.71$. Answer **(C)** is correct.

6. The total caloric value of a food is calculated by adding the calorie values for protein, carbohydrate and fat. What is the caloric value of 3.2 g of protein in kJ?

   A. 16.72 kJ
   B. 53.50 kJ
   C. 73.44 kJ
   D. 99.71 kJ
   E. 118.65 kJ

Answer: This question may be initially confusing because it does not tell you whether to use dark, milk or white chocolate. However, note that it is not actually about chocolate, but the caloric value of protein. This figure should be the same regardless of the type of chocolate—or, indeed, if you could calculate for protein in any food—since it is a question about protein, not chocolate. Choose any chocolate and use its data for this question. If you choose dark chocolate, there is a total of 598.43 kcal in 100 g of chocolate. The information under the table states that carbohydrates have 4 kcal per gram and fat has 9 kcal per gram. Thus to calculate the total calories from protein we subtract the calories from carbohydrates and fat: $598.43 - (45.9 \times 4) - (42.63 \times 9) = 31.16$ kcal. Next, calculate the number of calories per gram of protein: $31.16 \div 7.79 = 4$ kcal per gram. Calculate for 3.2 grams: $4 \times 3.2 = 12.8$; convert to kJ: $12.4 \times 4.18 = 53.50$ kJ. The correct answer is **(B)**.

7. Dark chocolate can be melted in cream to make a chocolate sauce. If 300 ml of chocolate sauce contains 60 g of dark chocolate and 815 kcal, how many calories are there per litre of cream?

   A. 996.29 kcal
   B. 1053.6 kcal
   C. 1196.9 kcal
   D. 1381.0 kcal
   E. 1519.8 kcal

Answer: First, find the number of calories in 60 g of dark chocolate: $0.6 \times 598.43 = 359.06$ kcal. There are 815 kcal in 300 ml of chocolate sauce; subtracting the calories from dark chocolate yields $815 - 359.06 = 455.94$ kcal in 300 ml of cream. Finally, calculate how many calories in 1 litre of cream: $455.94 \times 10 \div 3 = 1519.8$ kcal. The answer is **(E)**.

8. The chocolate shop introduces a new product: brownies made with 28% white chocolate, 43% milk chocolate and 29% dark chocolate. For one batch of 12 brownies, a total of 235 g of chocolate is used. What weight of dark chocolate is needed for 42 brownies?

   A. 238.53 g
   B. 267.15 g
   C. 290.08 g
   D. 313.22 g
   E. 568.45 g

Answer: Whilst there is a lot of new information in this question, note that the target is the weight of dark chocolate required for 42 brownies. Thus, you need only work with dark chocolate. First, calculate how much dark chocolate is needed to make one batch of 12 brownies, using the proportions of different chocolate types in the recipe: $235 \times 0.29 = 68.15$ g. Next calculate how many batches of brownies are needed for 42 brownies: $42 \div 12 = 3.5$ batches. Finally calculate how much dark chocolate is needed for 3.5 batches of brownies: $3.5 \times 68.16 = 238.53$ g. Answer **(A)** is correct.

Difficult Data

Some sets in the Quantitative Reasoning section may involve difficult data. Data may be difficult to work with because it is given in unusual or confusing formats, or because the data contains lots of bullet points and textual information. Difficult data is anything that is likely to make you spend more time than you should on the questions involved, or anything that looks a bit scary. When faced with difficult data, don't lose your nerve—continue working at the usual pace. If you take more time on questions with difficult data, or if you 'bottle' it, you have fallen for the difficult data trap.

If you start a new set and encounter data in a format you have never seen before, take a moment to catch your breath and see if you can get a quick handle on the format. If you struggle to understand how to read the data, **STOP**. Do not waste time on the set at this point in the section. Flag all the questions for review, and come back to the set on a second pass through the section. Such sets are relatively uncommon, but if you come back to them a second time, you will often find that your eyes take a different approach and unpack the data more easily. Such sets are designed to scare you, or make you freeze—wasting valuable time and missing out the marks in the sets with simpler data later in the section. Don't fall for this Quantitative trap!

To demonstrate these tips, work through the following four questions, which relate to the graph below. Try to answer each question in 30 seconds before reading the answer.

An architect records all the time she spends working, according to five main tasks, over the course of a week. The architect uses the data to make the circle graph shown below.

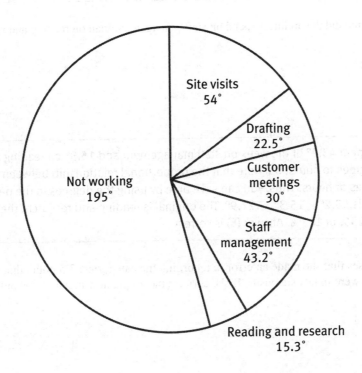

9. How much of the time when the architect was not working was she also not sleeping, if she slept for a total of 52.5 hours during the week?

    A. 36.1%
    B. 38.5%
    C. 40.9%
    D. 42.3%
    E. 44.7%

Answer: There are $24 \times 7 = 168$ hours in a week. The architect was not working for 195° out of 360° in the week, which is equivalent to $195° \div 360° = 0.5417$, or 54.17% of the week; that means the architect was not working for $0.5417 \times 168 = 91$ hours. If she slept for 52.5 hours, then there were $91 - 52.5 = 38.5$ hours in which she was not working and not sleeping. The architect therefore was not sleeping and not working for $38.5 \div 91 = 0.423$, or 42.3% of the time when she was not working. The correct answer is **(D)**. Note the two reasons this question was more challenging. First, we are not told the total number of hours in a week, though this is relatively straightforward to calculate. Second, all the data is given in degrees, out of a total of 360°, but this is not explained. You have to infer how the circle graph works, then divide by 360° to convert the data.

---

10. Drafting accounted for how much of the architect's time during the week?

    A. 7 hours
    B. 10.5 hours
    C. 12.5 hours
    D. 14 hours
    E. 22.5 hours

Answer: Drafting equals 22.5° of the 360° in the circle graph, which is 22.5° ÷ 360° = 0.0625, or 6.25%, of the graph. We know from the previous question that there are 168 hours in a week, so the architect spent 0.0625 × 168 = 10.5 hours drafting. The answer is **(B)**. Note that if this question came first in the set, it might have helped you figure out how the circle graph works a bit more quickly, since this question is much simpler than the first question in the set. If you struggle to understand the data on the first question in a set, you might try skipping it and going straight to the second question. It's quite common for relatively simpler questions to come later in a set, which will lead many test-takers to waste time on the initial, tougher question.

11. How much more time did the architect spend on staff management than on reading and research?
    - A. 92%
    - B. 117%
    - C. 142%
    - D. 167%
    - E. 182%

Answer: The architect spent 43.2° of the week on staff management and 15.3° on reading and research. You could convert these degrees to hours, but note that the proportional relationship between the two will be the same, whether in degrees or hours. Thus, you can save time by using the degrees in the percentage change formula. The difference is 43.2° − 15.3° = 27.9°. The original is reading and research; the percentage change is 27.9° ÷ 15.3° = 1.8235, or 182%. Answer **(E)** is correct.

12. The architect realises that she made an error in recording the categories: 3.5 hours that were recorded as customer meetings were in fact site visits. If she corrects the graph, how much of it should be site visits?
    - A. 46°
    - B. 57.5°
    - C. 61.5°
    - D. 64°
    - E. 67.5°

Answer: Site visits make up 54° in the original graph, so the answer must be greater than 54°; eliminate **(A)**. If, the architect spent 3.5 of the customer meeting hours on site visits, then we need to move the 3.5 hours from customer meetings to site visits and work out the new degrees for site visits. However, there is a shortcut— simply work out the degree equivalent of 3.5 hours, and add this amount to the degrees for site visits. 3.5 hours ÷ 168 hours = 0.020833, or 2.0833% of the week. Multiply by 360°: 0.020833 × 360° = 7.5°. Add this to the original degrees for site visits: 54° + 7.5° = 61.5°. The correct answer is **(C)**. Note that wrong answer trap **(B)** simply adds 3.5° to 54°, instead of converting 3.5 hours to degrees.

As these questions demonstrate, you must be prepared to check the data for each question, and to avoid common traps that are waiting for those who misread the data. You'll also need to improve your speed and accuracy with questions involving percentages—including percentage change—as these are incredibly common on the UKCAT. At Kaplan, we are sometimes surprised to find how many applicants to medical programmes are unable to work quickly and accurately with questions involving percentages—perhaps the skills involved are so basic they have been long forgotten, so they are worth practising in the run-up to Test Day.

Kaplan Timed Practice Set—*Tables and Difficult Data*

Set your timer for 2 minutes. Pace yourself, to ensure that you mark answers for all 4 questions.

The table includes information on waiting times across different departments at three hospitals in England, along with the national data, for a single year.

	A&E attendances				A&E attendances > 4 hours from arrival to admission, transfer or discharge		
	Type 1 Departments - Major A&E	Type 2 Departments - Single Specialty	Type 3 Departments - Other A&E/ Minor Injury Unit	Total attendances	Total Attendances > 4 hours	Percentage in 4 hours or less (Type 1)	Percentage in 4 hours or less (all)
England	1,265,406	47,250	614,634	1,927,290	199,075	84.6%	89.7%
Hospital A	11,362	2,113	2,256	15,731	3,373	70.8%	78.6%
Hospital B	16,887	1,581	5,103	23,571	3,515	80.2%	85.1%
Hospital C	10,973	0	0	10,973	1,323	87.9%	87.9%

13. What proportion of total attendances lasting more than 4 hours in England were at Hospital A?

    A. 1.17%
    B. 1.53%
    C. 1.69%
    D. 1.84%
    E. 1.95%

14. How many patients were seen in 4 hours or less at Hospital B?

    A. 18,903
    B. 19,445
    C. 19,987
    D. 20,059
    E. 20,131

15. The previous year in Hospital B, there were 21,973 total attendances. Of these, 14.2% were seen in more than 4 hours. What is the percentage increase in total attendances greater than 4 hours?

    A. 11.8%
    B. 12.7%
    C. 13.2%
    D. 13.9%
    E. 14.3%

16. How many patients admitted to type 1 departments were seen in more than 4 hours?

    A. 194,873
    B. 198,923
    C. 202,461
    D. 207,275
    E. 211,069

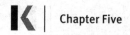

Kaplan Timed Practice Set—*Tables and Difficult Data* Answers and Explanations

This set includes an especially elaborate table, with column headings that might take quite a few seconds to understand. The table is also a bit unusual in that the figures for England as a whole are given in the top row, with the figures for three individual hospitals underneath. Hopefully, you were able to work with the table without too much complication or confusion. On the plus side, when you must confront such an elaborate table, you are unlikely to use very many cells from the table in answering any single question. In fact, most of the cells in the table were not needed to answer any of the questions in this set—indicating the importance of identifying what you need to solve before you go to the data.

13. (C)

First, identify the total number of attendances lasting more than 4 hours in England: 199,075. Next, find the total number of attendances lasting more than 4 hours at Hospital A: 3,373. Finally, calculate the proportion of attendances lasting more than 4 hours that took place at Hospital A: $3,373 \div 199,075 = 0.01694 = 1.69\%$. The answer is **(C)**.

14. (D)

According to the table, a total of 23,571 patients were seen in Hospital B, 85.1% of these patients were seen in less than 4 hours. Therefore, the total number of patients seen in 4 hours or less at Hospital B is: $23,571 \times 0.851 = 20,059$. Answer **(D)** is correct.

15. (B)

First calculate the total number of attendances greater than 4 hours the previous year: $21,973 \times 0.142 = 3,120$. Next, identify the total number of attendances greater than 4 hours in the current period: 3,515. Finally, calculate the percentage increase in total attendances greater than 4 hours: the difference is $3,515 - 3,120 = 395$; the percentage increase is $395 \div 3,120 = 0.1266 = 12.7\%$. The correct answer is **(B)**.

16. (A)

The total number of patients admitted to type 1 departments in England is 1,265,406. The table indicates that 84.6% of these were seen in 4 hours or less, so we know that $100\% - 84.6 = 15.4\%$ of patients were seen in more than 4 hours. Use this percentage to calculate the total number of patients admitted to type 1 departments in England in more than 4 hours: $1,265,406 \times 0.154 = 194,873$, answer **(A)**.

Remember

Many questions in the Quantitative section will involve percentages. You may have to simply find a percentage, or work backward from a percentage to find the part or the whole. The UKCAT's favourite formula is percentage change: be ready to use it several times on Test Day, and be prepared to rearrange the formula to solve for the original figure, the final figure, or the difference, as well as the percentage change.

Rates and Speed

The speed formula is the most commonly tested rate on the UKCAT. Be prepared to rearrange the formula to solve for any one of its constituent parts:

- $\text{Speed} = \dfrac{\text{Distance}}{\text{Time}}$

- $\text{Time} = \dfrac{\text{Distance}}{\text{Speed}}$

- $\text{Distance} = \text{Speed} \times \text{Time}$

Many questions involving the speed formula will introduce an extra step—and potential trap—by providing information in inconsistent units, or in units that are inconsistent with the units of the answer choices. To avoid mistakes on such questions, be sure to note the steps required to solve on your note-board. Include a conversion factor that will divide or multiply out the units that you don't need in the answer, so you are only left with the correct units. For instance, if you are given data in miles per minute $\left(\dfrac{\text{mi}}{\text{min}} \right)$, and you want an answer in miles per hour $\left(\dfrac{\text{mi}}{\text{hr}} \right)$, then multiply the original figure by $\dfrac{60\,\text{min}}{1\,\text{hr}}$, as this will eliminate the minutes and leave the hours in the denominator, where they belong. Conversion factors such as $\dfrac{60\,\text{min}}{1\,\text{hr}}$ can always be included in multiplication, so long as the amounts on the top and bottom of the fraction are equal—this is the same as multiplying by 1.

Be prepared as well for questions that may involve rates other than speed. Any two measurements could be combined into a rate, e.g. books per year, miles per gallon, pence per litre. Solving rate questions will usually involve working with fractions.

Here are four questions involving rates and speed, based on the map below. Try to answer each question in 30 seconds before moving on to the answer. Since you may answer some questions quickly, it is okay to spend a bit longer than 30 seconds on one or two that are very challenging—but try to mark an answer even for these in about a minute. Taking much longer as you practise will not help you prepare for UKCAT success.

Marco and Yasmin are going on a driving tour of Wales, with plans to visit the locations in the diagram.

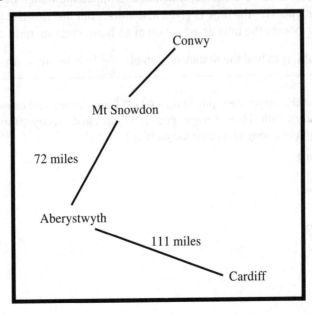

17. If they take 2.5 hours to drive from Cardiff to Aberystwyth without stopping, what is their speed?

    A. 29 mph
    B. 37 mph
    C. 44 mph
    D. 47 mph
    E. 49 mph

Answer: The unknown is speed, which equals distance divided by time. The distance from Cardiff to Aberystwyth is given in the map as 111 miles, and the time is given in the question as 2.5 hours. Thus, the speed $= 111$ mi $\div 2.5$ hr $= 44.4$ miles per hour, and the answer is **(C)**.

18. At a speed of 40 mph, what is the driving time from Aberystwyth to Mt Snowdon?

    A. 1 hour, 8 minutes
    B. 1 hour, 32 minutes
    C. 1 hour, 40 minutes
    D. 1 hour, 48 minutes
    E. 1 hour, 54 minutes

Answer: The unknown in this question is time, which equals distance divided by speed. The distance is given in the map as 72 miles, and the speed is given in the question as 40 mph. The time therefore equals 72 mi $\div 40$ mph $= 1.8$ hours. However, the answers give the time in hours and minutes, so subtract the hour and multiply by a conversion factor to find the remaining minutes: $0.8 \text{hr} \times \dfrac{60\,\text{min}}{1\,\text{hr}} = 48\,\text{min}.$ The total time for the drive from Aberystwyth to Mt Snowdon is therefore 1 hour, 48 minutes, and the answer is **(D)**.

19. How far is Conwy from Mt Snowdon, if the drive takes 52 minutes at a speed of 30 mph?

    A. 26 miles
    B. 32 miles
    C. 37 miles
    D. 44 miles
    E. 49 miles

Answer: The unknown in this question is distance, which equals speed multiplied by time. However, there is an added twist, as the units don't match—the time is given in minutes, but the speed is given in miles per hour. The quickest way to solve here is to write the time as a fraction of an hour: since an hour equals 60 minutes, write the time as $\dfrac{52}{60}$ hr. Then, multiply to find the distance: $30 \text{mph} \times \dfrac{52}{60} \text{hr} = 26 \text{miles}.$ Answer **(A)** is correct.

20. Yasmin switches on her MP3 player the moment they set off from Cardiff, and counts the songs played during their driving time to Aberystwyth. Their average speed is 37 mph, and exactly 40 songs play on the journey. What is the average length of a song played on the journey?

    A. 2.75 minutes per song
    B. 3 minutes per song
    C. 3.75 minutes per song
    D. 4 minutes per song
    E. 4.5 minutes per song

Answer: The answers are given in an unusual rate: minutes per song. Thus, start by finding the time required for the journey from Cardiff to Aberystwyth. Time equals distance divided by speed: 111 miles ÷ 37 mph = 3 hours. Since the answers are given in minutes, convert 3 hours into minutes: $3hrs \times \dfrac{60min}{1hr} = 180minutes$. Yasmin played 40 songs on the journey, so the rate of minutes per song is simply 180 minutes ÷ 40 songs = 4.5 minutes per song, answer **(E)**. While this question does involve an unusual rate, keeping an eye on the units involved—and converting at each step as required—is sufficient to get to the correct answer.

Kaplan Timed Practice Set—*Rates and Speed*

Set your timer for 2 minutes. Attempt to answer all 4 questions before time is up. If you have trouble with a question, try to eliminate any answers that seem too large or too small, based on the available data, and then make your best guess before moving on. Come back to any such troubling questions with any remaining time before the 2 minutes is up.

Doris, Mabel and Maud ride their mobility scooters from their sheltered accommodation to the shops, which are 3.5 km away. The mobility scooters normally travel at a constant speed of 10 km/hr.

21. How many minutes will it take the ladies to reach the shops?

    A. 21
    B. 24
    C. 28
    D. 33
    E. 35

22. On the way home, Mabel takes the scenic route. She arrives back at the sheltered accommodation 24 minutes after the others. How far did she travel on her journey home?

    A. 3.1 km
    B. 4.1 km
    C. 4.5 km
    D. 5.7 km
    E. 7.5 km

23. The next day, the battery on Maud's scooter is running low, and it takes her 37 minutes to reach the shops. At what speed is her mobility scooter now travelling?

    A. 4.8 km/hr
    B. 5.7 km/hr
    C. 6.3 km/hr
    D. 8.4 km/hr
    E. 9.5 km/hr

24. With a new battery, Maud's scooter can now travel at 14 km/hr. What is the percentage decrease in her journey time from the shops to the sheltered accommodation, compared to her initial journey?

    A. 15%
    B. 21%
    C. 29%
    D. 33%
    E. 35%

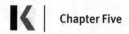

Kaplan Timed Practice Set—*Rates and Speed*: Answers and Explanations

Hopefully you were not surprised by the lack of visual data in this set. Whilst most sets in Quantitative Reasoning include at least one chart, graph or table, you are likely to see one or two sets that include no visual data. These may include brief textual information, which may provide essential, if limited, data. Sets with no visual data can generally be answered a bit more quickly than usual sets, and will tend to involve solving for a single rate or percentage. Your work from earlier questions in such sets will often prove useful and save time on later questions, so be sure to note the calculations—including any intermediate figures you came up with in finding the answers—on your noteboard.

21. (A)

This question involves straightforward use of the speed formula. The unknown in this question is time, which equals distance divided by speed: $T = D \div S$. The distance is 3.5 km and the speed is 10 km/hr, so divide: 3.5 km ÷ 10 km/hr = 0.35 hours. To convert to minutes, we multiply by 60: 0.35 × 60 = 21 minutes. The answer is therefore **(A)**.

22. (E)

The unknown in this question is distance, which equals speed multiplied by time: $D = S \times T$. Mabel's speed is 10 km/hr, and her time is 24 minutes more than the others, so add: 21 min + 24 min = 45 minutes, or 0.75 hours. Multiply to find Mabel's distance, taking the scenic route: 10 km/hr × 0.75 hours = 7.5 km. The correct answer is **(E)**.

23. (B)

In this question, the unknown is speed: $S = D \div T$. The distance is 3.5 km, and Maud's new time is 37 minutes, which equals $\frac{37}{60}$ hrs, or 0.617 hrs, if you divide out the fraction. To find Maud's new speed, divide: 3.5 km ÷ 0.617 hrs = 5.67 km/hr. The answer is therefore **(B)**.

24. (C)

This question is a little more complex, as it requires multiple steps: to find the percentage change in Maud's journey times, you must first calculate her new journey time with the new battery. Maud's original journey took 21 minutes. With the new battery, the journey time is now 3.5 km ÷ 14 km/hr = 0.25 hours, or 15 minutes. Remember, percentage change = difference ÷ original; her percentage decrease in journey time is the difference in the two times divided by the original time. The difference is 21 min − 15 min = 6 min, so the percentage change equals 6 min ÷ 21 min = 0.286, or 28.6%. This rounds up to 29%, so the correct answer is **(C)**.

Remember

A rate is a comparison of two measurements.

Examples: metres per second, miles per gallon, price per litre.

In a rate, *per* = division sign or fraction bar.

Virtually anything can be a unit of measurement in a rate on the UKCAT. Expect to see some odd units on Test Day.

Geometry

Geometry is likely to come up in at least a few questions in Quantitative Reasoning. Most geometry questions will involve common two-dimensional figures, such as circles, squares, rectangles and triangles. Be prepared to calculate the area, circumference or perimeter of such shapes; you might also be asked to find the length of a side, a diagonal, or the height of a triangle. Less commonly, you may be faced with unusual shapes—as in the set that follows. Many geometry questions will include diagrams, but others will not—look out for indications of shapes that will allow you to apply geometric rules and formulae. For example, you might notice that the text describes a rectangle, so you can use the properties of a rectangle to solve, e.g. two adjacent sides and the diagonal connecting them would form a triangle, so you could use Pythagoras' theorem to find the length of an unknown side, or of the diagonal.

If a question involves a diagram, look for any shapes that can help, keeping in mind that there may be more shapes in the diagram than are apparent at first glance. For example, a diagram of a house might include any number of rectangles, squares or triangles, depending which elements you combine into a larger shape.

When the data involves geometry, or elaborate figures that can be broken into smaller figures, sketching a quick copy of the diagram on your noteboard can be helpful—you can then add measurements and notations as you calculate. This will help to answer each question in the set, and will save time and frustration, since you are unable to write on the test paper itself.

Try working through the questions that accompany the diagram, allowing yourself 30 seconds for each question before reviewing the answer. Again, if a question is more time-consuming, you might allow yourself a bit longer, assuming that you have 'banked' time by answering quicker, earlier questions in less than 30 seconds each.

Flintborough Town Council is planning a new park. They prepare a scale model (2 m:1 km) to exhibit to the public. The model is 14 m long and 8 m wide, and is horizontally and vertically symmetrical.

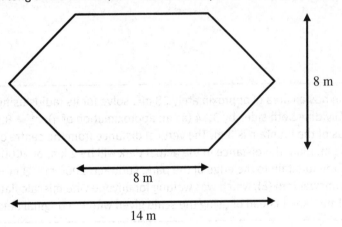

25. What is the area of the model?

    A. 64 m^2

    B. 80 m^2

    C. 88 m^2

    D. 96 m^2

    E. 102 m^2

Answer: This is a tricky area question, since the model will have to be divided into multiple smaller shapes whose area can be calculated, then added together. Thankfully, the model has horizontal and vertical symmetry, so it can be broken into several possible combinations of conventional shapes, which you can annotate after redrawing the figure on your scrap paper. Perhaps the simplest approach is to section off the centre portion into a square measuring 8 m on all sides, so this portion would have an area of 8 m × 8 m = 64 m². Since the actual area is larger, eliminate **(A)**. The remaining portions are triangles of equal area; these each have a base of 8 m and a height of 3 m, because 14 m − 8 m = 6 m, and half of this is equal to the height of each triangle. The area of a triangle is 0.5 × base × height, and since there are two equal triangles, their combined area is 2 × 0.5 × 8 m × 3 m = 24 m2. The total area is therefore 64 + 24 = 88 m²; the correct answer is therefore **(C)**.

---

26. The model is to be placed onto a rectangular board. What is the area of the board that will give a minimum border of 50 cm around the entire model?

    A. 72.25 m²
    B. 112.25 m²
    C. 123.25 m²
    D. 128 m²
    E. 135 m²

Answer: In order to ensure a border of 50 cm, or 0.5 m, around the model, a rectangular board would need to include an extra 0.5 m at each end of the model's longest vertical and horizontal measurements. Add in the extra 0.5 m: 14 + 0.5 + 0.5 = 15 m, and 8 + 0.5 + 0.5 = 9 m, so the area of the rectangular board must be 9 m × 15 m = 135 m². The answer is **(E)**.

---

27. A circular fountain, with an area of 28 m², is planned for the exact centre of the park. How far will it be from the edge of the fountain to the edge of the park, if the shortest possible distance is measured?

    A. 1961 m
    B. 1967 m
    C. 1991 m
    D. 1997 m
    E. 3997 m

Answer: Since the fountain has an area of approximately 28 m², solve for its radius using the formula for area of a circle: $\pi r^2 = 28$ m². Dividing both sides by 3.14 (as an approximation of π): $r^2 = 8.91$ m², or just a bit less than 9 m²; thus, the radius of the fountain is 3 m. The vertical distance from the centre of the model to the edge is 4 m; given the scale of 2 m:1 km, the distance in the actual park will be 2 km, or 2000 m. To solve for the distance from the edge of the fountain to the edge of the park, subtract: 2000 m − 3 m = 1997 m. The answer is therefore **(D)**. Note wrong answer trap **(E)**, which was waiting for anyone who miscalculated the distances in the actual park on a scale of 1 m:1 km, instead of using the scale given with the original data.

---

28. Once the park is built, a man runs around the perimeter at a speed of 15 km/hr. How many minutes does it take him to run around the perimeter of the park exactly once?

    A. 50 minutes
    B. 72 minutes
    C. 84 minutes
    D. 90 minutes
    E. 112 minutes

Answer: Once again, sketching out the figure on the noteboard is invaluable in breaking the model into shapes that are easier to use in calculating the perimeter of the park. If you divide the model into a central square and a triangle on each end in your work for Q. 25, you need only take one further step to find the remaining distances needed for the perimeter: divide each large triangle in half, forming two smaller triangles with a height of 3 m and a base of 4 m. Use Pythagoras's theorem to calculate the hypotenuse of this smaller triangle: $3^2 + 4^2 = h^2 = 9 + 16 = 25$. The hypotenuse is therefore 5 m.

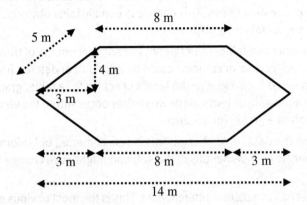

Sum up to find the total perimeter: 8 m + 8 m + 5 m + 5 m + 5 m + 5 m = 36 m. In the park, this distance equals 18 km. To solve for the runner's time, divide distance by speed: 18 km ÷ 15 km/hr = 1.2 hours. As the answers are in minutes, multiply: 1.2 hr × 60 min = 72 min, so the correct answer is **(B)**.

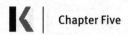

Changing Data

Quantitative Reasoning data can also be difficult because it changes from question to question. In recent years, the UKCAT has included one or two sets in each Quantitative section with changing data. In these sets, the data changes between some or all of the questions. There are a few basic ways in which the data can change:

- The first few questions have one table/chart/graph, which is replaced by a completely different table/chart/graph for the final question or two. This change is usually fairly obvious, but you need to be aware of the possibility so you are not taken by surprise.

- The first few questions have one table/chart/graph, but some elements of the data change for one or more later questions. For example: rows or columns could be added to or deleted from a table; lines or bars could be added to or deleted from a graph; the labels or scales for a table, graph or chart could change. These changes can be more subtle, particularly when they occur within the visual data, or when it's a change to the axis labels of a graph, for instance.

- The text above or below the data could change. This is less common, but information added or deleted in a later question could alter the fundamentals of the set, and might even change the approach you must take to solve for the answer.

- Each question in the set has completely different data. This is the most obvious example of changing data, and also appears to be the most common. In this case, it's not so much a set as four individual questions, each with unique data, which could be in a variety of formats and usually on completely unrelated topics. However, it is still useful to think of these as a set of 4, since they come as a group of 4 individual questions.

Our best advice is not to worry about changing data. It will be very obvious if you have 4 individual questions, each with different data, which is the most common. For example, the first question might have a table, the second might have no visual data (text only), the third might have a different table, and the fourth, only text. However, you must take care to try to keep your timing close to 30 seconds per question. It's easier to spend an extra 10–15 seconds per question when each question has different data, since you have to read any text and ensure a basic understanding of the table/chart/graph, in addition to working out what the question is asking for and doing the maths. Compare this to your work on a set with the same data for 4 questions – you may briefly orient yourself to the data before starting the first question, but normally you can rely on it being the same, so you effectively save time on the final three questions in the set. If each question has different data, then you are at risk for spending quite a bit of extra time per question, so avoid falling for this trap.

It is possible that you will see a set where only part of the data changes (second point above) or where the entire table/chart/graph changes (first point above) on a later question. If you encounter either of these cases, then you may not be able to use your work from previous questions on later questions in the set. You might also have to calculate based on different cells from the table or data points from a graph, depending what has been added or deleted.

Again, the bottom line: Try not to worry about changing data. If you notice a change, then you need only work out the relevant bits required to answer the next question. If things have changed partially but fundamentally, try not to think too much about it, beyond what you need for the next question; remember, changing data is meant to throw you off your game. Don't let it succeed!

Attack the questions that start with the data at the top of the next page, allowing yourself 30 seconds for each question before reviewing the answer. If a question is more time-consuming, you might allow yourself a bit longer, assuming that you have 'banked' time by answering quicker, easier questions in less than 30 seconds each.

During an afternoon shift, a factory manufactures several different batches of shampoo, listed in the left-hand column. Each batch of shampoo contains one or more types of colouring, and one or more types of scent.

Colourings and scents are liquid ingredients; they can be diluted by adding more water or strengthened by adding more pure colouring or scent.

The figures for colouring and scent are the percentage purity (e.g., 70% means 70% pure, with the remaining 30% made up of water) of the colouring/scent solution, followed by the amount of colouring/scent solution used per 10 litres of shampoo in the batch.

Each different type of shampoo is designated by a number; the letter that follows each number indicates the batch, in the order that batches are made each day. The first batch of each day is A; to avoid confusion, the letters I and O are omitted from the batch sequence.

Ingredients marked with a dash were not used in that shampoo/batch.

Shampoo/Batch	Blue Colouring	Yellow Colouring	Scent A307	Scent A311	Scent B401
31/L	–	70% 150 ml	18% 40 ml	–	35% 84 ml
33/J	60% 125 ml	12% 60 ml	–	55% 72 ml	–
33/M	56% 134 ml	90% 8 ml	–	42% 90 ml	–
35/K	40% 96 ml	–	85% 36 ml	–	–
35/N	32% 120 ml	–	45% 68 ml	–	–

29. What is the proportion of pure blue colouring to pure yellow colouring in 33/J?
    A. 12:125
    B. 12:25
    C. 25:24
    D. 25:12
    E. 125:12

Answer: Every 10 litres of batch 33/J contains 125 ml of blue colouring solution that is 60% pure and 60 ml of yellow colouring solution that is 12% pure. Thus, every 10 litres of 33/J contains 0.6×125 ml $= 75$ ml of pure blue colouring, and 0.12×60 ml $= 7.2$ ml of pure yellow colouring. The ratio of pure blue colouring to pure yellow colouring is 75:7.2, or 10.4167:1. From this point, there are three approaches to determine the correct answer. First, you could test the values of the answer choices with the calculator, omitting those that are clearly too small; for example, answers (A) and (B) are each less than 1. Second, you could deduce that the left-hand number in the proportion has to be a little more than 10 times the right-hand number. Finally, you could rewrite 75:7.2 as 750:72, then reduce both sides by a factor of 6, reducing the proportion to its simplest form, 125:12. Whichever approach you took, answer **(E)** is correct.

During an afternoon shift, a factory manufactures several different batches of shampoo, listed in the left-hand column. Each batch of shampoo contains one or more types of colouring, and one or more types of scent.

Colourings and scents are liquid ingredients; they can be diluted by adding more water or strengthened by adding more pure colouring or scent.

The figures for colouring and scent are the percentage purity (e.g., 70% means 70% pure, with the remaining 30% made up of water) of the colouring/scent solution, followed by the amount of colouring/scent solution used per 10 litres of shampoo in the batch.

Each different type of shampoo is designated by a number; the letter that follows each number indicates the batch, in the order that batches are made each day. The first batch of each day is A; to avoid confusion, the letters I and O are omitted from the batch sequence.

Ingredients marked with a dash were not used in that shampoo/batch.

Shampoo/Batch	Blue Colouring	Yellow Colouring	Scent A307	Scent A311	Scent B401
31/L	–	70% 150 ml	18% 40 ml	–	35% 84 ml
33/J	60% 125 ml	12% 60 ml	–	55% 72 ml	–
33/M	56% 134 ml	90% 8 ml	–	42% 90 ml	–
35/K	40% 96 ml	–	85% 36 ml	–	–
35/N	32% 120 ml	–	45% 68 ml	–	–

30. At the end of the shift, the supervisor notices that both batches of shampoo 33 were made with the wrong strength of Scent A311 solution. Instead of 55% and 42%, the strengths of the solutions used should have been 65% and 52%, respectively. What total amount of pure (100% strength) Scent A311 must be added batches J and M?

    A. 7.2 ml
    B. 11.4 ml
    C. 12.9 ml
    D. 16.2 ml
    E. 19.3 ml

Answer: Batch 33/J was made with 72 ml of 55% pure Scent A311 solution, which contains 0.55×72 ml = 39.6 ml of pure Scent A311. However, this batch should have been made with 72 ml of 65% pure Scent A311 solution, or 0.65×72 ml = 46.8 ml of pure Scent A311. Thus, $46.8 - 39.6 = 7.2$ ml of pure Scent A311 must be added to batch 33/J.

Batch 33/M was made with 90 ml of 42% pure Scent A311 solution, which contains 0.42×90 ml = 37.8 ml of pure Scent A311. However, this batch should have been made with 90 ml of 52% pure Scent A311 solution, or 0.52×90 ml = 46.8 ml of pure Scent A311. Thus, $46.8 - 37.8 = 9$ ml of pure Scent A311 solution must be added to batch 33/M.

Therefore, the total amount of pure Scent A311 that must be added to batches J and M is $7.2 + 9 = 16.2$ ml, answer **(D)**.

During an afternoon shift, a factory manufactures several different batches of shampoo, listed in the left-hand column. Each batch of shampoo contains one or more types of colouring, and one or more types of scent.

Colourings and scents are liquid ingredients; they can be diluted by adding more water or strengthened by adding more pure colouring or scent.

The figures for colouring and scent are the percentage purity (e.g., 70% means 70% pure, with the remaining 30% made up of water) of the colouring/scent solution, followed by the amount of colouring/scent solution used per 10 litres of shampoo in the batch.

Each different type of shampoo is designated by a number; the letter that follows each number indicates the batch, in the order that batches are made each day. The first batch of each day is A; to avoid confusion, the letters I and O are omitted from the batch sequence.

Ingredients marked with a dash were not used in that shampoo/batch.

Shampoo/Batch	Blue Colouring	Yellow Colouring	Scent A307	Scent A311	Scent B401
31/L	–	70% 150 ml	18% 40 ml	–	35% 84 ml
33/M	56% 134 ml	90% 8 ml	–	42% 90 ml	–
35/K	40% 96 ml	–	85% 36 ml	–	–
35/N	32% 120 ml	–	45% 68 ml	–	–
37/J	63% 81 ml	30% 91 ml	–	–	68% 70 ml

31. If 1250 litres of shampoo were made in each batch, how many litres of pure blue colouring were used?
    A. 20.56 L
    B. 25.36 L
    C. 28.36 L
    D. 30.56 L
    E. 59.66 L

Answer: The data from the previous two questions has changed. Take a few seconds to scan and see what's different. The most important thing is to confirm that the information above the table is identical; a quick scan reveals that it is. Note that in this case, the meaning of the percentages and volumes in the table is defined in this earlier text; if the text above the table had changed, then the percentage or the volumes (or both) could have meant something entirely different. Since it hasn't, you can proceed with the next question. This question asks for the total amount of pure blue colouring used, in litres, if 1250 litres of shampoo were made in each batch. The data in the table gives the amount of blue colouring solution used per 10 litres of shampoo, so you must work out the amount of pure blue colouring per 10 litres in each batch, then add these and multiply the total by 125 (1250 ÷ 10):

$$33/M: 0.56 \times 134 \text{ ml} = 75.04 \text{ ml}$$
$$35/K: 0.4 \times 96 \text{ ml} = 38.4 \text{ ml}$$
$$35/N: 0.32 \times 120 \text{ ml} = 38.4 \text{ ml}$$
$$37/J: 0.63 \times 81 \text{ ml} = 51.03 \text{ ml}$$

Total pure blue colouring in 10 L of each batch = 75.04 ml + 38.4 ml + 38.4 ml + 51.03 ml = 202.87 ml
Total pure blue colouring in 1250 L of each batch = 202.87 ml × 125 = 25,358.75 ml
Note that the answers are given in litres, so divide by 1000: 25,358.75 ml ÷ 1000 = 25.36 L. Answer **(B)** is correct.

During an afternoon shift, a factory manufactures several different batches of shampoo, listed in the left-hand column. Each batch of shampoo contains one or more types of colouring, and one or more types of scent.

Colourings and scents are liquid ingredients; they can be diluted by adding more water or strengthened by adding more pure colouring or scent.

The figures for colouring and scent are the percentage purity (e.g., 70% means 70% pure, with the remaining 30% made up of water) of the colouring/scent solution, followed by the amount of colouring/scent solution used per 10 litres of shampoo in the batch.

Each different type of shampoo is designated by a number; the letter that follows each number indicates the batch, in the order that batches are made each day. The first batch of each day is A; to avoid confusion, the letters I and O are omitted from the batch sequence.

Ingredients marked with a dash were not used in that shampoo/batch.

Shampoo/Batch	Blue Colouring	Yellow Colouring	Scent A307	Scent A311	Scent B401
31/L	–	70% 150 ml	18% 40 ml	–	35% 84 ml
33/M	56% 134 ml	90% 8 ml	–	42% 90 ml	–
35/K	40% 96 ml	–	85% 36 ml	–	–
35/N	32% 120 ml	–	45% 68 ml	–	–
37/J	63% 81 ml	30% 91 ml	–	–	68% 70 ml

32. The first batch of shampoo made by the evening shift, batch P, is not labelled properly. If batch P was made with 65 ml of yellow colouring solution (42% pure) per 10 litres of shampoo, then it is most consistent with which of the other shampoo batches?

    A. 31/L
    B. 33/M
    C. 35/K
    D. 35/N
    E. 37/J

Answer: Only three of the five batches in the table contain yellow colouring; 35/K and 35/N do not, so eliminate them straightaway.

Batch P was made with 65 ml of 42% pure yellow colouring solution per 10 litres of shampoo. Thus, there was 0.42 × 65 ml = 27.3 ml of pure yellow colouring in every 10 litres of batch P. Check the amounts of pure yellow colouring in the three remaining answer choices:

    31/L: 0.7 × 150 ml = 105 ml
    33/M: 0.9 × 8 ml = 7.2 ml
    37/J: 0.3 × 91 ml = 27.3 ml

Batch P contains an identical amount of pure yellow colouring to batch 37/J, so those two batches are the most consistent. The correct answer is **(E)**.

Kaplan Timed Practice Set—*Geometry and Changing Data*

Remember, it's only 2 minutes to complete this set. Pace yourself, so you can finish all 4 questions before time is up.

The shark tank at an aquarium has a viewing window with a height of 5 m and a length of 20 m. The tank extends backwards by 3 m. The tank is filed to 50 cm below the brim with water, and there is nothing covering its top.

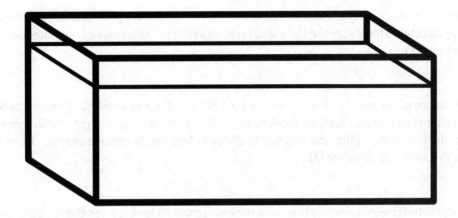

33. What is the volume of water in the tank?
    A. 243 m^3
    B. 250 m^3
    C. 270 m^3
    D. 293 m^3
    E. 300 m^3

34. On a very hot day, 6 m^3 of water evaporates from the tank. What is the percentage change in the depth of the water?
    A. 2%
    B. 4%
    C. 5%
    D. 6%
    E. 9%

35. The shark is 2 m long. It starts with its tail touching one end of the tank and swims at a constant speed of 200 cm per second until its head touches the far side of the tank. How long does it take to traverse the tank?
    A. 5.4 seconds
    B. 7.2 seconds
    C. 8.4 seconds
    D. 9 seconds
    E. 10 seconds

36. The aquarium owners wish to make the glass algae-proof. They must coat the inside and outside of the tank with mould-proofer, which costs £17 per pot. Each pot covers 25 m^2 of glass. How much will it cost to algae-proof the inside of the tank in its entirety?
    A. £187
    B. £204
    C. £221
    D. £272
    E. £289

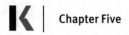

Kaplan Timed Practice Set—*Geometry and Changing Data*: Answers and Explanations

These questions were certainly more challenging than those earlier in this chapter. Even on a set with geometry and changing data, you can expect to find at least one or two questions that can be answered fairly quickly. So don't despair if you found it difficult to finish—it's meant to be!

33. (C)

Volume of water in the tank = length × width × height = 20 m × 3 m × 4.5 m = 270 m³, and the answer is **(C)**. If you mistakenly calculated the volume of the entire tank, rather than the volume of the water, you would have fallen for answer trap **(E)**.

34. (A)

The area of the surface of the tank is 20 m × 3 m = 60 m². If the volume of water has dropped by 6 m³, then the depth of water that evaporated must be 6 m³/60 m² = 0.1 m. Percentage change = difference ÷ original, and the original depth of water in the tank was 4.5 m; divide to find the percentage change: 0.1 m ÷ 4.5 m = 0.0222, or 2%. The answer is therefore **(A)**.

35. (D)

The unknown here is the time required for the shark to swim across its tank, so use the speed formula to solve: Time = Distance ÷ Speed. The shark's speed is given as 200 cm/sec, which equals 2 m/sec. Since the shark is 2 m long and starts with its tail touching one wall of the tank, the shark does not swim the total distance of 20 m, but rather swims 20 m − 2 m = 18 m. To solve, plug these figures into the speed formula: Time = 18 m ÷ 2 m/sec = 9 sec. The correct answer is **(D)**.

36. (B)

Drawing a quick sketch of the plan of the tank would help to ensure that you don't miss out each segment of glass that must be algae-proofed:

```
              ┌─────────────────────────────┐
              │        Back 20 × 5          │
    ┌─────────┼─────────────────────────────┼─────────┐
    │ Side    │                             │ Side    │
    │ 3 × 5   │      Bottom 20 × 3          │ 3 × 5   │
    └─────────┼─────────────────────────────┼─────────┘
              │        Back 20 × 5          │
              └─────────────────────────────┘
```

The total area to be covered is the bottom, plus two sides, plus the front and back, which are also equal. The total area of these is (20 × 3) + 2(20 × 5) + 2(3 × 5) = 60 + 200 + 30 = 290 m². Divide to find the number of pots required: 290 m² ÷ 25 m² per pot = 11.6. This means that 12 pots of mould-proofer are needed, giving a total cost of 12 × £17 = £204, answer **(B)**.

Score Higher Online

As you practise online, keep an eye out for geometry questions without diagrams.

If you are given dimensions that describe a standard shape—such as a square, circle, rectangle or cube—be prepared to use the appropriate geometry formula.

You may also find it helpful to sketch the shape on your noteboard.

Keeping Perspective—Quantitative Reasoning

Well done! You have now looked at the examples of the common types of data, questions and challenges that are found in the Quantitative Reasoning section, and practised the strategies necessary to work through all of these systematically and efficiently. You are about to tackle a Quantitative Reasoning quiz, completing five sets under timed conditions. By eyeballing, estimating and minimising the maths wherever possible, you should have enough time to attempt—and to mark an answer for—every question in the Kaplan UKCAT quiz.

Remember to be aware of questions that seem overly complicated or that you are struggling to complete, and get used to guessing an answer, marking for review, and moving on—just as you will do on Test Day—to ensure you submit answers for as many questions as possible.

Students who are less familiar with the test format may find themselves bogged down on an especially difficult or time-consuming question, missing the opportunity to answer questions later in the section that may have earned them more marks and a higher overall score.

Before beginning the Kaplan UKCAT quiz, take a few moments to review some of Kaplan's tips that will help you maximise your performance on the quiz—and also on Test Day:

Not every question requires complex calculations. Several questions in any given Quantitative section can be answered by simply reading data, by eyeballing or estimating, or by making a straightforward calculation involving just one or two steps.

Three-part formulae pop up again and again. Confidence in setting up and solving three-part formulae is essential to success in this section. The most common formulae are speed, mean and percentage change—which may be used alone or in combination.

Use the noteboard. Making notes on the noteboard can help to maintain accuracy when setting up calculations and solving, and will also help on questions involving figures, where a rough sketch onto which you can fill in measurements, etc., as they are calculated will save time and reduce the chance of making simple mistakes. Use scrap paper as you continue to practise to simulate the noteboard, rather than writing directly on the questions themselves—you won't be able to do so on Test Day.

Take care with related concepts. As some of these examples have shown, it is easy to get caught up in questions and to not notice simple shifts in focus such as percentages vs real numbers, generalising specific cases to larger populations, etc. It is important to maintain awareness of this whilst powering through the section.

Eliminate. Elimination of wrong answers—those that are too small/large, those that are in the wrong units, those that are odd when the answer must be even, etc.—will help to minimise maths and find the fastest route to the correct answer.

Check your Kaplan Online Centre and the UKCAT website for details of any test changes in the year you sit the exam. The Quantitative section has not undergone any significant changes in a number of years, but that does not mean that there won't be test changes in the year you sit the UKCAT. Be sure to check for these ahead of time, to minimise the risk of any rude surprises on Test Day.

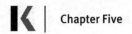

Chapter 5 Kaplan UKCAT Quiz

Set your timer for 13 minutes. Try to evaluate all 20 statements and questions, and mark an answer for each before time is up. If a statement is difficult, try to eliminate one answer and then make your best guess, so you can keep to 2 minutes per set.

The fare structures of five taxi companies are indicated in the table.

Taxi Company	Base Price	Price per mile	Price per min	Luggage
1	£3.50	£1.55	£0.20	–
2	£5.00	£1.99	–	£3 per bag
3	–	£2.50	£0.48	–
4	£2.00	£1.75	£0.35	£5 per bag
5	–	–	£1.14	£4

37. How much more does it cost to travel 4.7 miles in 35 minutes, 54 seconds with Taxi Company 4 compared to Taxi Company 3?

   A. £4.89
   B. £5.09
   C. £5.78
   D. £6.19
   E. £6.76

38. Taxi Company 2 buys a new luxury vehicle for its fleet. The base price of a journey needs to be increased so that a 15-mile journey costs 10% more. What is the new base price?

   A. £7.49
   B. £8.10
   C. £8.49
   D. £8.89
   E. £9.19

39. After getting a puncture, a car from Taxi Company 5 is stopped for 32 minutes while the tyre is changed. If the total cost of the journey is £67.55 and the driver agrees to reimburse the waiting time, what proportion of the total price is reimbursed?

   A. 49.9%
   B. 54.0%
   C. 57.1%
   D. 60.4%
   E. 65.7%

40. Cars from Taxi Company 2 and Taxi Company 5 both depart simultaneously traveling at a constant 25 miles per hour without any luggage. How long would it take for the prices of both journeys to be identical, in minutes and seconds?

   A. 8 minutes, 43 seconds
   B. 9 minutes, 12 seconds
   C. 11 minutes, 51 seconds
   D. 14 minutes, 22 seconds
   E. 16 minutes, 8 seconds

Mrs Tiwari runs a clothes shop. She buys the dresses as she needs more stock, paying £130 for batches of ten dresses, and sells each dress for £25.

41. If Mrs Tiwari sells 17 dresses, what profit has she made per dress?

   A. £7.96
   B. £8.75
   C. £9.18
   D. £9.71
   E. £9.98

42. In a summer sale, Mrs Tiwari advertises a 15% discount on all items. What is the percentage change in profit on a sale dress compared to a non-sale dress, assuming all dresses in stock are sold?

   A. 15%
   B. 22%
   C. 24%
   D. 27%
   E. 31%

43. Mrs Tiwari exports 40 dresses to a shop in Belgium at full price. She must pay a customs tax of 12% on the first £500 paid to her, and 8% of any further money she receives on the sale of the dresses. What is the total profit that she makes on these dresses?

   A. £380
   B. £420
   C. £445
   D. £475
   E. £520

44. The Belgian shop sells each dress for 32 euros. The exchange rate is £1:1.12 euro. What is the difference in price for a dress between the Belgian shop and Mrs Tiwari's shop during the sale?

   A. £6.86
   B. £7.32
   C. £8.04
   D. £8.20
   E. £9.12

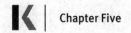

Paul's Paints are running a deal on white, blue and red paint. Blue paint costs £6.20 per litre, red paint £5.51 per litre and white paint £2.11 per litre. They will mix the paints in equal parts (1:1 mixture) to create new colours, as shown. Each mixture costs £3 extra for the time taken, plus £1.59 to clean the machine.

	Blue	Red	White
Blue	Blue	Purple	Pale Blue
Red	Purple	Red	Pink
White	Pale Blue	Pink	White

To improve sales, Paul offers to further mix 2 parts of each colour created with 1 part of either blue, red or white paint to make seven new colours. The extra charges for time and cleaning remain the same as for the simple mixtures.

	Pale Blue	Pink	Purple
Blue	Cornflower	Mauve	Indigo
Red	Mauve	Rose	Violet
White	Sky	Blush	Mauve

45.   Niamh wishes to buy 5 litres of pink paint. How much will it cost her?

   A.   £19.05
   B.   £21.05
   C.   £23.64
   D.   £27.45
   E.   £38.10

46.   Yosuke purchases 3 litres of cornflower paint. What is the total cost?

   A.   £6.31
   B.   £7.32
   C.   £8.04
   D.   £14.51
   E.   £19.10

47.   A litre of paint will cover 1.5 m². Magali's bedroom is 3 m × 5 m, and the ceiling is 2.5 m high. She wishes to paint the walls in mauve and the ceiling in white. How many litres of paint does she require?

   A.   26 L
   B.   27 L
   C.   36 L
   D.   37 L
   E.   42 L

48.   Chris is very bored in the shop one day, and decides to experiment. He mixes 6 litres of indigo paint with twice as much mauve paint, and then adds 3 litres each of rose, blush and sky coloured paint. How much would 1 litre of the resulting colour cost, excluding time and cleaning costs?

   A.   £3.64
   B.   £4.61
   C.   £6.92
   D.   £13.64
   E.   £14.92

Twice each year – in April and October – staff at the zoo complete a census of all the animals that they are responsible for.

Results of the census from the last two counts at the Reptile House are shown below.

	October	April
Alligators	6	7
Lizards	202	183
Snakes	198	223
Tortoises	94	89
Turtles	64	39

49. How many more lizards and turtles were there in October than in April?

    A. 8.1%
    B. 8.8%
    C. 16.5%
    D. 19.8%
    E. 44.0%

According to a study by the World Health Organization, 7 million people worldwide were killed by air pollution in 2012; 40% of these people lived in the Western Pacific region, which includes China.

In 2012, air pollution was attributed to a higher number of deaths per capita in China – 172 deaths per 100,000 people – than in any other country.

Population of China (2012): 1.351 billion

50. How many people in countries in the Western Pacific region (excluding China) were killed by air pollution in 2012?

    A. 476,280
    B. 785,465
    C. 2,014,535
    D. 2,323,720
    E. 2,800,000

The densities of some common liquids at certain temperatures are given below.

Substance	Temperature (°C)	Density (kg/m^3)
Glycerine	25	1259
Sea water	25	1025
Turpentine	25	868.2
Water (pure)	4	1000

51. How much greater is the density of glycerine than the density of turpentine, in g/cm3, assuming equal volumes of both liquids are at a constant temperature of 25°C?

   A. 0.003908
   B. 0.3908
   C. 3.908
   D. 390.8
   E. 390,800

In any leap year, an extra day (29th February) is added at the end of February. Thus, a leap year has 366 days, whilst a normal year has 365 days.

Any year divisible by 4 is a leap year, except those that are divisible by 100 but not 400. For example, 1600 was a leap year, but 1700 and 1800 were not. Years divisible by 100 are known as century years.

William Shakespeare was born in April 1564 (exact date unknown) and died 23rd April 1616. The 400th anniversary of Shakespeare's death was celebrated on 23rd April 2016.

52. Exactly how many days passed from Shakespeare's death to the 400th anniversary (counting from the day after he died, up through and including the day of the 400th anniversary)?

   A. 146,000
   B. 146,096
   C. 146,097
   D. 146,099
   E. 146,100

The following graph shows the number of pupils, divided by sex, in each class for AS-level subjects at a sixth-form college.

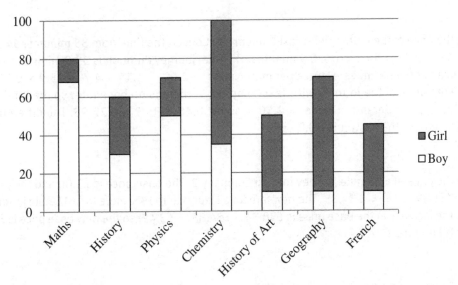

53. How many more boys study Chemistry than girls study Maths?

 A. 23
 B. 25
 C. 30
 D. 35
 E. 37

54. What percentage of History of Art students are girls?

 A. 50%
 B. 60%
 C. 70%
 D. 80%
 E. 90%

55. Half of all Economics students are boys, and there are 10 more girls studying Economics than French. What is the total number of Economics students?

 A. 45
 B. 70
 C. 90
 D. 110
 E. 115

56. Half of the girls studying Chemistry also study Biology, and one-third of the girls studying Geography also study Biology; there are 10 more girls who study Biology, who do not also study Chemistry or Geography. How many boys study Biology, if there are two-thirds as many boys as girls studying Biology?

 A. 29
 B. 35
 C. 42
 D. 63
 E. 95

STOP. IF YOU FINISH BEFORE TIME IS UP, CHECK ANY QUESTIONS YOU HAVE MARKED FOR REVIEW. YOU MAY GO BACK TO QUESTIONS IN THIS QUIZ ONLY.

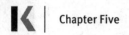

Chapter 5 Kaplan UKCAT Quiz: Answers and Explanations

37. (D)

First, calculate the price of the journey with Taxi Company 4. Convert the time from 35 minutes, 54 seconds to just minutes: 54 seconds = 54 ÷ 60 = 0.9 minutes. The total journey duration is 35.9 minutes. The total cost is base rate + price per mile × miles + price per min × mins = 2.00 + 1.75 × 4.7 + 35.9 × 0.35 = £22.79. Next, calculate the price of the journey with Taxi Company 3: there is no base rate, so the total cost is price per mile × miles + price per min × mins = 2.50 × 4.7 + 0.48 × 35.9 = £28.98. The difference in price is 28.98 – 22.79 = £6.19. The answer is **(D)**.

38. (C)

First, calculate the price of a 15-mile journey for Taxi Company 2. The base price is £5.00 and the price per mile is £1.99: £5 + (£1.99 × 15) = £34.85. The new fare for a luxury car is 10% more for a 15-mile journey: £34.85 × 1.1 = £38.34. The increase in the base price is £38.34 – £34.85 = £3.49, so the new base price is £3.49 + £5 = £8.49. Answer **(C)** is correct.

39. (B)

Taxi Company 5 charges £1.14 per minute; while it is stopped for 32 minutes, the cost incurred is: 32 × £1.14 = £36.48. The total cost of the journey is £67.55, meaning that £36.48 ÷ £67.55 = 54.0% of the total price is reimbursed. The correct answer is **(B)**.

40. (E)

In order to answer this question, calculate the price per minute for both taxis. First, convert the speed to miles per minute: 25 miles per hour = 25 ÷ 60 = 0.416 miles per minute. The car from Taxi Company 2 costs £1.99 per mile, plus the £5.00 base rate; the price per minute is £1.99 × 0.416 = £0.83 per minute, plus the £5.00 base rate. The car from Taxi Company 5 charges £1.14 per minute, without a base rate. If x is the unknown number of minutes, then we must solve the equation: 5.00 + 0.83x = 1.14x; 0.31x = 5.00 and x = 16.13 minutes. 16.13 minutes = 16 minutes + 0.13 × 60 seconds = 16 minutes, 8 seconds. The correct answer is **(E)**.

41. (D)

Mrs Tiwari must have bought two batches of dresses in order to have sold 17, so she has paid 2 × £130 = £260. She earned 17 × £25 = £425 from the sale of the 17 dresses. £425 – £260 = £165 profit. Divide to find the profit per dress sold: £165 ÷ 17 = £9.71. The answer is **(D)**.

42. (E)

The tempting answer trap here is 15%, as that is the discount mentioned in the question. However, only the sale price of the dress has changed; the cost price has not, so Mrs Tiwari's profit will have changed by more than 15%. To solve, use the percentage change formula, which first requires you to find the original profit per dress, and the difference in profit per dress during the summer sale. If all stock is sold, then the cost of a dress is £130 ÷ 10 = £13, and the profit (at the original price) is £25 – £13 = £12. During the summer sale, a customer would pay 0.85 × £25 = £21.25 per dress, leaving a profit of £21.25 – £13 = £8.25. Subtract to find the difference in profit during the summer sale: £12 – £8.25 = £3.75. Divide to find the percentage change: £3.75 ÷ £12 = 0.3125, or 31%. The correct answer is **(E)**.

43. (A)

40 dresses sold at full price means that Mrs Tiwari will be paid 40 × £25 = £1000. She must pay 12% of the first £500: 0.12 × 500 = 60. She must also pay 8% of the second £500: 0.08 × 500 = 40. Sum these figures to find the total due in customs tax: £60 + £40 = £100. She will also have paid 4 × £130 = £520 to buy the dresses in the first place, so her total profit is £1000 – £620 = £380. The answer is therefore **(A)**.

44. (B)

The final question asks for the difference in price between the Belgian shop and Mrs Tiwari's shop during the sale. We already calculated the sale price in the second question: £21.25; if you noted this on your noteboard, then you would not have to work it out again here. Next, calculate the Belgian sale price in pounds: 32 euros ÷ 1.12 euros/pound = £28.57. Finally, subtract for the difference: £28.57 − £21.25 = £7.32, answer **(B)**.

45. (C)

Pink paint is made from equal parts of Red and White paint. Red paint costs £5.51, and White paint £2.11, and 1 litre of each will mix to make 2 litres of Pink paint, with a cost of £5.51 + £2.11 = £7.62. Since Niamh wants 5 L of Pink paint, and 5 L = 2 L × 2.5, multiply the cost of 2 L by 2.5 to find the cost of 5 L: £7.62 × 2.5 = £19.05. Don't forget to factor in the extra £3 for time and £1.59 for cleaning costs, resulting in a total of £23.64. The answer is **(C)**.

46. (E)

According to the data, Cornflower paint is one part Blue and two parts Pale Blue (which itself is one part Blue and one part White). 3 litres of Cornflower paint is therefore made up of 1 litre of White paint and 2 litres of Blue paint. The cost of this would be £2.11 + (2 × £6.20) = £14.51. With the additional costs of time and cleaning, the total price is £19.10, so the answer is **(E)**.

47. (D)

The colours in this question are not important, as we only need to calculate the total amount of paint needed, making this question more straightforward than it might appear at first glance. A noteboard sketch of Magali's room will help find the correct answer quickly:

The total area is therefore 2(3 × 2.5) + 2(5 × 2.5) + (3 × 5) = 15 + 25 + 15 = 55 m². Divide to find the litres required: 55 m² ÷ 1.5 m²/L = 36.7 L. Magali will need 37 litres, answer **(D)**.

48. (B)

At first glance, this question looks like it will involve a great deal of calculation, and therefore it is probably best to guess an answer, mark it for review, and move on, so you can maximise the time that you have to spend on questions where you can find correct answers more quickly. If you had time to solve this question when you came back to it at the end of the Kaplan UKCAT quiz, the fastest way is to note the number of litres of each colour used in the mixture:

- Indigo: 6 L = 4 L Blue + 2 L Red
- Mauve: 12 L = 4 L Blue + 4 L Red + 4 L White
- Rose: 3 L = 2 L Red + 1 L White
- Blush: 3 L = 1 L Red + 2 L White
- Sky: 3 L = 2 L White + 1 L Blue

Sum to find the total litres of the three basic colours, and then multiply for the cost for each:

- Red = 2 L + 4 L + 2 L + 1 L = 9 L; 9 L × £5.51/L = £49.59
- Blue = 4 L + 4 L + 1 L = 9 L; 9 L × £6.20/L = £55.80
- White = 4 L + 1 L + 2 L + 2 L = 9 L; 9 L × £2.11/L = £18.99

Add these three for the total cost, then divide by 27 for the cost per litre: £49.59 + £55.80 + £18.99 = £124.38; £124.38 ÷ 27 L = £4.61 per litre. The correct answer is **(B)**.

49. (D)

There were 202 + 64 = 266 lizards and turtles in October, and 183 + 39 = 222 lizards and turtles in April, a difference of 44 lizards and turtles. However, the answers are percentages; to calculate 44 as a percentage of 222, divide: 44 ÷ 222 = 0.198, or 19.8% more lizards and turtles in October than in April. The correct answer is **(D)**. Note that wrong answer trap **(C)** mistakenly calculates 22 as a percentage of 266, the figure for October. That's the figure for percentage decrease from October to April – but that's not what's asked for here.

50. (A)

The total number of people killed by air pollution in the Western Pacific region in 2012 is 40% of 7 million, or 0.4 × 7,000,000 = 2,800,000. To solve, we must work out the number of people killed by air pollution in China, then subtract from 2,800,000. Air pollution caused 172 deaths per 100,000 people in China in 2012; think of this figure as a fraction (172/100,000), which must be multiplied by the population of China (1,351,000,000). Before multiplying, reduce 100,000 from the denominator and from the population of China: 13,510 × 172 = 2,323,720. That's the number of people in China killed by air pollution in 2012; subtract from the original figure for the number of people killed by air pollution in the other Western Pacific countries: 2,800,000 – 2,323,720 = 476,280. Answer **(A)** is correct.

51. (B)

The difference between the density of glycerine and the density of turpentine, in kg/m^3, is 1259 – 868.2 = 390.8. There are 1000 g in a kg, and a million cm^3 in 1 m^3; thus, you must multiply by 1000 and divide by a million – or, multiply by 0.001 – to convert from kg/m^3 to g/cm^3: 390.8 × 0.001 = 0.3908. Answer **(B)** is correct.

52. (C)

Four hundred years have passed, from the day after Shakespeare died to the 400th anniversary date; if these were all normal years, that would be a total of 400 × 365 = 146,000 days. However, that does not include the leap days. In any given period of 100 years, there would be a leap day every fourth year, except in the century year – 1700, 1800, etc. Thus, there would normally be 24 leap days in a period of 100 years, unless the century year is divisible by 400 – 1600, 2000, etc – in which case there would be 25 leap days. This period of 400 years includes four century years – 1700, 1800, 1900 and 2000 – so there would be three hundred-year periods with 24 leap days, and one – the one include the year 2000 – that with 25 leap days. Therefore, the total number of leap days is (24 × 3) + 25 = 72 + 25 = 97. The total number of days, then, is 146,000 + 97 = 146,097. Answer **(C)** is correct.

53. (A)

This first question is a great candidate for eyeballing. Scanning the graph shows us that girls are in grey, and boys in white. The scale on the y-axis goes up in increments of 20. Approximately 35 boys study Chemistry, and approximately 12 girls study Maths, so the answer is 35 – 12 = 23. The answer is **(A)**.

54. (D)

Another reasonably straightforward question, allowing you to bank time for the more complex questions in the Kaplan UKCAT quiz. The graph shows that a total of 50 students study History of Art, and that 40 of these are girls: $\frac{40}{50} = 0.8$, or 80%, of History of Art students are girls. The answer is therefore **(D)**.

55. (C)

The graph shows that 35 girls study French, so there must be $35 + 10 = 45$ girls studying Economics. If these 45 girls $= 50\%$ of the Economics students, then there must be 45 boys studying Economics, and the total number of Economics students is $45 \times 2 = 90$. The correct answer is **(C)**.

56. (C)

The final question in this set is a bit more complicated, so make a note of the various figures involved on your noteboard as you work. There are approximately 66 girls studying Chemistry, so there are $66 \times 0.5 = 33$ girls who study both Chemistry and Biology. There are approximately 60 girls studying Geography, so there are $60 \times 0.333 = 20$ girls who study both Geography and Biology. Adding in the 10 further girls who study Biology, but neither Chemistry nor Geography, there are a total of $33 + 20 + 10 = 63$ girls who study Biology. The number of boys studying Biology is two-thirds the number of girls, so there are $63 \times 0.667 = 42$ boys studying Biology. The answer is **(C)**.

Abstract Reasoning

LEARNING OBJECTIVES

In this section, you'll learn to:

- Explain the breakdown of the Abstract Reasoning section of the UKCAT
- Scan sets and identify patterns in Type 1 and Type 4 questions
- Vary your approach and identify progressions in Type 2 and Type 3 questions

---

The Task

Abstract Reasoning is the fourth scored subtest on the UKCAT. The Abstract section consists of 55 items, which must be answered in 13 minutes. Most Abstract items are in the same format, known as Type 1: they come in sets of 5, with a corresponding Set A and Set B. The test shapes appear one at a time, to the right of Sets A and B. You must evaluate whether the test shapes belong to Set A, Set B or Neither. As with the other subtests, there is 1 minute to read the instructions. This allows 1 minute to complete each set, and it makes the Abstract section the most time-constrained subtest on the UKCAT. Thus, it's essential to approach the Abstract questions with a time-saving strategy in mind.

You will see a small number of Abstract questions in three additional Abstract question types (Type 2, Type 3 and Type 4) on Test Day. The official practice tests include one set of Type 4 (5 questions) and another set with a mix of Type 2 and Type 3: two Type 2 questions and three Type 3 questions. This distribution of question types in an Abstract section has been consistent for a few years now, and we expect it is likely to be the same distribution you will encounter on Test Day.

As a result, you should focus your Abstract preparations on Type 1, since these items account for 9 of 11 sets in the Abstract section; note as well that Type 4—one further set on Test Day—is very similar to Type 1. It is worth practising the other two types as well, but you will get very few marks from Type 2 and Type 3 questions, and they are much harder to answer correctly within the allotted time, for reasons that will soon become clear.

Be sure to check your Kaplan Online Centre for an update as to the exact test format (and any additional Kaplan UKCAT test tips and practice questions) in the year you take the test.

The Format

Each Type 1 set is composed of a Set A and a Set B. Set A and Set B both contain six 'boxes'. In Set A, each of the boxes will share one or more attributes. This shared attribute for Set A is termed 'the pattern'. Likewise, Set B's six boxes will also have one or more shared attributes, and Set B will have its own unique pattern. Note that Set A and Set B can never have the exact same pattern. The difference may be quite subtle; nevertheless, there will always be a difference between Set A and Set B.

Each Abstract Reasoning 'test shape' is a single box containing various shapes within it. The answer choices for Type 1 questions are always the same: Set A, Set B or Neither. These answers require you to evaluate the test shapes according to the patterns in Sets A and B:

Set A: The test shape fits the pattern for Set A exactly, but not Set B.
Set B: The test shape fits the pattern for Set B exactly, but not Set A.
Neither: Three possibilities may lead to an answer of Neither:

- the test shape does not fit the pattern for either Set A or B;
- the test shape only partially fits the pattern for Set A or B; or
- the test shape fits the patterns for both Set A and Set B.

Type 1 is the only Abstract question type that has answer choices in this format. The format for the other Abstract question types will be explained later in the chapter. The skills you will develop in attacking Type 1 questions will be extremely useful in attacking the other question types—but it is easier to learn these skills by focusing on a single question type. So we'll start with the most common one.

The Challenges

The most obvious challenge in Abstract Reasoning is timing: 55 questions in 13 minutes makes this the fastest paced subsection on the UKCAT. Many test-takers will simply take too long searching for patterns, or will spend a large amount of time on one particular set, and will not finish the section.

The other major challenge in the Abstract section is finding the patterns. No test-takers will have learned any visual pattern finding techniques in school. Some test-takers may feel this is a skill they are either lucky enough to be born with or not. The truth is that visual pattern finding is a skill that can be learned and developed with an understanding of what kind of patterns to look for and with sufficient practice.

Kaplan Top Tips for Abstract Reasoning

1. Don't start with the test shape

There are several good reasons not to start with the test shape:

- *The test shape doesn't help you find the pattern.* The test shape may not have the pattern for either set, so you will waste valuable time if you try to use the test shape to find the pattern.
- *Marks come from finding patterns, not matching.* Occasionally there will be overlap between the patterns for Set A and Set B. A test shape may even look very similar to a box in one of the sets, but actually fit the pattern for the other set. If you try to simply match the test shapes to a similar-looking box in one of the sets, you will waste time and very likely lose marks.

2. Check the simplest box first

This is a fantastic approach that will dramatically improve your pattern finding skills for two reasons:

- *Distracting shapes are minimised.* Not all shapes in the boxes have to be of any relevance to the patterns. Shapes that are not part of the pattern are 'distractors'. The box containing the fewest number of items will have the fewest distractors, and thus will help you focus in on the true pattern.

- *Even the simplest box contains the pattern.* If the simplest box contains only one shape, your task becomes much more straightforward. For example, if a box contains a single shaded triangle in a corner of the box, you now have a clue that the pattern is either about triangles, a shaded shape, or arrangement in the corner. By checking the other boxes in the set for these same characteristics, you will find the pattern quickly.

3. Learn to search the pattern categories

Once you know what types of patterns are common on the UKCAT, you will spot patterns with ease. Basic patterns involve:

Types—a particular type of shape.

Features—the colour, size and number of a shape.

Arrangement—the position of shapes within the box, as well as relative to each other.

Most UKCAT patterns use one or two of these categories, while some of the most difficult patterns may involve all. Patterns for Set A and Set B will often use the same pattern category. However, the patterns do not necessarily have to be related.

4. If unsure, move on

Spending too much time on one pattern means that you will run out of time and miss easy marks at the end of the section. You should spend no more than 1 minute on each set, which normally includes 30 seconds to find both patterns, then 5 seconds to evaluate each test shape. If you haven't seen the patterns after 45 seconds, it is unlikely that you will see the patterns with more time. At this point, it is crucial to take a guess and mark these questions for review.

The best Abstract test-takers are ruthless in moving forward to finish the section. If you follow the timing guidelines precisely, you will have 2 minutes at the end of the section to return for a second look at the difficult sets you have marked for review. It is quite common for patterns to become obvious with a fresh look.

Don't feel bad if you don't see every pattern. Even Abstract experts will encounter one or two difficult patterns they can't quite figure out! Often you can get more (if not all) of the questions in a set correct based on a partial pattern—more on this later.

5. Make the most of the Abstract sets in this book

As you practise with this book, always try to find the pattern and answer the questions within the 1 minute per set guideline. After your timed practice, come back to any sets you found difficult or impossible the first time round, and see if you can get the pattern with a little more time and fresh eyes. Then check the explanations for the pattern. The explanations may also include tips on pattern finding techniques that you will find helpful on later questions.

Score Higher Online

It's essential to ensure you have the most up-to-date information about the Abstract question types, and the approximate balance of question types in the Abstract section in the year you sit the UKCAT. We expect this may be something of a developing situation, as the balance of Abstract question types has shifted on an annual basis in recent years. Be sure to check your Kaplan Online Centre and the test-maker's website, so you are not caught out by unexpected test changes on Test Day.

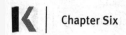
Kaplan Timed Practice Set—*Try the Kaplan Top Tips*

Set your timer for 1 minute. Write down answers for the 5 test shapes before time is up!

Set A   Set B

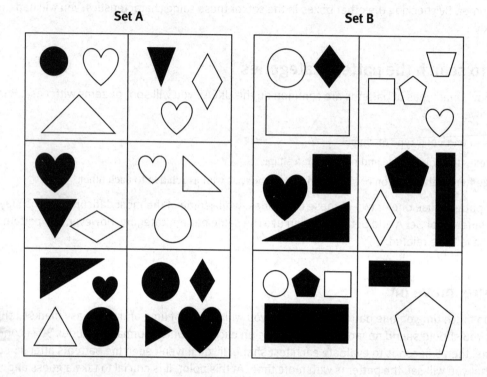

Test Shapes

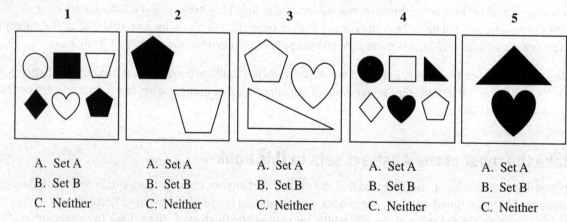

1	2	3	4	5
A. Set A	A. Set A	A. Set A	A. Set A	A. Set A
B. Set B	B. Set B	B. Set B	B. Set B	B. Set B
C. Neither	C. Neither	C. Neither	C. Neither	C. Neither

Remember

On Test Day, you will see the test shapes one at a time, to the right of Set B. In this book, we have printed all 5 test shapes for each set below Set A and Set B, to facilitate easier and speedier practising. You will have to click through the test shapes on Test Day, which will take a few seconds more.

Whether practising with this book or with a computer-based UKCAT, you might want to cover the test shapes with your hand until you find the pattern. This will help you to focus on Sets A and B, and ensure that you do not let the test shape distract you from finding the patterns.

Kaplan Timed Practice Set—*Try the Kaplan Top Tips*: Answers and Explanations

If you found the patterns—well done! If not, don't fret—you're just getting started. In either case, you will want to review the approach to this set using the Kaplan Abstract top tips.

The simplest box in either set is the lower-right box in Set B, which contains a rectangle and a pentagon. Now, check this against the pattern categories. The pattern may involve the type of shape (rectangle, pentagon or both) or a feature of the shape (it could be something like straight sides on all shapes in the box, or that the rectangle must be black and the pentagon white). Check the other boxes in Set B, and you'll find there is a rectangle in every box – remembering that squares are also rectangles—though the colour of the rectangle can be black or white; the arrangement of the rectangle varies. Notice that a pentagon does not appear in every box in Set B, so it is a distractor shape – the pentagon isn't part of the pattern. Thus, the pattern in Set B appears to be that there is a rectangle in every box; this is a simple type of shape pattern. Now, examine Set A and look for a similar pattern. Every box in Set A contains a triangle and a heart. This is the pattern for Set A.

1. (B)
The first test shape contains a square, which is a type of rectangle, so it fits the pattern for Set B. Note that the test shape also contains a heart, but no triangle; if there were both a heart and a triangle, then it would also fit the pattern for Set A. It doesn't, so the answer is **(B)**.

2. (C)
This test shape contains a pentagon and a trapezium. As a result, it lacks the shapes required for the pattern for either set. The answer is therefore **(C)**. Notice, though, that if someone who didn't find the pattern in Set B might easily have clicked **(B)** here, since the pentagon is a common distractor shape in Set B, but never appears in Set A. That's why we call them distractors—they obscure the pattern, and can lead you into a wrong answer trap.

3. (A)
This test shape includes a triangle and a heart, so it fits the pattern for Set A.

4. (C)
This test shape contains a triangle and a heart, so it belongs to Set A. However, it also contains a square, so it also belongs to Set B. Since it fits the pattern for both sets, it belongs exclusively to neither.

5. (A)
The last test shape has a triangle and a heart, so it belongs to Set A.

Don't worry if you didn't find this pattern straightaway. With more practice, you will improve with speed as you develop 'trained eyes' of your own.

There was an additional challenge in this set, in the middle left box of Set B. Notice that this box includes a square (fitting the pattern for Set B), but also a triangle and a heart. Thus, if this box had reappeared as a test shape, the answer would have been **(C)**, since it fits the pattern for both sets. However, it is perfectly fair for the UKCAT to give you a box in the original sets that fits both patterns, because that box fits the pattern in the set where it appears. This does happen on occasion, so it is worth being aware so you are not thrown off course when you see something similar in future.

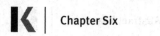

Multiple Categories

Many of the UKCAT Abstract patterns will only involve a pattern from one category. The first practice set was a classic pattern involving type of shape, and just the sort of pattern that you should have at the forefront of your mind when attacking new Abstract sets. Other patterns may involve two or more basic categories. Adding on layers of patterns is one way that an Abstract pattern can become more difficult.

Keep in mind, though, that you are likely to see only one or two really overly complex patterns on Test Day. Don't be drawn into the trap of overinvesting your time to make sure you haven't missed every aspect of the pattern. If the pattern seems simple, it probably is!

Let's have a look at the other pattern categories and how they might be combined on Test Day with another example set. Take 30 seconds to find the patterns.

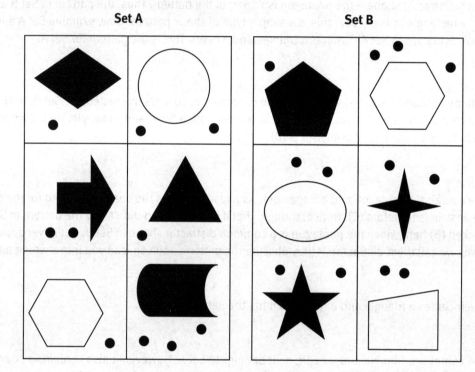

At first glance the pair of sets here seems very similar; the simplest box in each set contains a large shape with one small black circle.

There are actually two ways to use the simplest box in each set. The first is to compare the simplest box in Set A with other boxes in Set A. The second is to compare the simplest box in Set A with the simplest box in Set B. How are they different? For example, looking at the upper left -hand box in each set, you can see that the main difference is in how the shapes are arranged within the box. In Set A, the large shape is above the small black circles; in Set B, the small black circles are arranged above the large shape.

This pattern combines all of our basic categories. We have a type of shape pattern—each box has to contain small circles. Other features are important too. There is a colour element because all the small circles are shaded black. Number and size are also included as there is one large shape in each box. The pattern in how these shapes are arranged is the crucial difference between Set A and Set B.

Consider each of the test shapes in turn. Spend no more than 30 seconds total on the 5 test shapes, and be sure to mark an answer for each.

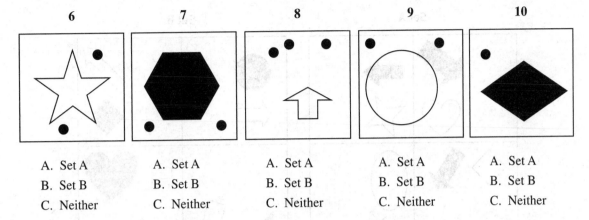

6	7	8	9	10
A. Set A	A. Set A	A. Set A	A. Set A	A. Set A
B. Set B	B. Set B	B. Set B	B. Set B	B. Set B
C. Neither	C. Neither	C. Neither	C. Neither	C. Neither

Answers and Explanations

6. (C)

The first test shape has small black circles above and below the large shape. The answer is therefore **(C)**.

7. (A)

This test shape has a large shape and small black circles below it. The answer is **(A)**.

8. (C)

This test shape has three small black circles; however, there is no big shape. This test shape belongs to neither set; thus, the correct answer is **(C)**. If you hadn't seen the arrangement pattern, you could have still earned this mark by simply noticing that a large shape was required for both Sets A and B. The good news is that there are many marks, like this one, that you can pick up even if you haven't spotted the entire pattern.

9. (B)

This test shape has a large shape with small black circles above it. The answer is **(B)**.

10. (B)

The last test shape looks very similar to a box in Set A. This would potentially trap a student who was trying to match the test shapes to individual boxes in Set A or Set B. Having identified the pattern, this one is quick, straightforward work—the correct answer is **(B)**.

Let's try working through another set on the next page.

Set your timer for 1 minute. Try to find the patterns below in 30 seconds. If you don't spot the patterns after 45 seconds, move on to the test shapes and take a guess.

Set A   **Set B**

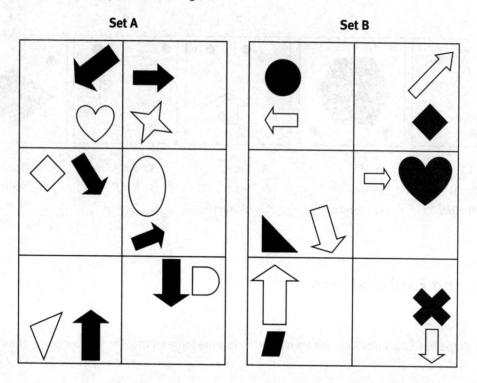

Test Shapes

| 11 | 12 | 13 | 14 | 15 |

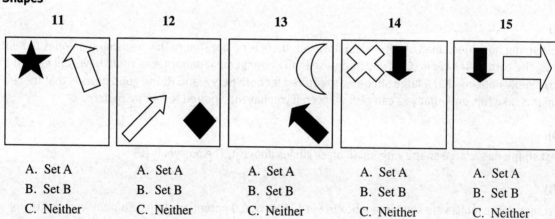

A. Set A
B. Set B
C. Neither

A. Set A
B. Set B
C. Neither

A. Set A
B. Set B
C. Neither

A. Set A
B. Set B
C. Neither

A. Set A
B. Set B
C. Neither

Answers and Explanations

If you looked for the box with the fewest number of items in Sets A and B, you'll have noticed that all the boxes in both sets have 2 shapes—so there isn't a 'simplest' box in either. And this is indeed part of the pattern: both Set A and Set B have exactly 2 shapes in each box. In Set A, there is a black arrow and another white shape in each box; in Set B, there is a white arrow and another black shape in each box. You may have checked the test shapes based on this partial pattern, in which case you would have answered three questions correctly – and got two incorrect. This is a good example of a partial pattern – they can be effective, certainly much more effective than blind guessing when you can't 'see' the whole pattern. But you may have noticed something more in common within each set.

To find the rest of the pattern, check for common categories first. There is one type of shape—an arrow—in every box in both Set A and Set B; the second shape could be anything. We have already dealt with colour; consider other shape features (such as size) and the arrangement of the shapes in each box to find the difference between the two sets. In both sets, both shapes in each box are arranged in the same half (or same side) of the box. In Set A, the black arrow always points towards the empty half of the box; in Set B, the white arrow always points towards the full half of the box. You could also describe this as the black arrow in Set A pointing to the other side of the box and the white arrow in Set B pointing to the same side of the box containing the shapes – the key is to see that the direction of the arrow depends on the arrangement of the two shapes in each pattern.

11. (B)

The first test shape has a black star and a white arrow in the top half of the box, and the arrow is pointing towards the top of the box. This test shape belongs to **(B)**.

12. (C)

This test shape has a black diamond and a white arrow in the bottom half of the box, but the arrow is pointing towards the top of the box, not the bottom. As such, the test shape does not fit the pattern for Set B. The colours are not right for it to fit into Set A. Thus, it belongs to neither set.

13. (A)

Here, there are a white crescent and black arrow in the right half of the box; the arrow is pointing to the upper left, so it belongs to **(A)**.

14. (A)

This test shape has a white cross next to a black arrow in the top half of the box; the black arrow is pointing down. This fits the pattern for Set A.

15. (C)

This test shape includes two arrows! Don't panic, and remember that each pattern is defined by an arrow, plus any other shape of the other colour. Thus, it is theoretically possible to have a second arrow as the other shape, even though this did not occur in either of the original sets. Remember, we've already seen one answer matching each pattern with a second shape (the star and the crescent) that were not present in the original sets.

The pattern for Set A requires that the black arrow point towards the empty half of the box, as the black arrow does here; there also needs to be another white shape, which we have here. So this test shape fits the pattern for Set A. The pattern for Set B requires that the white arrow point towards the full half of the box, as the white arrow does here; there also needs to be another black shape, which we have here. Thus, the test shape also fits the pattern for Set B. Since it can fit into both patterns, it belongs to neither. The answer is **(C)**.

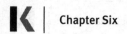

Kaplan Timed Practice Set—*Try the Kaplan Top Tips*

Set your timer for 1 minute. Write down answers for the 5 test shapes before time is up!

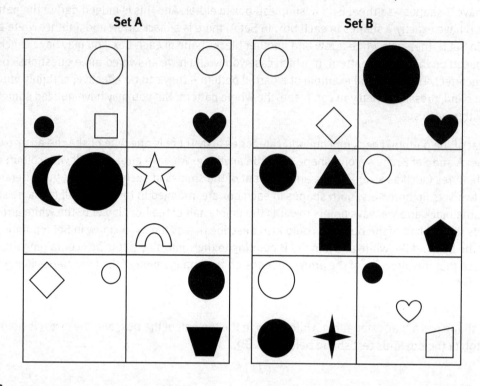

Set A

Set B

Test Shapes

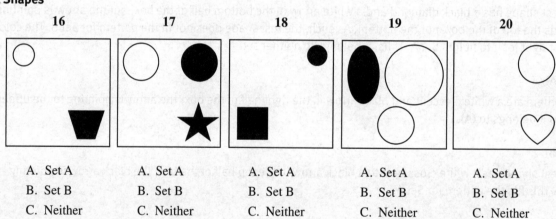

| 16 | 17 | 18 | 19 | 20 |

16.
A. Set A
B. Set B
C. Neither

17.
A. Set A
B. Set B
C. Neither

18.
A. Set A
B. Set B
C. Neither

19.
A. Set A
B. Set B
C. Neither

20.
A. Set A
B. Set B
C. Neither

Kaplan Timed Practice Set—*Abstract Basics*: Answers and Explanations

Starting with the simplest box leads to the marks once again here. The simplest boxes in Set A and Set B contain two shapes – a circle and one other shape. Comparing these within each set, you will notice that each box in Set A has a circle in the upper right-hand corner of the box, while in Set B the circle is in the upper left-hand corner of the box. There's one further element to the pattern, which is perhaps most easily noticed by comparing the two boxes in each set that have the same shapes: the circle and diamond, or the circle and heart. In Set A, the second shape is in an adjacent corner; in Set B, the second shape is in the corner diagonally opposite the circle. Note that some boxes in each original set include distractor shapes, such as the black circle in the lower left-hand corner in the upper-left box in Set A and the heart in the centre of the lower-right box in Set B. These distractors are meant to make it harder to see the pattern, but they are not part of the pattern, as they do not apply to every box in the set.

16. (B)

The first test shape contains a circle in the upper-left hand corner of the box and another shape in the lower-right hand corner, so the correct answer is **(B)**.

17. (C)

This test shape has a circle in the upper-right hand corner with another shape in an adjacent corner, so it fits the pattern for Set A. However, the test shape also has a circle in the upper-left hand corner with another shape in the lower-right corner, so it also fits the pattern for Set B. Thus, it belongs to neither set exclusively. Answer **(C)** is correct.

18. (C)

This test shape has a circle in the upper-right hand corner. For it to fit into Set A, it would need another shape in either the upper-left corner or the lower-right corner. However, the only other shape is in the lower-left corner. Thus, the test shape belongs to neither set.

19. (A)

This test shape has a circle in the upper-right hand corner and an oval in an adjacent corner, so it belongs to Set A. Note that the other circle at the bottom is not in a corner, so it is a distractor shape with no bearing on the patterns.

20. (A)

This test shape has a circle in the upper-right hand corner and a heart in an adjacent corner, so it fits the pattern for Set A.

Basic Patterns Review

Training your eyes to quickly spot the basic Abstract patterns is vital to achieving a good score on Test Day. Take a moment to commit the basic patterns to memory:

Type of shape
Features of shapes:
- Number—an absolute number of items or of a particular shape
- Colour—the shading of shapes
- Size—the size of shapes

Arrangement: the position of shapes within the box as well as relative to each other.

Now we'll move on to consider the various factors that can make a pattern complex.

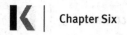

Complex Patterns

The patterns seen so far have been relatively simple. The majority of sets on Test Day will have relatively simple patterns, and you can achieve a respectable score by ensuring that you work your way through the entire section picking up all of the easy points. Many UKCAT test-takers are unable to finish the section, due to their inability to find the simple patterns quickly—the more you can do so, the greater advantage you will have over the competition.

Complex patterns are just as vulnerable to strategy, and to a methodical approach by 'trained eyes' that know how to spot them. Be careful, though, as some 'trained eyes' become obsessed with finding complex patterns, and look for complexity in all sets; as a result, they run the risk of not being able to finish the section. So bear in mind that most sets are not complex, and don't fret when you find a pattern that seems too easy, or simple or obvious to be correct. If a pattern seems simple or obvious—that's almost always because it is!

Complex patterns present many different twists. Let us take a look at a few of the most common, and most challenging, examples that you may encounter on Test Day.

Counting

Number patterns can be very complex. While a basic number pattern includes counting numbers of shapes (e.g. 2 triangles in each box), a more complex number pattern can involve counting other features. Instead of number of shapes, you might have to count the number of sides, intersections, 'spaces', angles or even the number of times you have to take your pencil off the page to draw a shape within a box.

To further complicate matters, a number pattern can also be about whether you have an even or an odd number of something, though this is less common.

Once test-takers know that the sets can contain these sorts of patterns, they suddenly start to see a lot of the tough patterns. However, this comes with a big downside—students start launching into counting everything in a set right away and end up wasting time. You must find a balance. The best approach is to look for basic patterns first, and consider counting if and only if you haven't been able to find a basic pattern.

Remember that the vast majority of number patterns will be relatively simple; the more you practise, the more these basic number patterns will almost seem to 'jump out' when you encounter them. In this exercise, we'll look at a basic number pattern, followed by a more advanced one, to help you train your eyes.

Take 30 seconds to find the patterns below, and another 30 seconds to assess the test shapes.

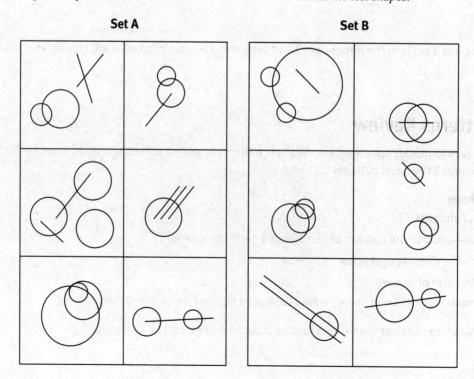

Set A   Set B

Test Shapes

21	22	23	24	25
A. Set A	A. Set A	A. Set A	A. Set A	A. Set A
B. Set B	B. Set B	B. Set B	B. Set B	B. Set B
C. Neither	C. Neither	C. Neither	C. Neither	C. Neither

Answers and Explanations

You will have noticed the various numbers of circles and lines in the boxes in both sets. Counting the circles or lines proves problematic, since there isn't a fixed number of either in Set A or Set B. Remember, you can count anything in the box, including the 'crossovers' or intersection points. Each box in Set A includes 3 intersection points, while each box in Set B includes 4 intersection points.

Consider as well whether type of shape (circles or lines) is essential to either pattern: Note that there is one box in each set that contains only circles; all the other boxes have some combination of circles and lines. This means that each box in Set A and Set B must contain a circle; lines can be part of the pattern in both sets, but they are not required.

Note how quickly you can assess the test shapes once you have found these patterns.

21. (B)
The first test shape has 4 intersections, so belongs to Set B.

22. (C)
There are 6 intersections in this test shape, so it belongs to neither set.

23. (A)
This test shape contains 3 intersections, so it belongs to Set A.

24. (B)
This test shape has 4 intersections. Therefore it belongs to Set B.

25. (C)
There isn't a circle in this test shape, and there are only 2 intersections. This test shape belongs to neither set.

Once again, take 30 seconds to find the patterns below, and another 30 seconds to assess the test shapes. If you need a bit longer to find the patterns, you can take up to a minute to do so, but you must assess the test shapes quickly.

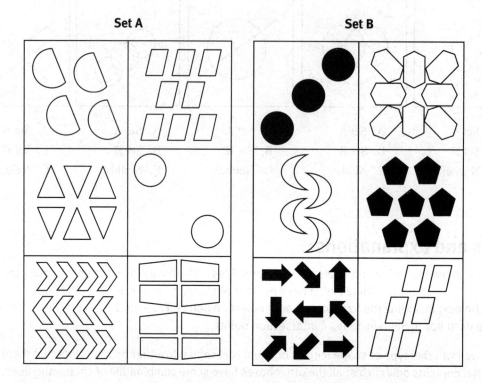

Test Shapes

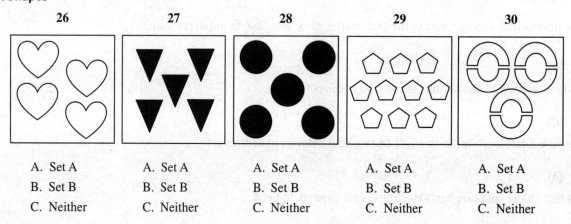

26	27	28	29	30
A. Set A	A. Set A	A. Set A	A. Set A	A. Set A
B. Set B	B. Set B	B. Set B	B. Set B	B. Set B
C. Neither	C. Neither	C. Neither	C. Neither	C. Neither

Answers and Explanations

You may have noticed a few things straightaway about these sets. Each box in each set contains multiple copies of the same shape, with a unique type of shape in every box. Also, all the shapes in Set A are white; in Set B, all the shapes in a box are either white or black. These points may seem 'obvious' – but be sure to note them on Test Day, as even the obvious elements are going to be part of the pattern. Whenever you see different types of shapes, consider whether any numbers are involved in the pattern. That's the case in Set A, where the number of shapes in each box is double the number of sides on the shape. Thus, when a box contains triangles, there are six triangles; when a box includes hexagons, there are 12 hexagons; when there are circles, with the circumference counting as one side, there are two circles. As a result, there's always an even number of white shapes in Set A.

Contrast this with Set B, which appears to have a more complicated pattern. It might be easiest to see if you compare the boxes that have the same types of shapes: Set B has three black circles (compared to two white circles in Set A), and eight white hexagons (compared to 12 white hexagons in Set A). Therefore, in Set B, the number of shapes equals the number of sides on the shape plus 2. Also, in Set B, if there's an odd number of sides, the shapes are black; if there's an even number of sides, the shapes are white. Note that there is an overlap in the rules – if there is an even number of white shapes in a test shape, it could fit either pattern – you'll have to check the maths based on the number of sides.

26. (C)

The first test shape includes 4 white hearts. Since it's an even number, it could fit both patterns. A heart has 2 sides, so doubling the number of sides (2×2) equals the number of hearts, fitting the pattern for Set A. However, adding two to the number of sides ($2 + 2$) also equals the number of hearts, fitting the pattern for Set B. Since the test shape fits both patterns, it belongs exclusively to neither. Answer **(C)** is correct.

27. (B)

This test shape contains 5 black triangles. There is an odd number of black shapes, which fits the first part of the pattern for B. A triangle has 3 sides, so the number of triangles equals the number of sides on a triangle plus 2, fitting the maths for Set B. Answer **(B)** is correct.

28. (C)

This test shape features 5 black circles. There is an odd number of black shapes, which fits the first part of the pattern for Set B. However, the maths do not add up: a circle has one side, and the rule in Set B is two plus the number of sides. So there should be 3 circles ($2 + 1$), not 5. As a result, the test shape does not fit into Set B. To fit into Set A, the test shape would need 2 white circles (2×1). Thus, the answer is **(C)**.

29. (A)

This test shape includes 10 white pentagons. There are 5 sides on a pentagon, and the number of pentagons is double the number of sides of a pentagon (2×5), so the test shape belongs to Set A.

30. (B)

This test shape contains 6 white rainbows. Each rainbow has 4 sides, and the number of rainbows is two more than the number of sides on a rainbow ($2 + 4$), so the test shape fits into Set B.

This set was quite challenging, but notice how quickly it became apparent that there were number issues. Particularly in Set A, where it was clear that each box had a different number of the same white shape, but no shapes were repeated in different boxes. Thus, it could not be a shape or colour pattern; the size and arrangement of the shapes did not seem to be an issue—it had to be a number pattern.

This is a good example of a number pattern tending to 'jump out'—they tend to be fairly obvious, either because there is the same number of something in every box (e.g. two triangles) or because the other differences in a set are minimal. Trust your eyes to see the obvious number patterns, and don't fall for the trap of counting everything in every set, or counting more frequently than necessary.

If you are really stuck finding a pattern, it most likely isn't a number pattern, anyway. It's probably an arrangement pattern. Let's look at some of the issues with complex arrangements.

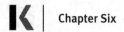

Complex Arrangement

Arrangement patterns can be very difficult to spot, since there are so many varieties of possible arrangement. A pattern may depend on the arrangement of a single shape, the arrangement of a single type or colour of shape, or the arrangement of all the shapes in the box. Look for arrangement patterns when you do not spot any basic patterns that are especially simple or obvious.

There are two broad categories of arrangement patterns:

- Absolute—a single shape or type/colour of shape is in a fixed position. Examples: circles in the corners; black shapes in the top half of the box; quadrilateral inside a curved shape.
- Relative—a single shape or type/colour of shape is positioned relative to another single shape or type/colour of shape. Examples: white shapes to the left of black shapes; circles above triangles; three smiley faces in a row.

Occasionally you will encounter a more unusual geometric arrangement. For example, the shapes may be arranged with some kind of symmetry (either within the individual shapes, or in the way they are grouped in the box), or there may be a clockwise or anticlockwise arrangement. Be prepared to mentally rotate or flip the shapes or the individual boxes to test for these uncommon possibilities when you suspect they may be in play.

Note that in the examples of relative arrangement, the shapes that define the pattern (e.g. circles above triangles) could be anywhere in the box, and there could be any number of distractor shapes present in the set or the test shapes. Note as well that any of the basic categories that do not define an arrangement pattern (type of shape, colour, size, number) can be distractors, which is why it can be so difficult to spot arrangement patterns.

In this exercise, you will attack two challenging arrangement patterns—one absolute, one relative. Try to keep to the recommended timing for each set. If you struggle, try to spot the difference between Set A and Set B. Finding this distinction will help you to find the patterns in both sets.

See if you can find the patterns in Set A and Set B in 30 seconds. Take another 30 seconds to assess the test shapes.

Set A

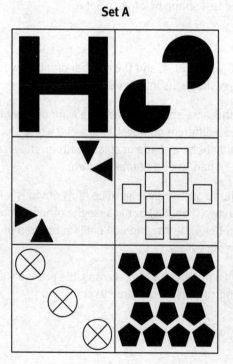

Set B

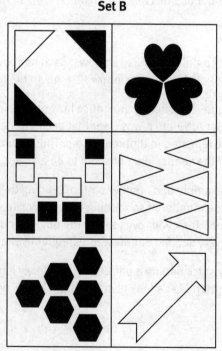

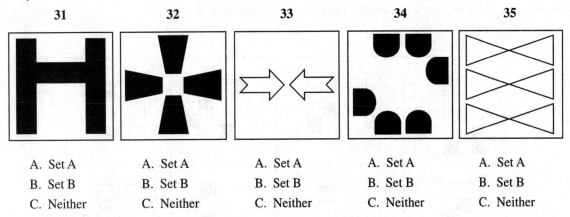

Test Shapes

31	32	33	34	35

A. Set A
B. Set B
C. Neither

A. Set A
B. Set B
C. Neither

A. Set A
B. Set B
C. Neither

A. Set A
B. Set B
C. Neither

A. Set A
B. Set B
C. Neither

Answers and Explanations

You will have noticed that each box contains black or white shapes; if there is more than one shape in the box, the same shape is repeated. In Set A, all the shapes in each box are the same colour; in Set B, they may be different colours. However, there is a lot of variation within each set, which indicates that the patterns aren't about colour or type of shape. The patterns are in fact about arrangement, along lines of symmetry. If you fold a box (each overall figure) in half along a line of symmetry (horizontal, vertical or diagonal), all the shapes will line up exactly. In Set A, there are two lines of symmetry in each box. In Set B, there is one line of symmetry in each box. Note that these lines can be horizontal, vertical or diagonal –check the test shapes carefully, so you don't miss any lines of symmetry.

31. (B)

The first test shape is somewhat similar to the upper-left box in Set A, but the central bar in the H has been moved up, so that it resembles goalposts. This figure has only a vertical line of symmetry; it fits the pattern for Set B.

32. (C)

This figure can be folded along the horizontal axis, the vertical axis or either diagonal axis, so it has four lines of symmetry. It belongs to neither set.

33. (A)

This test shape can be folded along the horizontal axis or the vertical axis. It has two lines of symmetry, so it fits the pattern for Set A.

34. (C)

If you fold this test shape along any potential line of symmetry – horizontal, vertical or diagonal – there are two shapes that do not line up. There aren't any lines of symmetry. The answer is **(C)**.

35. (A)

This test shape has horizontal and vertical lines of symmetry, but no diagonal symmetry. It belongs to Set A.

Take a minute to find the patterns and assess the test shapes. If you need more than 30 seconds to find the patterns, then try to move more quickly when you come to the test shapes.

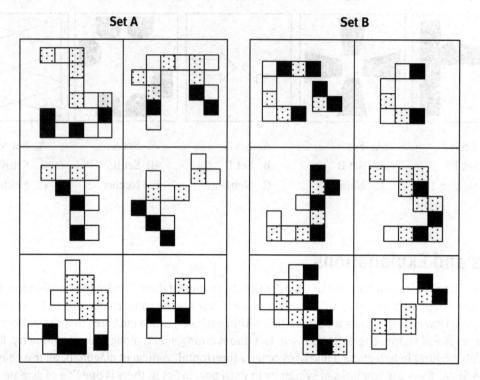

Test Shapes

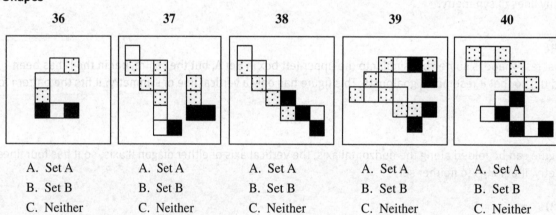

36	**37**	**38**	**39**	**40**
A. Set A	A. Set A	A. Set A	A. Set A	A. Set A
B. Set B	B. Set B	B. Set B	B. Set B	B. Set B
C. Neither	C. Neither	C. Neither	C. Neither	C. Neither

Answers and Explanations

All the boxes in each set include small squares that are white, black or dotted. The squares have been arranged into figures—some boxes have all the squares in a single figure, some have multiple figures. The number of squares in each box in each set is different; some have an even number, some have an odd number. When you do not notice a number pattern straightaway, it is likely that the pattern does not involve number. In this case, it is all about arrangement; specifically, within each box, one group of shaded squares are positioned relative to another group of shaded squares. In Set A, the dotted squares are arranged above the black squares. In Set B, the white squares are arranged to the left of the black squares. The extra shading in each set (white squares in Set A; dotted squares in Set B) is a distractor—it's irrelevant to the pattern.

36. (A)

The first test shape has all the dotted squares above the black squares, so it belongs to Set A.

37. (C)

All the dotted squares are above the black squares in this test shape, so it fits the pattern for Set A. However, all the white squares are to the left of the black squares, so it also fit the pattern for Set B. Since it fits both patterns, it belongs exclusively to neither set.

38. (C)

Not all the dotted squares in this figure are above the black square—some are in the same rows—so it cannot fit the pattern for Set A. Not all the white squares are to the left of the black squares—one white square is to the right of black squares—so it cannot fit the pattern for Set B. The answer is **(C)**.

39. (B)

All the white squares are to the left of the black squares, so this test shape belongs to Set B.

40. (A)

All the dotted squares are above the black squares, so the figure fits the pattern for Set A.

Remember

Sometimes it is easier to see the pattern if you start with Set B.

In this set, the relative arrangement of the white and black squares in Set B may have been easier to 'see' than the relative arrangement of the dotted and black squares in Set A.

Don't hesitate to start with Set B, or to move on to Set B when you find yourself struggling to find anything resembling a pattern in Set A.

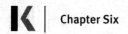

Kaplan Timed Practice Set—*Complex Arrangement*

Set your timer for 1 minute. Write down answers for the 5 test shapes before time is up!

Set A   **Set B**

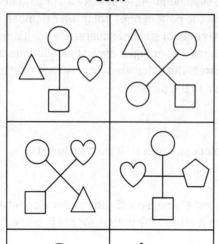
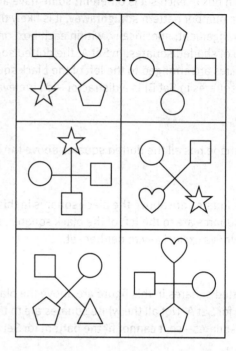

Test Shapes

41	42	43	44	45

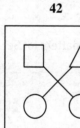
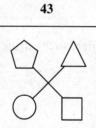
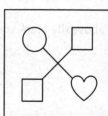
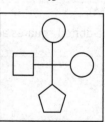

A. Set A
B. Set B
C. Neither

A. Set A
B. Set B
C. Neither

A. Set A
B. Set B
C. Neither

A. Set A
B. Set B
C. Neither

A. Set A
B. Set B
C. Neither

Kaplan Timed Practice Set—*Complex Arrangement*: Answers and Explanations

Each box in each set contains four white shapes, connected by two lines that form a cross. There are various shapes at the ends of the lines, but all boxes in each set include a circle and a square. The difference between the two sets is the arrangement of these two shapes. In Set A, the circle is always directly above the square; in Set B, the circle is always directly across from the square. Note that whether the circle and square are connected by a line is not part of the pattern.

41. (A)

This first test shape includes a circle directly above a square, so it fits the pattern for Set A.

42. (C)

This test shape has a square directly above a circle, rather than a circle above a square, so it does not fit into Set A. The test shape has a circle directly across from a circle, rather than a circle across from a square, so it does not fit into Set B. As a result, it fits into neither set.

43. (B)

This test shape contains a circle directly across from a square, so it belongs to Set B.

44. (C)

This test shape has a circle directly above a square, so it fits the pattern for Set A. However, it also has a circle directly across from a square, so it also fits the pattern for Set B. Since the test shape fits into both patterns, it belongs exclusively to neither. Answer **(C)** is correct.

45. (B)

This test shape includes a circle directly across from a square, so it fits the pattern for Set B.

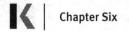

Conditional Patterns

A further way that the UKCAT makes patterns more complex is with conditional characteristics. Conditionals are patterns in which a characteristic of one item in the box dictates a characteristic of another item in the box. For example, you might see a pattern where each box contains a circle and a square, with this conditional: if the circle is shaded, it is positioned above the square; if the circle is not shaded, it is positioned below the square. The pattern in the other set might then be the opposite, or it might be a similar but slightly different conditional—for example, it might involve shading and positioning of shapes that are different from the shapes in Set A. Conditionals can be time-consuming to identify, and even more time-consuming in evaluating answer choices, since you will have to apply the conditionals from Set A and Set B to every test shape.

There are two hints for spotting conditionals. First, if you see arrows, consider if the direction they are pointing is related to the position, shading or type of shape of another shape (or shapes) in the box. Second, if two sets seem almost identical, and you have already checked for an arrangement pattern—check for conditionals.

Remember, conditional patterns are really rather rare on the UKCAT, so only look for them if you can't find anything else.

Take 30 seconds to find the conditional pattern in the set below. Make a note of the pattern on your scrap paper, then spend no more than 30 seconds evaluating the test shapes.

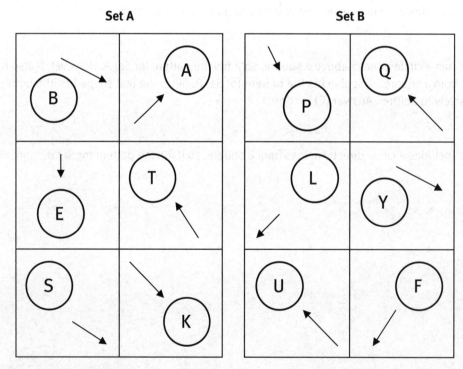

Test Shapes

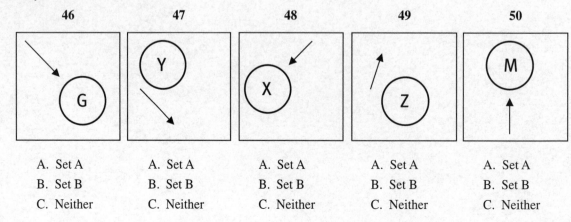

46	47	48	49	50
A. Set A	A. Set A	A. Set A	A. Set A	A. Set A
B. Set B	B. Set B	B. Set B	B. Set B	B. Set B
C. Neither	C. Neither	C. Neither	C. Neither	C. Neither

Answers and Explanations

The most obvious part of the pattern that you will notice straightaway is that all boxes in both sets have an arrow and a circle containing a letter. So the difference between the sets must involve the letters inside the circles, some of which are straight and some of which are curved letters. Since each box also contains an arrow, consider whether the direction of the arrow corresponds to the letter inside the circle. In Set A, if the arrow points at the circle, the letter is straight. If the arrow doesn't point at the circle, the letter inside has curves. The pattern for Set B is the exact opposite: the arrow points at circles with curved letters and not at those containing straight letters.

46. (B)

The first test shape has an arrow pointing at a curved letter. This fits into Set B.

47. (B)

The letter here is straight, and the arrow points away from it. This also belongs to Set B.

48. (A)

The arrow points at a circle containing a straight letter. The correct answer is (A).

49. (B)

The arrow doesn't point at a circle containing a straight letter. The answer must be (B).

50. (A)

The arrow is pointing at a circle containing a straight letter. This corresponds to Set A.

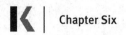
Kaplan Timed Practice Set—*Conditional Patterns*

Set your timer for 1 minute. Write down answers for the 5 test shapes before time is up!

Set A

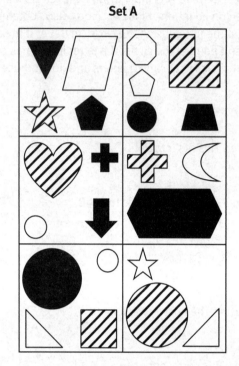

Set B

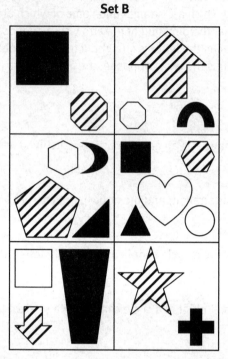

Test Shapes

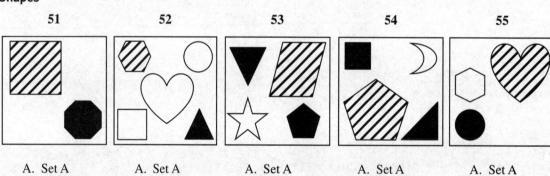

51	52	53	54	55
A. Set A	A. Set A	A. Set A	A. Set A	A. Set A
B. Set B	B. Set B	B. Set B	B. Set B	B. Set B
C. Neither	C. Neither	C. Neither	C. Neither	C. Neither

Kaplan Timed Practice Set—*Conditional Patterns*: Answers and Explanations

All the boxes include a striped shape, suggesting that the stripes might be essential to the pattern. In this case, it might be better to start with Set B, since two of the boxes contain only two shapes. The upper-left box in Set B has a large black square and a smaller striped octagon; the lower-right box in Set B has a large striped star and a smaller black cross. Two other boxes in Set B have the largest shape striped: the arrow (upper-right box) and the pentagon (middle-left box). In the three boxes in Set B where the largest shape is striped, there is a black shape in the lower-right corner of the box. In the other three boxes in Set B, the shape with the most sides is striped (octagon in the upper-left box, hexagon in the middle-right box, and arrow in the lower-left box); if the shape with the most sides is striped in Set B, then, there is a square in the upper-left corner of the box.

In Set A, there are similar conditionals. Three boxes in Set A have the largest shape striped: the L-shape (upper-right box), the heart (middle-left box) and the circle (lower-right box). In Set A, if the largest shape is striped, there is a circle in the lower-left corner. The other three boxes in Set A have the shape with the most sides striped (star, cross, square). If the shape with the most sides is striped in Set A, there is a white shape in the upper-right corner of the box.

You might make a quick note of the conditionals before proceeding. You would want to do the same on your noteboard on Test Day, as it is very easy to mix up the conditionals when working quickly.

Set A

largest shape striped → circle LL

most sides striped → white UR

Set B

largest shape striped → black LR

most sides striped → square UL

51. (B)

In the first test shape, the largest shape is a striped square, and there is black octagon in the lower-right corner. This fits the pattern for Set B.

52. (A)

This test shape has a striped hexagon; the largest shape is a white heart. The striped hexagon has the most sides, so it is the controlling shape. If the shape with the most sides is striped, we would expect to see a white shape in the upper-right corner (in Set A) or a square in the upper-left corner (in Set B). This test shape has a white circle in the upper-right and a hexagon in the upper-left, so it fits the pattern for Set A. Note that if there was a square instead of a hexagon in the upper-left, the test shape would also fit the pattern for Set B.

53. (B)

The largest shape is a striped parallelogram; the shape with the most sides is a white star. If the largest shape is striped, we expect to see a circle in the lower-left corner (in Set A) or a black shape in the lower-right corner (in Set B). There isn't a circle in this box, but there is a black pentagon in the lower-right corner. The test shape belongs to Set B.

54. (C)

The largest shape in this box is a striped pentagon, which is also the shape with the most sides. Thus, any of the conditionals from either set could apply. In this case, we have a white crescent in the upper-right corner, matching the pattern for Set A. However, we also have a square in the upper-left corner and a black shape in the lower-right corner, matching both conditionals for Set B. Since the test shape matches both patterns, it belongs exclusively to neither set.

55. (A)

The shape with the most sides is the white pentagon; the largest shape is the striped heart in the upper-right corner. There is a circle in the lower-left corner, so the test shape belongs to Set A.

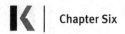

Finding Partial Patterns

If, after learning about all the common and complex patterns, you find yourself seeing more patterns but running out of time, you are not alone. With newly trained eyes, looking for patterns can be a systematic but very time-consuming process, and the temptation to keep searching until you find every minor nuance in every pattern is irresistible. This may lead you to proceed through Abstract sets at a slower pace, which will result in a lower score. However, as you practice more and more, your speed will improve and you'll find that you can find most, if not all, patterns, rather quickly and accurately.

Once you've become relatively quick, you'll still need to learn when to give up. Almost every UKCAT test is going to contain one or two horrendously difficult patterns that are going to stump even the most brilliant Abstract Reasoning test-takers. The best approach with these sets is to spend up to a minute finding part of the pattern, then use this partial pattern to assess the test shapes. Often, you can eliminate Set A or Set B as a possible answer based on a partial pattern, leaving you with a 50–50 guess. These are good odds, and certainly better than guessing blindly—or panicking and wasting time—on a very hard set.

Take no longer than 1 minute, and see if you can find part of a pattern in the set below.

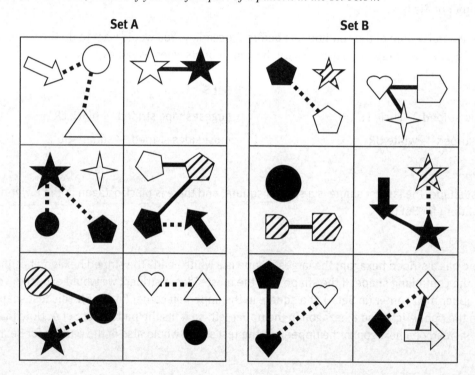

Answer

These sets have lots of different shapes, with unusual shadings, connected by dashed and straight lines. Don't panic, and start with the simplest box first. In Set A, the upper right-hand box has two stars connected by a solid line. Is that pattern repeated elsewhere in the set? Yes—there are two identical shapes connected by a straight line in the middle right and lower left boxes. Compare to the simplest box in Set B; the upper right box has three white shapes—a pentagon, heart and star—all connected by solid lines. Check the other boxes to see if this is a pattern: the lower right box has a white diamond and arrow connected by a solid line; the boxes above and to the left of it each have two black shapes connected by a solid line. Thus, the partial pattern is that the same types of shapes are connected by solid lines in Set A, and the same colour shapes are connected by solid lines in Set B. If that's all you've seen, you can actually make some good eliminations when you move on to the test shapes.

Take 30 seconds to evaluate the test shapes, and make your best guess based on the partial pattern.

Test Shapes

56	57	58	59	60
A. Set A	A. Set A	A. Set A	A. Set A	A. Set A
B. Set B	B. Set B	B. Set B	B. Set B	B. Set B
C. Neither	C. Neither	C. Neither	C. Neither	C. Neither

Answers and Explanations

Based on the partial pattern, the two white arrows in the first test shape should be connected by a solid line in Set A (because they are the same shape) and also in Set B (because they are the same colour); as such, this test shape cannot fit into either set. The second test shape has two black shapes connected by a solid line, which fits the pattern for Set B; because the two pentagons are not connected by a solid line, it doesn't fit the pattern for Set A, so the answer must be **(B)**. The third test shape has two circles connected by a solid line; the circles are different colours, so the answer must be **(A)**. The fourth test shape does not fit either set, as it has two different shapes of different colour connected by a solid line; the answer must be **(C)**. The final test shape does not have a solid line, but two different shapes of the same colour are connected by a dotted line. This cannot fit the pattern for Set B, so it's a 50–50 guess between **(A)** and **(C)**.

Even if you only found part of the partial patterns—say, only the detail involving solid lines connecting shapes of the same type in Set A—that would be enough to get the third test shape correct, and to eliminate **(A)** as an answer choice for the first, second and fourth test shapes (as all of these include identical shapes that are not connected by a solid line). You would have to guess randomly on the final test shape, but would still be able to pick up 2 or 3 marks from the 5 available in this set—far more than you'd get by guessing randomly on all 5 test shapes, or by leaving them unanswered.

For the record: This pattern is incredibly complex, involving many features as well as arrangements. In Set A, if shapes are of the same shading, they are connected with a dotted line. If the shapes are of the same type, they are connected with a solid line. Shapes that aren't the same colour or the same shape as another in the box are not connected. In Set B, if the shapes are of the same type, they are connected with a dotted line. If they are the same colour, they are connected by a solid line. Other shapes are not connected. Thus, the final test shape fits into Set A, as it features two different white shapes connected by a dotted line.

Score Higher Online

Even with the sharpest Abstract skills, you may occasionally encounter a set that is so unusual or difficult that you can't see the pattern, even after a minute.

If you can't find the pattern and are not sure of what to guess, flag all items for review.

Come back to the set on a second pass through the section. You will often find that with fresh eyes, something will 'jump out' that you did not notice the first time.

Kaplan Timed Practice Set—*Finding Partial Patterns*

Set your timer for 1 minute. Do your best to find a partial pattern—if not the complete pattern—for each set before the minute is up. It is okay to take the full minute to find the patterns, as this is a very advanced set. If you do so, then give yourself no more than 30 seconds to mark answers for all 5 test shapes. If unsure, eliminate based on a partial pattern and make a guess.

Set A **Set B**

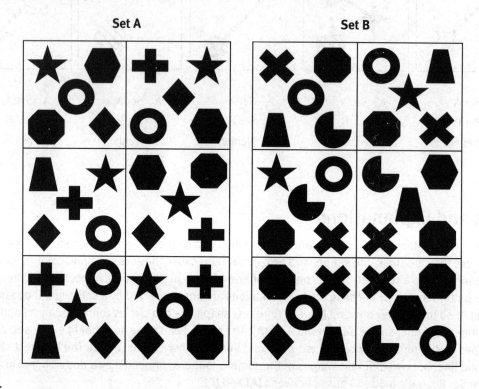

Test Shapes

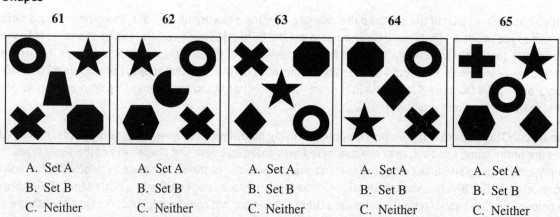

61	62	63	64	65
A. Set A	A. Set A	A. Set A	A. Set A	A. Set A
B. Set B	B. Set B	B. Set B	B. Set B	B. Set B
C. Neither	C. Neither	C. Neither	C. Neither	C. Neither

Kaplan Timed Practice Set—*Finding Partial Patterns*: Answers and Explanations

There are a lot of distractor shapes in this set, and it's impossible to start with the box with the fewest shapes, since each box in each set contains five black shapes, one in each corner and one in the centre. These are key aspects to each pattern, but they are not distinct—you must look for the differences between the two patterns, based on what appears in every box in each set. As soon as you notice that a shape is missing in a box, you can mentally cross it off the list, as it cannot be part of the pattern. Thus, there are two shapes in each set that are part of the pattern: the star and the diamond in Set A, and the cross and the octagon in Set B. There is a further element of arrangement in each set: in Set A, the star is always above the diamond; in Set B, the octagon and cross are always next to each other.

61. (B)

This first test shape includes a cross and an octagon next to each other in the bottom row, so it fits the pattern for Set B.

62. (C)

This test shape includes a star, but no diamond, so it cannot fit the pattern for Set A. It also includes a cross, but no octagon, so it cannot fit the pattern for Set B. The test shape fits into neither set.

63. (C)

This test shape has a star above a diamond, so it belongs to Set A. However, it also has a cross next to an octagon, so it also belongs to Set B. Since the test shape belongs to both sets, it fits exclusively into neither. The answer is **(C)**.

64. (C)

This test shape includes a star, a diamond, a cross and an octagon. However, the diamond is above the star, so it does not belong to Set A; the octagon is next to the ring, not the cross, so it does not belong to Set B. Thus, it belongs to neither set.

65. (A)

Suppose you had identified the shapes that define each pattern – the star and diamond in Set A, and the cross and octagon in Set B – but not the arrangement of these shapes in each pattern. In that case, you would very likely have still selected the correct answers for the first and last test shapes, since they fit the patterns for Set B and Set A, respectively. The three test shapes that fit neither set would have been more challenging – though they were challenging enough with the full pattern in mind! Even so, by comparing the three middle test shapes to Set A and Set B based solely on the star and diamond defining Set A and the cross and octagon defining B, you would likely have noted that test shape 62 lacked a diamond and octagon, so it belongs to neither set, and that test shapes 63 and 64 had all 4 shapes, so you would likely have picked **(C)** anyway, even though you would not have worked out the distinction between 63 (fits both patterns exactly) and 64 (right shapes but wrong arrangement in both patterns).

This goes to show the power of partial patterns on the UKCAT. With sets as complex as these, there may be some element (likely to do with arrangement) that you simply won't see, or won't be able to work out, even if you invest a full minute or two in looking for it. Don't worry—make your best guess based on what you can see. You'll find more often than not that a partial pattern is enough to pick up most (if not all) of the marks on a complex set.

The most important thing to remember about complex sets is timing: You still have only 1 minute total to find the patterns and click the answers for all 5 test shapes. If you work more quickly on the simple to moderate difficulty patterns, then you would have a bit of extra time for the few harder sets that you will encounter. However, it is essential that you do not go over 1 minute per set on average on your first pass through the section, otherwise you risk running out of time. This means that if you are ahead for timing, you might be able to spend up to 90 seconds on a complex set, allowing up to a minute to find the patterns. But you simply cannot take any longer than a minute for pattern-finding on any one set, or you are going to miss out marks at the end of the section— and very likely, the marks that you miss will have been a lot easier if you had got to them.

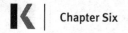

Other Abstract Question Types

The other three Abstract question types each have 4 answer choices, and each answer choice is a test shape. Thus, your skills at assessing test shapes and finding the common features—and to do so quickly—will continue to be essential.

Type 4 Questions

Type 4 questions are virtually identical to Type 1 questions. The key differences:

- You will be asked to select the test shape that fits the pattern for one of the sets.
- The answer choices are 4 test shapes.

Thus, any time you see Set A and Set B, you should start by finding the patterns. Be sure to read each question to check whether it is asking about Set A or Set B. Any answers that fit neither pattern will be incorrect. Since each question will ask about one set, an answer that fits both patterns must be correct, since it can belong equally to Set A or Set B. Such answers are less common—most answers will fit exclusively into Set A or Set B, or they will fit neither set.

Give yourself 30 seconds to find the patterns in Set A and Set B, then 30 seconds to answer the 5 questions that follow.

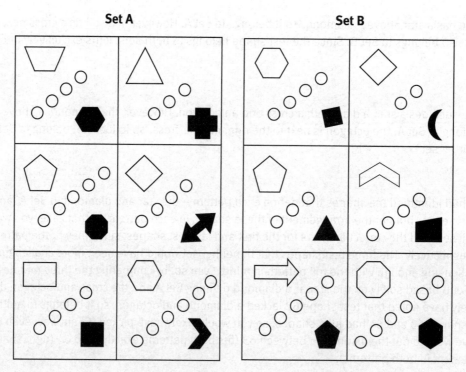

66. Which of the following test shapes belongs in Set A?

   A. 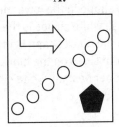 B. 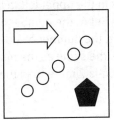 C. 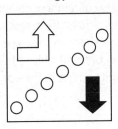 D.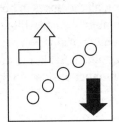

67. Which of the following test shapes belongs in Set A?

   A.  B. 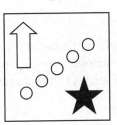 C.  D.

68. Which of the following test shapes belongs in Set B?

   A. 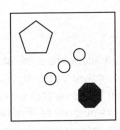 B. 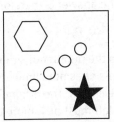 C. 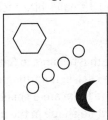 D.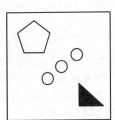

69. Which of the following test shapes belongs in Set B?

   A. 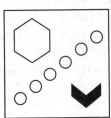 B. 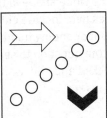 C. 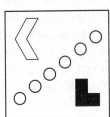 D.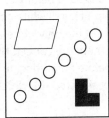

70. Which of the following test shapes belongs in Set A?

   A. 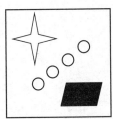 B. 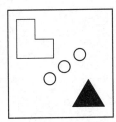 C. 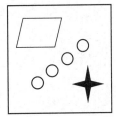 D.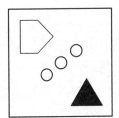

Answers and Explanations

In this set, all the boxes in both sets contain a white shape in the upper left, a black shape in the lower right, and a number of small white circles across the diagonal. In Set A, the number of small white circles is the same as the number of sides on the white shape in the upper left; the number of sides on the black shape is irrelevant to the pattern. In Set B, the number of small white circles is the same as the number of sides on the black shape, and the number of sides on the white shape in the upper left is 2 more than the number of small white circles.

66. (A)

The first question asks about Set A, so compare the number of sides on the shape in the upper left of each box to the number of small white circles. The only answer choice that gives an equal number for both of these is **(A)**, in which there are 7 small white circles and 7 sides on the white arrow in the upper left. Hence, answer **(A)** is correct.

67. (D)

This question asks for a test shape that belongs to Set A, so the number of sides on the white shape in the upper left must be the same as the number of small white circles on the diagonal. The only answer choices in which these numbers are equal is **(D)**, with 2 small white circles on the diagonal and 2 sides on the white crescent in the upper left, so **(D)** is correct.

68. (D)

For a test shape to belong to Set B, the number of sides on the black shape must be equal to the number of small white circles on the diagonal. The options here include either 3 or 4 small white circles on the diagonal, but the number of sides on the black shape only corresponds to the number of small white circles in **(D)**, in which there are a black triangle and 3 small white circles. The answer is therefore **(D)**.

69. (B)

This question asks for a test shape that belongs to Set B, so the number of sides on the black shape must be equal to the number of small white circles; unfortunately, this does not eliminate any answers, as both versions of the black shape have 6 sides, and there are 6 small white circles. The other element to the pattern in Set B is that the number of sides of the white shape in the upper left must be 2 more than the number of small white circles, so the correct answer will have 8 sides on the white shape in the upper left. The only choice that has an 8-sided white shape in the upper left is **(B)**, so **(B)** is correct.

70. (C)

For a test shape to belong to Set A, the number of sides on the white shape in the upper left must be equal to the number of small white circles on the diagonal. The choices here include either 3 or 4 white circles on the diagonal, but the only white shape in the upper left with a corresponding number of sides is the parallelogram in **(C)**; **(C)** is therefore correct. Note the importance of checking the question to see whether it is asking about Set A or Set B before answering. In this question, if you hadn't checked and had assumed it was Set B, you would have incorrectly selected **(D)**, which fits the pattern for Set B.

Kaplan Timed Practice Set—*Type 4 Questions*

Set your timer for 1 minute. Mark an answer for all 5 questions before time is up.

Set A

Set B

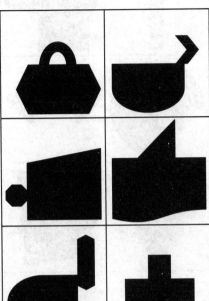
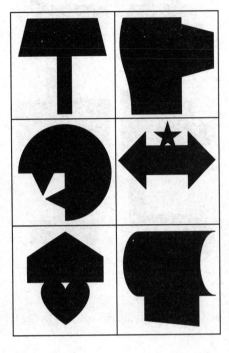

71. Which of the following test shapes belongs in Set A?

    A.   **B.**   **C.**   **D.**

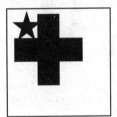

72. Which of the following test shapes belongs in Set A?

    A.   **B.**   **C.**   **D.**

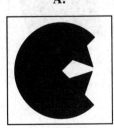
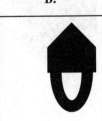
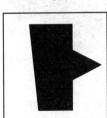
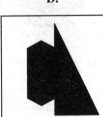

Set A   **Set B**

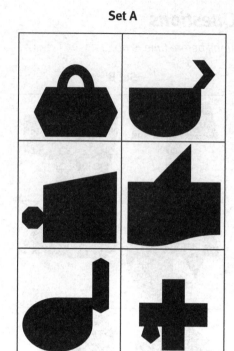 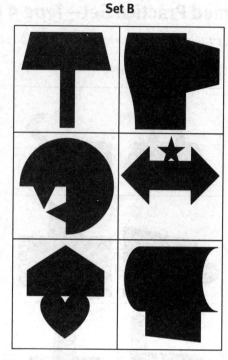

73. Which of the following test shapes belongs in Set B?

    A.   B.   C.   D.

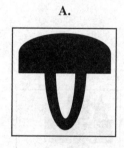 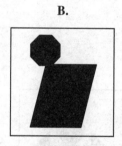 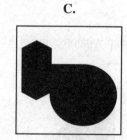 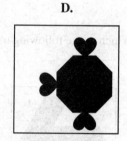

74. Which of the following test shapes belongs in Set B?

    A.   B.   C.   D.

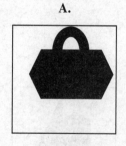 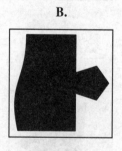 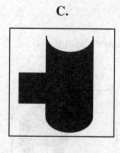 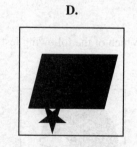

75. Which of the following test shapes belongs in Set A?

    A.   B.   C.   D.

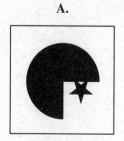  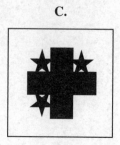 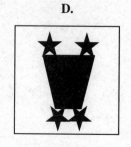

Kaplan Timed Practice Set—*Type 4 Questions*: Answers and Explanations

All the boxes in both sets include multiple shapes that are 'stuck together' to make a single large black figure. The types of shape vary widely within each set, and the overall figures they form are quite large – so the pattern cannot involve type of shape or features such as colour or size. However, the key distinction in the sets is the arrangement of the overall figure within the box. In Set A, most of the figure is in the bottom half of the box; in Set B, most of the figure is in the top half of the box. On Test Day, you might make a brief note on your noteboard (e.g. 'A = btm; B = top') to ensure you don't invert the patterns when assessing the test shapes.

71. (C)

The first question asks about Set A, which requires most of the figure formed by the joined up shapes to appear in the bottom half of the box. Almost all of the double-headed arrow in **(C)** is in the bottom half of the box; all the other test shapes are evenly split between top and bottom halves of the box, or the figures are mostly in the top half of the box. Answer **(C)** is correct.

72. (D)

Again, you must find the test shape that fits the pattern for Set A – the one with most of the figure in the bottom half of the box. The large triangle in **(D)** is mostly in the bottom half of the box; the hexagon joined to the triangle is also (if just slightly) more in the bottom than the top half of the box. The correct answer is **(D)**.

73. (A)

This question asks for the test shape that belongs to Set B, which means that it must have most of the figure in the top half of the box. The only test shape that is arranged in this way is **(A)**.

74. (A)

Set B requires the large black figure to be arranged so that most of it is in the top half of the box. Three of the test shapes are clearly mostly in the bottom half of the box, whilst **(A)** is almost entirely in the top half of the box. **(A)** is correct. NB that even though **(A)** repeats a figure from Set A, the actual shapes and figures are irrelevant to the patterns – it is simply a question of whether the figure is arranged in the top half (Set B) or bottom half (Set A) of the box.

75. (B)

This question asks about Set A, which means that most of the figure must be in the bottom half of the box. All the test shapes have stars joined to a larger central shape, but three of the resulting figures are mostly in the top half of the box. Answer **(B)** is mostly in the bottom, so it is correct.

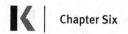

Type 2 and Type 3 Questions

Instead of patterns, Type 2 and Type 3 Abstract questions involve progressions—so you must choose the answer that best completes the progression. Progressions involve the same categories as patterns: types of shapes, features of shapes and arrangements. In the official UKCAT practice questions for Type 2 and Type 3, most elements of the progressions involve arrangement and colour, so students generally find that it's a bit easier to 'see' the progressions than it is to see the patterns.

Each Type 2 question will present a series of 4 boxes in a single row. You are asked to select the answer that completes the series. Thus, you must choose the test shape that correctly comes fifth in the progression.

Each Type 3 question will present two pairs of boxes. The first pair of boxes features a progression, in which there are a number of changes from the first box to the second box. The second pair of boxes will have the same progression, only the second box in the second pair is blank; you must choose the test shape that correctly completes it.

Here are some Kaplan UKCAT top tips for Type 2 and Type 3 questions:

- Patterns are about what is the same in the boxes. Progressions are about what is different in the boxes.
- These questions appear individually, not in sets of 5. This means you have only 12 seconds per question, so you must work quickly and eliminate ruthlessly. Thus, as soon as you note one element of the progression, eliminate the answer choices that do not present this correctly.
- Do not attempt to identify all elements of the progression before checking the answer choices. Doing so makes each question take a minute or longer.

You will now have a chance to practise a few Type 2 questions, followed by a few Type 3 questions. Afterward, there will be a timed set including a mix of Type 2 and Type 3 questions. In the initial practice, prioritise accuracy over speed, so you can learn the question format. Finding progressions feels a bit different to finding patterns; you need to get a good sense of it before attempting timed practice.

Type 2 Practice

76.   Which figure completes the series?

A.	B.	C.	D.

   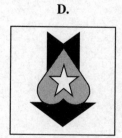

Answer—Question 76

The small shape at the front of each box becomes the medium middle shape in the next box, while the medium middle shape enlarges and moves to the back, and the large back shape becomes the small front shape. The colour is relative to position, so that the front shape is always grey, the middle shape white, and the back shape black. The middle shape is always flipped vertically from its usual orientation. Thus, the correct answer will have a small grey star in front, a white heart pointing upwards in the middle, and a large black arrow pointing upwards in the back. **(C)** is correct.

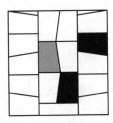 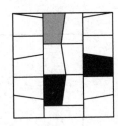 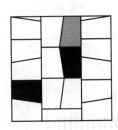 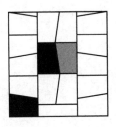

77. Which figure completes the series?

A.   **B.**   **C.**   **D.**

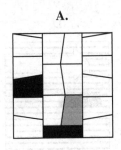 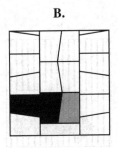 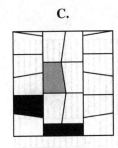 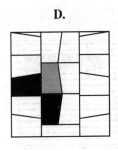

Answer—Question 77

Each box consists of a field of shapes, almost entirely the same quadrilateral, with the appearance of a stained glass window. There are three coloured segments – two black, one grey – that move throughout the shapes. Given that there are so many shapes, and the arrangement is somewhat irregular, it can be tough to see the sequence quickly. Remember, you would only have 12 seconds to answer this question on Test Day; questions as elaborate as this one are designed to make you waste time and miss easier marks elsewhere. In this case, the best approach is to track one of the coloured shapes, work out where it should be in the correct answers, and eliminate the answers with the shape in the wrong position. Hopefully, you can get to the answer swiftly without having to check all three coloured shapes. The grey shape is the most distinct; it moves up the centre-left column of shapes, then over one shape and down the centre-right column. Thus, the grey shape in the correct answer would be the centre-right shape immediately above the narrow rectangle at the bottom of the box. Eliminate **(C)** and **(D)**. The lower black shading moves leftwards across the shapes, then snakes down to the bottom row in the fourth box. Hence, it follows that this black shading would move to the bottom rectangle in the correct answer. Answer **(A)** is correct.

For the record: The upper black shading moves down, then leftwards across a middle row of shapes, always moving to the next shape across (or down, when it cannot go across) that shares a side. Thus, it moves from the centre-left shape in the fourth box to the third quadrilateral in the leftmost column in the correct answer. Note that this shading always moves to a shape with a common side, so it cannot jump down to the fourth quadrilateral in the leftmost column, as this one does not border the centre-left black shape in the fourth box.

Type 3 Practice

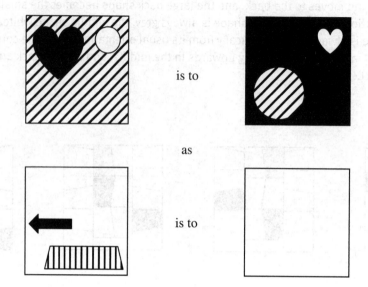

is to

as

is to

78. Which figure completes the statement?

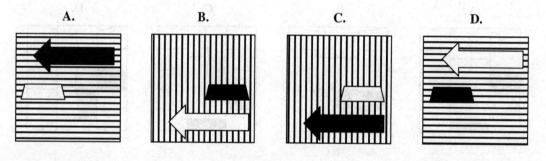

A.　　　　　　　B.　　　　　　　C.　　　　　　　D.

Answer—Question 78

In the first row, the small shape is in the same position in both boxes, and also the same colour; only the type of shape has switched. The small shape in the second row is a black arrow at the middle-left of the box; thus, the small shape in the correct answer must be a black trapezium at the middle-left. Eliminate **(A)** and **(C)**. The large shape stays on the same side of the box but swaps vertically to the other side of the box, whilst also switching type of shape with the small shape. The second row starts with a large trapezium in the lower-right of the box, so the correct answer must have a large arrow at the upper-right of the box. Answer **(D)** is correct.

For the record: Note that the background of the first box in each row swaps colours with the large shape; any stripes rotate 90° clockwise. These details would also help to identify **(D)** as the correct answer. In this case, there were more details in the sequence than required to eliminate the incorrect answers. On Test Day, be careful not to do any more work than required on Type 3 questions—check the answers (and eliminate any that are incorrect) as soon as you spot one detail in the sequence.

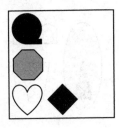

is to

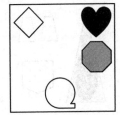

as

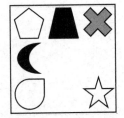

is to

79. Which figure completes the statement?

A. **B.** **C.** **D.**

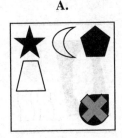 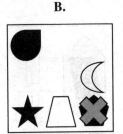 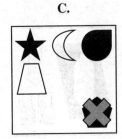 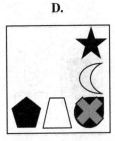

Answer—Question 79

In the first row, the grey shape moves directly across the box, retaining its colour, whilst the shape that is originally white moves to the opposite corner and becomes black. The shapes that are originally black swap places and become white. The second row may seem more complicated at first glance, since there are six shapes instead of four, but apply the same rules carefully, to avoid errors that might lead to a wrong answer trap. The grey shape, the cross, moves directly across the box to the lower-right corner. All the white shapes move to opposite corners and become black, so the star should be in the upper-left corner, the teardrop in the upper-right, and the pentagon in the lower-right. Answer **(C)** is correct.

For the record: Note that the shapes that were originally black must swap places whilst also becoming white. If you started with this detail of the sequence, you would have eliminated **(B)** and **(D)** before checking the three shapes that were originally white.

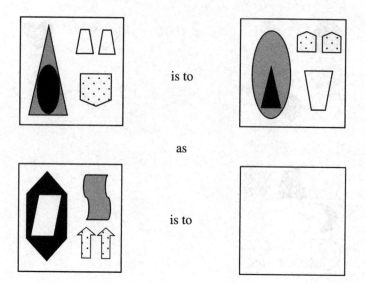

80. Which figure completes the statement?

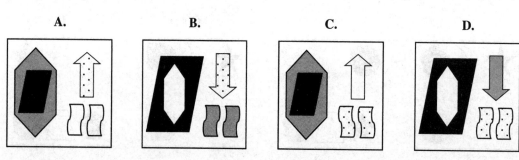

Answer—Question 80

The two shapes at the left switch size and position in the first row, so that the medium-sized inside shape in the first box becomes the large shape in the second box, and vice versa; these two shapes also switch shading. Thus, the large black hexagon at the left of the first box in the second row must become the medium inside shape in the correct answer; since the original medium inside shape is white, the medium-sized hexagon must also be white. Eliminate **(A)** and **(C)**. The shapes at the right switch position, top and bottom, and retain their original shading; the single medium-sized shape becomes two smaller shapes, and the two smaller shapes become one medium-sized shape. Answer **(B)** is correct.

Kaplan Timed Practice Set—*Type 2 and Type 3 Questions*

Set your timer for 1 minute. Try to mark answers for all 5 questions before time is up. If you need a bit longer, you might allow an additional 30 seconds to finish the set.

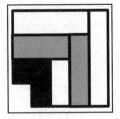 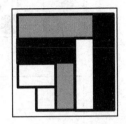 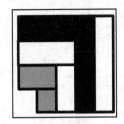 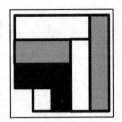

81. Which figure completes the series?

    A.   **B.**   **C.**   **D.**

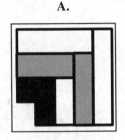 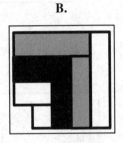 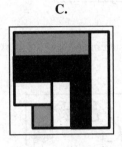 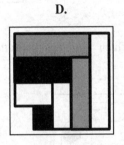

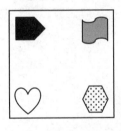 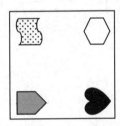 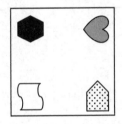 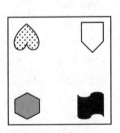

82. Which figure completes the series?

    A.   **B.**   **C.**   **D.**

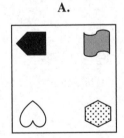 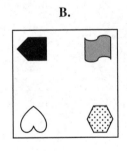 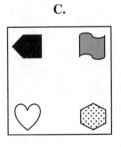 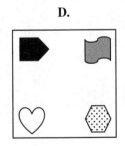

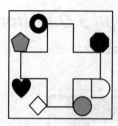 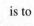 is to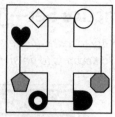

as

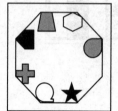 is to

83. Which figure completes the statement?

A.	B.	C.	D.

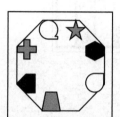 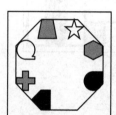 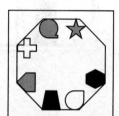 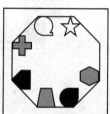

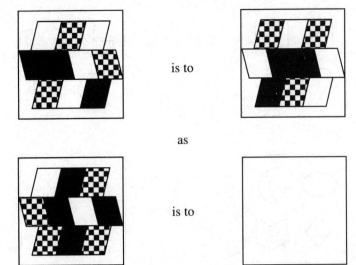

is to

as

is to

84. Which figure completes the statement?

A.   **B.**   **C.**   **D.**

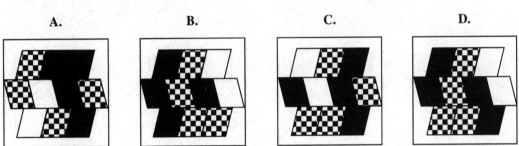

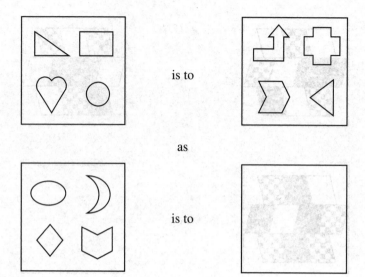

is to

as

is to

85. Which figure completes the statement?

A.   B.   C.   D.

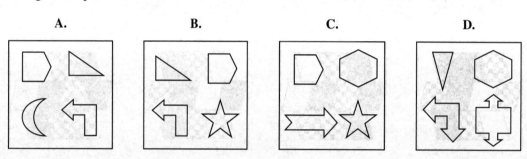

Kaplan Timed Practice Set—*Type 2 and Type 3 Questions*: Answers and Explanations

81. (D)

The figure in each step of the sequence is made up of seven rectangles, which are white, black or grey. The three shadings move vertically up the three horizontal rectangles at the left side of the figure, with the top shading moving to the bottom of these three positions. The shadings of these three rectangles in the fourth step match the shadings in the first step, indicating that the cycle repeats every three steps. Thus, the shadings of these three rectangles in the fifth step—the correct answer—will match the second step. Eliminate **(A)**. The shadings of the other four rectangles move horizontally to the left with each step; since there are four rectangles and four shadings, this cycle repeats every four steps. As a result, the shadings of these four rectangles in the fifth step will match the first step: black, white, grey, white. Answer **(D)** is correct.

82. (B)

The shapes rotate around the corners of the box, moving one position anticlockwise with each step of the sequence; their colours move one shape anticlockwise at the same time, so that the heart's colour moves to the hexagon in the next step, the hexagon's colour moves to the flag, and so on. Since there are four shapes and four colours, the cycle repeats every four steps. As a result, the shapes and colours are in the same corners of the box in the fifth step—the correct answer—as in the first step. However, the orientation of the shapes is not necessarily the same. Note that the pentagon moves from the upper-left corner to the lower-left in the first two steps without rotating; we can see that the flag and the hexagon do the same in subsequent steps. Thus, the upside-down heart in the upper-left corner of the fourth step must move to the lower-left corner without rotating in the fifth step. Eliminate **(C)** and **(D)**. The only difference in the remaining answers is the orientation of the hexagon. In the initial steps, the heart moves from the lower-left corner to the lower-right corner whilst also rotating 90° anticlockwise; the pentagon and the flag make similar rotations when making the same move in subsequent steps. The hexagon must therefore rotate 90° anticlockwise from the fourth step to the fifth. The correct answer is **(B)**.

83. (A)

In the first box, the cross is surrounded by seven small shapes located at its outer vertices; the eighth position (the upper-right outer vertex in the first box) is effectively blank. In the second box, all the shapes have moved; note that all the shapes that were originally on the left are still on the left, and all those originally on the right are still on the right. This indicates that the shapes have moved within their half of the box; you can analyse each half of the box independently. In the left half, all the shapes retain the same colour from the first box to the second; the upper shapes and lower shapes have simply swapped places vertically. In the right half of the first box, the four positions (clockwise from the top) are blank, octagon, D-shape, circle; in the second box, each moves one position clockwise, so the circle takes the blank space, the blank space takes the octagon's space, and so on. The colours have also rotated one position clockwise within the three shapes in the right half. In the second row, the large background figure is an octagon instead of a cross, with the small shapes arranged inside the eight vertices of the octagon. Since the eight positions for the small shapes are paired vertically—very similar to the first row—the same logic applies. The small shapes in the left half of the box must swap positions vertically, whilst retaining their original colours. Eliminate **(B)** and **(C)**. The shapes in the right half of the box must rotate one position clockwise, which means the star will move to the top position, replaced in the bottom position by the blank space. The colours in the right half of the box must also rotate clockwise, so that the star is grey, the hexagon black and the teardrop white. Answer **(A)** is correct.

84. (C)

The figure in each box consists of ten parallelograms: three in the top row, four in the middle row and three in the bottom row. Some are white; some are black; some are chequered. It might be simplest to think of the ten parallelograms as a blank (white) surface, across which the black and chequered segments move. In the first row, the black segments move one parallelogram to the right from the first box to the second. In the second row, then, the black parallelogram in the top row should move from the middle position to the right position, whilst the black parallelogram in the bottom row moves in the same way (from the bottom-middle to bottom-right). The black parallelogram in the middle-left position in the middle row should move to the middle-right position, whilst the black parallelogram in the rightmost position in the middle row should move to the leftmost position. Only **(C)** has the black parallelograms in the correct positions; **(C)** is correct.

For the record: The chequered parallelograms move one position anticlockwise around the outside of the figure (all but the two middle positions in the middle row). Any position not covered by a black or chequered segment is white (blank), so there is no 'logic' to the white segments – they are not moving.

85. (D)

Each box contains 4 white shapes, and the shapes in the 1st and 2nd boxes are entirely different. This means that the type of shape cannot be part of the progression. Compare the shapes in the same relative position in the top two boxes: the upper-left shape changes from a triangle to a bent arrow, the upper-right shape changes from a rectangle to a cross, the lower-right shape changes from a circle to a triangle, and the lower-left shape changes from a heart to a chevron. Each shape in the second box in the top row, then, has three times as many sides as the shape in the same position in the first box. The shapes in the first box in the bottom row (going clockwise, starting in the upper-left) have 1, 2, 6 and 4 sides, respectively, so the shapes in the correct answer must have 3, 6, 18 and 12 sides. The correct answer is therefore **(D)**.

For the record: Answer **(C)** is a trap answer; each shape in **(C)** has 4 more sides than the corresponding shape in the same position in the first box in the bottom row. Whilst this is a logical progression, it is not the same as the progression in the top row. You must first find the progression in the top row, then apply it to the bottom row to work out the correct answer.

Remember

The pace is quite different in Type 2 and Type 3 questions. In Type 1 and Type 4, you can use the fact that the questions come in sets of 5 to your advantage; taking time to find the pattern before attacking the test shapes will yield most of the marks in this section. In Type 2 and Type 3 questions, do your best to pick up any marks that are achievable in 15–20 seconds (at most!) per question. Any longer, and you may run out of time for remaining sets in the section.

Keeping Perspective—Abstract Reasoning

You are about to complete a timed Kaplan UKCAT Abstract Reasoning quiz, consisting of 6 sets with 5 test shapes each. Pace yourself, and spend no more than 1 minute per set. Even if you find yourself running out of time near the end, make your best guess based on any partial patterns you can find. It is essential that you get in the mindset of marking an answer for every question, and that you practise doing so as you complete several sets under UKCAT time pressure.

Before you begin the quiz, let's review the Kaplan top tips for Abstract mastery.

Know the common pattern categories. There are only so many building blocks for the patterns that the UKCAT can present on Test Day. Eventually you will develop an 'eye' for all of them. Be sure to consider the types of shapes, features of shapes and arrangement when you first examine each set.

Start with the simplest box in each set. Since the simplest box in each set must contain the pattern, starting with this box will prevent you from becoming lost in distractor shapes and allow you to quickly eliminate pattern categories.

Search for simple patterns first. Don't assume every set is going to be high difficulty. The truth is that you will see many straightforward sets on Test Day. Picking up all (or most) of these marks will ensure you do very well in the Abstract section.

If an aspect of a set seems very unusual, it's probably part of the pattern. If you do see an unusual feature, focus in on it. It is unlikely to have been included to distract you and is almost certainly part of the pattern.

Type 2 and Type 3 questions are about progressions, not patterns. Progressions are about what is different from one box to the next, so these are generally a bit easier to spot than patterns. However, don't fall for the common trap of identifying all elements of a progression before checking the answers. As soon as you see one element of the progression—a change in colour, or a rotation or 'moving' shape—go straight to the answers and eliminate those that do not match that element. The progression in most Type 2 and Type 3 questions will have 4 or more elements, but you can answer virtually any of them by finding only 2 or 3 elements of the progression. Don't do any work beyond the minimum necessary to determine the correct answer.

Be ruthless in moving forward. The wisest test-taker knows when a set has been designed to trap test-takers into wasting time. If you've spent a minute on a set, take a guess and move on. Mark the questions for review and, instead of feeling upset that you couldn't see the pattern, feel happy that you didn't fall into the trap of wasting time, as so many other test-takers will have done.

Chapter 6 Kaplan UKCAT Quiz

Set your timer for 7 minutes. Try to evaluate all 30 items and mark an answer for each before time is up. If a pattern is difficult, don't spend much more than a minute; mark an answer, make your best guess and move on to the other sets. Use any time remaining to come back to sets where you had difficulty in spotting the pattern.

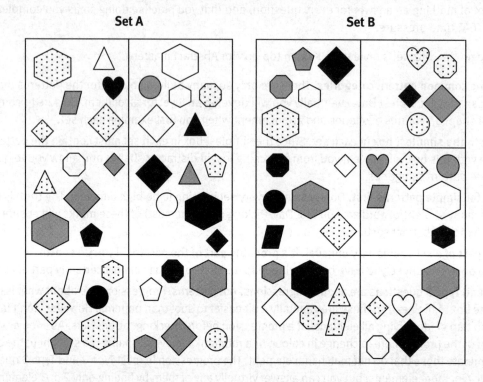

Set A   Set B

Test Shapes

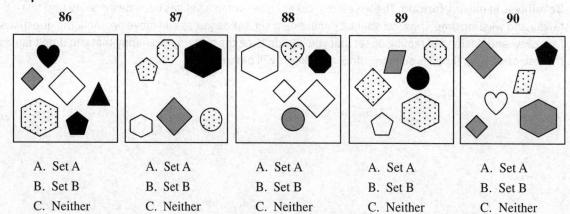

| 86 | 87 | 88 | 89 | 90 |

A. Set A	A. Set A	A. Set A	A. Set A	A. Set A
B. Set B	B. Set B	B. Set B	B. Set B	B. Set B
C. Neither	C. Neither	C. Neither	C. Neither	C. Neither

Set A	Set B
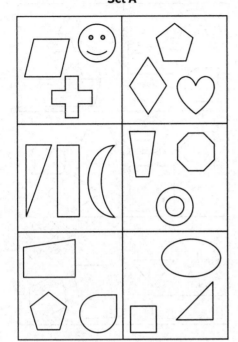	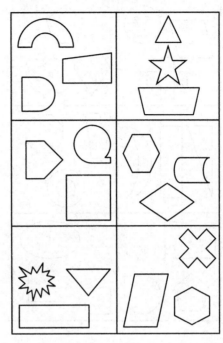

91. Which of the following test shapes belongs in Set A?

A.	B.	C.	D.
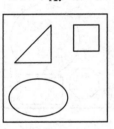	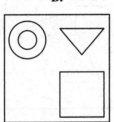	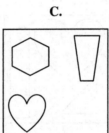	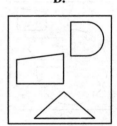

92. Which of the following test shapes belongs in Set B?

A.	B.	C.	D.
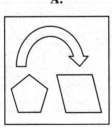	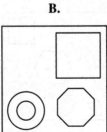	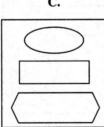	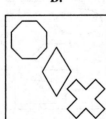

Set A   **Set B**

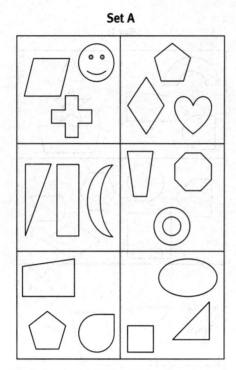 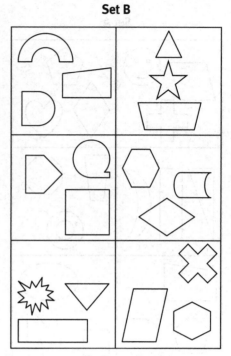

93.   Which of the following test shapes belongs in Set A?

A.   B.   C.   D.

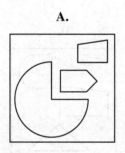 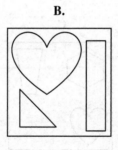 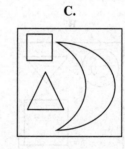 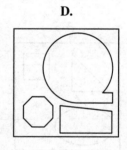

94.   Which of the following test shapes belongs in Set B?

A.   B.   C.   D.

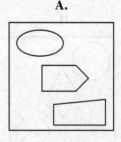 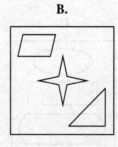 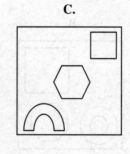 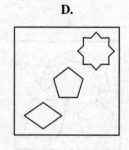

95.   Which of the following test shapes belongs in Set B?

A.   B.   C.   D.

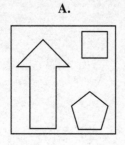 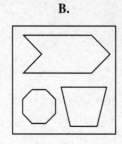 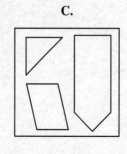 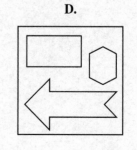

Set A

Set B

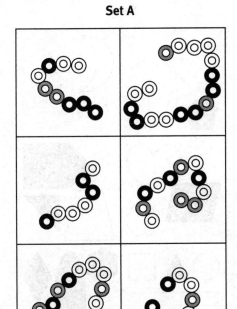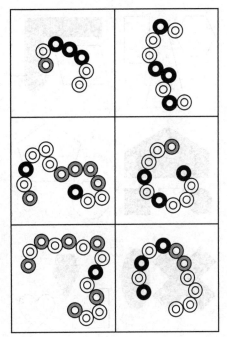

Test Shapes

96	97	98	99	100

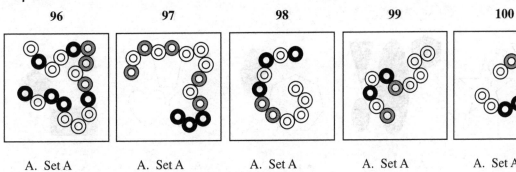

A. Set A	A. Set A	A. Set A	A. Set A	A. Set A
B. Set B	B. Set B	B. Set B	B. Set B	B. Set B
C. Neither	C. Neither	C. Neither	C. Neither	C. Neither

Set A

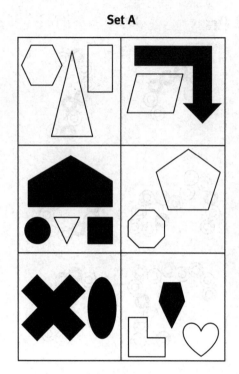

Set B

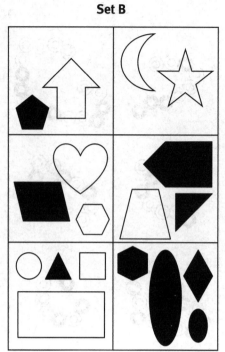

Test Shapes

101	102	103	104	105

A. Set A
B. Set B
C. Neither

A. Set A
B. Set B
C. Neither

A. Set A
B. Set B
C. Neither

A. Set A
B. Set B
C. Neither

A. Set A
B. Set B
C. Neither

Set A   **Set B**

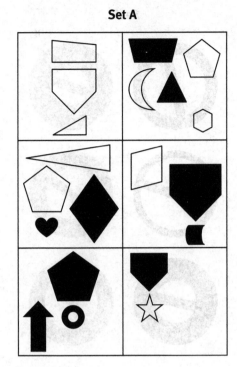
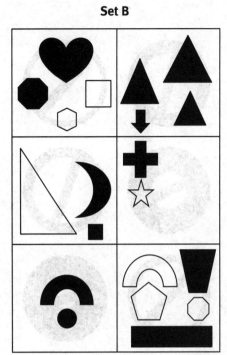

Test Shapes

106	107	108	109	110

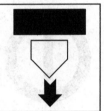
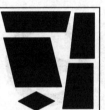
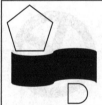

106	107	108	109	110
A. Set A	A. Set A	A. Set A	A. Set A	A. Set A
B. Set B	B. Set B	B. Set B	B. Set B	B. Set B
C. Neither	C. Neither	C. Neither	C. Neither	C. Neither

Set A   **Set B**

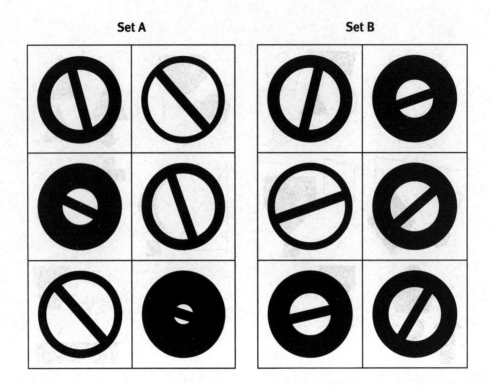

Test Shapes

111	112	113	114	115

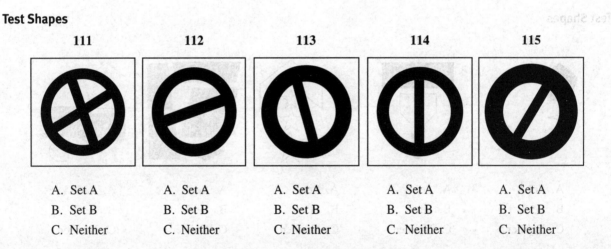

A. Set A   A. Set A   A. Set A   A. Set A   A. Set A
B. Set B   B. Set B   B. Set B   B. Set B   B. Set B
C. Neither C. Neither C. Neither C. Neither C. Neither

STOP. IF YOU FINISH BEFORE TIME IS UP, CHECK ANY QUESTIONS YOU HAVE MARKED FOR REVIEW. YOU MAY GO BACK TO QUESTIONS IN THIS QUIZ ONLY.

Chapter 6 Kaplan UKCAT Quiz: Answers and Explanations

86. (B)

All the boxes contain six shapes: a medium-sized hexagon and diamond, a smaller version of one of those shapes, with three further smaller shapes. None of the smaller shapes is repeated in the same box, and none of the smaller shapes (besides the hexagon/diamond) appears in every box in either set. The patterns are all about colour. In Set A, the larger hexagon and diamond are the same colour, and they match the smaller version of the hexagon/diamond; the other three smaller shapes in the box are different colours (white, black, grey, dotted). In Set B, the two larger shapes and the smaller hexagon/diamond are three different colours (white, black, grey, dotted); the other three smaller shapes are all the same, fourth colour.

The smaller shapes in the first test shape are a grey diamond and three black shapes: a heart, a triangle and a pentagon. The two larger shapes are a dotted hexagon and a white diamond. With these colours, the test shape belongs to Set B.

87. (B)

Three of the smaller shapes – the octagon, the pentagon and the circle – are dotted, whilst the small hexagon is white. The large hexagon is black, and the large diamond is grey. This test shape fits the pattern for Set B.

88. (A)

The large hexagon and diamond are white, matching the smaller diamond. The other three small shapes are a dotted heart, a black octagon and a grey circle. This test shape belongs to Set A.

89. (C)

The large hexagon and diamond are dotted, matching the small octagon. The other three small shapes are a grey parallelogram, a black circle and a white pentagon. There isn't a smaller hexagon or diamond, so the test shape cannot belong to Set A or Set B.

90. (A)

The large hexagon and diamond are grey, matching the smaller diamond. The other three small shapes are a white heart, a dotted parallelogram and a black pentagon, fitting the pattern for Set A.

91. (D)

All the boxes contain three white shapes; one shape in each box is a quadrilateral. In Set A, the quadrilateral is to the left of a curved shape. In Set B, the quadrilateral is below a concave shape.

The first question asks about Set A, so the quadrilateral should be to the left of the curved shape. In three of the answers, the curved shape is to the left of the quadrilateral. The quadrilateral in **(D)** is to the left of the D-shape, so it fits the pattern for Set A. Answer **(D)** is correct.

92. (A)

This question asks for a test shape that belongs to Set B, so the correct answer must have a quadrilateral below a concave shape. The curved arrow in **(A)** is concave, and the parallelogram is below it. The correct answer is **(A)**.

93. (C)

For a test shape to belong to Set A, there must be a quadrilateral to the left of a curved shape. The square in **(C)** is to the left of the crescent. The answer is therefore **(C)**.

94. (D)

This question asks for a test shape that belongs to Set B. Find the test shape with a quadrilateral below a concave shape. The diamond in **(D)** is below the 8-pointed star, so **(D)** is correct.

95. (B)

Three of the test shapes (all but **(C)**) include a concave shape; only **(B)** has the quadrilateral below the concave shape. **(B)** is therefore correct. NB that in wrong answer trap **(A)**, the square would be considered to be above the arrow, since the top of the square is slightly higher in the box than the top of the arrow. A subtle but essential distinction.

96. (B)

Each box contains a single figure made up of several rings, which are white, black or grey. All three colours appear in all the boxes (except the middle-left box of Set A), so you may be tempted to count the number of rings of each colour in each box, or the number of rings of each colour that are grouped together, but this will not yield a pattern in either set. Instead, the pattern is about the arrangement of some of the white rings. In Set A, the rings in the upper-right part of the figure are white; in Set B, the rings in the lower-right part of the figure are white. In each set, one or more white rings in the relevant position are all that is required for the pattern.

The first test shape has white rings in the lower-right part of the figure, so it belongs to Set B.

97. (A)

This test shape has white rings in the upper-right part of the figure, so it belongs to Set A.

98. (B)

The lower-right end of this figure consists of white rings, fitting the pattern for Set B.

99. (A)

The upper-right end of this figure consists of white rings, fitting the pattern for Set A.

100. (C)

The upper-left and lower-left ends of this figure are white rings; the upper-right and lower-right portions of the figure are grey and black, respectively. Since there are no white rings in the upper-right or the lower-right part of the figure, it belongs to neither set.

101. (A)

The total number of sides in each box in Set A is 13. The total number of sides in each box in Set B is 12.

The first test shape includes a star and a triangle, with a total of 13 sides. It belongs to Set A.

102. (C)

This box contains a hexagon, a triangle and two ovals. The total number of sides is 11. The test shape belongs to neither set.

103. (B)

The heptagon and pentagon in this box have a total of 12 sides. The answer is **(B)**.

104. (C)

This box includes an octagon, a trapezium and a heart. The total number of sides is 14. The answer is **(C)**.

105. (A)

This test shape features a pentagon and two quadrilaterals, with a total of 13 sides. The answer is **(A)**.

106. (C)

The simplest box in Set A contains a black pentagon above a smaller white star. The simplest boxes in Set B contain a black arch above a smaller black circle and a black cross above a smaller white star. In Set A, then, the smallest shape is directly below a pentagon. In Set B, the smallest shape is directly below a black shape. Note that the other shapes, and the colours of the shapes, are distractors.

The first test shape includes a small white star below a larger black pentagon. Since the smallest shape is below a pentagon, it fits the pattern for Set A. However, the smallest shape is below a black shape, so it also fits the pattern for Set B. The answer is therefore **(C)**.

107. (A)

The smallest shape, the black arrows, is directly below a white pentagon. The test shape belongs to Set A.

108. (C)

There are no pentagons, so the test shape cannot belong to Set A. There are no black shapes, so the test shape cannot belong to Set B. It belongs to neither set.

109. (B)

The smallest shape is the black diamond, directly below a black parallelogram. The test shape belongs to Set B.

110. (B)

The white D-shape is the smallest shape in this test shape. Since the D-shape is below a black shape, the test shape fits the pattern for Set B.

111. (C)

The sets here are very similar looking—remember to consider an arrangement pattern when the sets contain identical shapes. The lines in Set A are downward-sloping, while the lines in Set B are upward-sloping. The first test shape has two crossed lines. This is clearly different from Set A and Set B, so the correct answer is **(C)**.

112. (B)

This test shape has a line that slopes upward. The correct answer is **(B)**.

113. (A)

The downward-sloping line means this test shape belongs to Set A.

114. (C)

The line in this shape is vertical, so it cannot belong to either set. The answer is **(C)**.

115. (B)

This test shape has an upward-sloping line, so the answer is **(B)**.

Situational Judgement

The Task

Situational Judgement is the fifth and final section of the UKCAT. Unlike the previous four sections, you do not receive a scaled score from 300 to 900 in Situational Judgement; instead, you are assessed from Band 1 to Band 4. The band reflects the degree to which the answers you chose match the correct answers as determined by a panel of medical experts: Band 1 means that most of your answers were the same as the panel of medical experts; Band 4 means that very few of your answers were the same. Thus, the task in Situational Judgement is to pick the same answer as the panel of medical experts. You have 26 minutes to answer 68 items, so you must work very quickly.

The Format

The Situational Judgement section consists of 21 scenarios, each accompanied by 2 to 6 items. The scenarios are drawn from real-life clinical and educational situations, and you must consider how a doctor, dentist or student would respond in the circumstances described. Most scenarios will involve a conflict between what a clinician or student is meant to be doing and an interfering issue that arises. The interfering issue could be a problematic behaviour by a patient or a fellow student or clinician, or a 'life issue' that could make it difficult to carry on as normal.

The first part of the section—just over slightly half of the items—are appropriateness questions, in which you must assess whether possible responses to the situation in the scenario are appropriate or inappropriate. The final part of the section—just under half of the items—are importance questions, in which you must decide whether a series of factors are important or not important in deciding how to respond to the scenario.

Both types of questions include four answer choices, so you must choose a side: appropriate/inappropriate, or important/not important. There is no middle option. Also, you must consider each possible response/factor independently of the others in the scenario. This means that each answer choice can be correct more than once in a given scenario. In fact, when you review the Situational Judgement scenarios in the official UKCAT practice materials, you'll notice that some scenarios have the same correct answer for all possible responses. Thus, it's essential that you consider each response on its own, without any regard for which answers have already been correct in that same scenario.

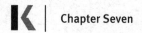

The Challenges

The most obvious challenge in Situational Judgement is timing: 68 questions and 21 scenarios in 26 minutes means that you have only about 30 seconds to read each scenario, and 10–15 seconds to answer each question. If you work any more slowly, you will run out of time.

The other major challenge in Situational Judgement is the fact that the correct answers are based on principles of medical professionalism that are well known and 'obvious' to the medical experts who have decided the correct answers, but are likely far from obvious to the vast majority of UKCAT test-takers, who are mostly sixth-formers with limited medical experience. Even so, you are likely to have at least a vague awareness of some of these issues, and you can sharpen this relatively easily as you practise ahead of your UKCAT Test Day.

Whilst it is true that none of the items requires 'medical or procedural knowledge' (in the words of the UKCAT test-maker), you will find it difficult to score in Band 1 or Band 2 unless you familiarise yourself with the principles of medical professionalism. In this sense, Situational Judgement is the only section of the UKCAT with very specific content that you must revise before Test Day in order to achieve a high score.

Kaplan Top Tips for Situational Judgement

1. Read the scenario first

This may seem like an obvious point, but we have found that many students initially approach Situational Judgement using their well-honed Verbal Reasoning instincts and go right to the first response option, and then scan the scenario for support. There's a real temptation to do so, as Situational Judgement uses the same visual interface as Verbal Reasoning, with the scenario on the left -hand side of the screen and the response options one at a time on the right-hand side. However, you must always read the scenario before attempting the first response, as you must understand the conflicting issues involved before deciding on appropriateness or importance. If you try to rush and only scan the scenarios, you are highly likely to miss out essential words that could make a huge difference to your understanding of the scenario. It shouldn't take more than 20–30 seconds to read each scenario, so practise for this timing—and for always reading the scenario first—as you revise.

2. Choose a side

As you read each of the response options, get used to making a 'snap judgement' and choosing a side. Decide quickly if the response is appropriate or inappropriate, or if a factor is important or not important. While there will be a few responses or factors that will be very tough to assess quickly, even for the most experienced of medical professionals, the vast majority are relatively straightforward, and you will save valuable time—and maximise your marks—by practising and preparing to choose a side quickly and confidently as often as possible.

3. Know when it's OK to choose (B) or (C)

Unlike in the other sections of the UKCAT, the four answer choices in Situational Judgement do not have an equal probability of being correct. In the official Situational Judgement practice materials from the UKCAT Consortium, answers **(A)** and **(D)** are correct about 70% of the time, and answers **(B)** and **(C)** are correct about 30% of the time. This means that, most of the time, simply choosing a side will be sufficient to get to the correct answer. The partial marking is likely to help with this as well. It is not entirely clear how the partial marking works—the test-maker has provided no information on this—however, the most logical possibility is that you receive partial marks for giving an answer that is close to the correct answer. For example, if the correct answer is **(C)** and you choose **(D)**, then you would get partial marks for choosing **(D)**.

It is OK to choose **(B)** or **(C)** when the response is less than optimal for some reason, and when the possible negative consequences of that response are not severe. If the negative consequences could be severe, then the correct answer is **(D)**.

4. Learn the key principles of medical professionalism

You will have plenty of time to learn and practise these in real-life settings as you proceed through your medical or dental education, and in your early career as a clinician. However, you are expected to have a basic knowledge of the key principles of medical professionalism in order to obtain a respectable score in Situational Judgement on the UKCAT.

There are two key ways to build your knowledge of these key principles:

1. **Review all the official Situational Judgement practice questions and answers**. This includes all questions in the online UKCAT practice tests available on the UKCAT website, as well as the questions in the official UKCAT practice app. Be sure to download and work through the questions in the UKCAT Official Guide, a PDF that is available on the UKCAT website. This PDF repeats many of the same questions from the app, but in a great format for reading through the official questions and worked answers, so you can start to understand why the correct answers are correct.

2. **Download and review the free booklet *Good Medical Practice*, available from the General Medical Council website.** All the key principles of medical professionalism are drawn from this 40-page booklet. Copies are normally given out to medical students as part of their medical education, so you will get a head start on learning its contents as you prepare for the UKCAT. Whilst this booklet is not explicitly mentioned in the worked answers to the official Situational Judgement questions, you will notice many references to the content of the booklet, and the occasional reference to the General Medical Council. The more time you invest learning these key principles, the more confident and prepared you will be for Situational Judgement questions on Test Day.

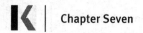

Kaplan Timed Practice Set—*Try the Kaplan Top Tips*

Set your timer for 90 seconds. Mark answers for all 5 questions before time is up!

> Lucy is a medical student at the university hospital. Several of the consultants have just returned from a leaving lunch for one of their colleagues. Lucy notices one of the consultants, Dr Perkins, struggling to maintain his balance in the corridor. Dr Perkins stumbles into Lucy, and she can smell whisky on his breath. Lucy asks if everything is all right, and Dr Perkins says he is in a rush, as he has a patient waiting on the operating table.

How **appropriate** are each of the following responses by **Lucy** in this situation?

1. Take Dr Perkins to one side and suggest he is not in a fit state to interact with patients

    A. A very appropriate thing to do
    B. Appropriate, but not ideal
    C. Inappropriate, but not awful
    D. A very inappropriate thing to do

2. Inform the patient that the surgery will not take place

    A. A very appropriate thing to do
    B. Appropriate, but not ideal
    C. Inappropriate, but not awful
    D. A very inappropriate thing to do

3. Email a formal complaint against Dr Perkins to the hospital chairman

    A. A very appropriate thing to do
    B. Appropriate, but not ideal
    C. Inappropriate, but not awful
    D. A very inappropriate thing to do

4. Seek immediate advice from the consultant that supervises her work at the hospital

    A. A very appropriate thing to do
    B. Appropriate, but not ideal
    C. Inappropriate, but not awful
    D. A very inappropriate thing to do

5. Check with the surgical nurse to determine whether Dr Perkins is actually about to perform surgery

    A. A very appropriate thing to do
    B. Appropriate, but not ideal
    C. Inappropriate, but not awful
    D. A very inappropriate thing to do

Kaplan Timed Practice Set—*Try the Kaplan Top Tips*: Answers and Explanations

How did you get on with your first timed set? If you worked efficiently, you should have been able to read the scenario and assess all 5 response options in 90 seconds. If you struggled here, be sure to try to spend no more than 30 seconds reading the scenario in the upcoming sets in this chapter. You'll also want to keep to no more than 10-15 seconds per response option—if you are taking longer to deliberate, then you will miss out quite a lot of items at the end of the section. We'll cover a few more tips to help with pacing in this chapter. For now, here are the worked answers for this first set.

1. (A)

Since it is very clear to Lucy that Dr Perkins is under the influence of alcohol, then it would be just as clear to any patients that he encounters in his current state. Thus, it is highly appropriate for Lucy to take him to one side and suggest that he should avoid interacting with patients. A medical student might feel uncomfortable addressing this issue with a consultant, but Dr Perkins's behaviour here is especially egregious. There is a real risk to public confidence in the profession, not to mention to the patient's life if the doctor were to perform surgery—so Lucy would be entirely correct to intervene in this manner.

2. (D)

It would seriously undermine the patient's confidence in the medical profession to hear from a medical student, rather than a doctor in charge of the patient's care, that a surgery will not take place. This response option is therefore highly inappropriate.

3. (D)

Responses that involve formal complaints or written complaints are usually considered very inappropriate. This response is especially so, as there is no guarantee that the hospital chairman would read the email or be able to do anything about it before Dr Perkins heads into the operating theatre. This response does nothing to address the real risk to patient safety and the patient's confidence in the profession, and is not a local solution.

4. (A)

It is always very appropriate for a medical professional to seek advice from a senior colleague, and even more so in the case of a medical student who is encountering an ethically perilous situation for the first time.

5. (B)

This response is not inappropriate, as the surgical nurse is a good person to confirm this detail for Lucy. However, it's less than ideal, as determining whether Dr Perkins actually has a patient scheduled for surgery does nothing to address the fact that the doctor is not in a fit state to see patients.

Score Higher Online

Situational Judgement tends to change slightly from year to year—for example, the overall number of questions or passages may vary slightly in 2018 from last year's exam.

Check your Kaplan Online Centre in June for the latest test updates, which will include any changes to the Situational Judgement section. These changes are usually announced by the test-maker in early May; we'll need to review all the official practice questions to confirm the extent of the changes and give you the most accurate info in the online update.

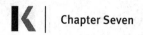

Appropriateness Scenarios

In the first half of the Situational Judgement section, you will be asked to decide the appropriateness of possible responses to the scenario. You must assess each option in an Appropriateness scenario independently of the others. Thus, you should not assume that each answer choice will be used once, or that there will be one best response among the options given. A scenario could have a series of possible responses that are all very appropriate, or all very inappropriate, or some mix of the two.

You must decide on the appropriateness of the possible responses based on the details in the scenario, and evaluate these according to the principles of medical professionalism. Some of the key principles that come up again and again in Situational Judgement include:

- Doctors and medical students must not do anything to undermine public confidence in the profession, and must act promptly to address a situation in which public confidence in the profession is at risk.
- Doctors and medical students must never act or imply that they have knowledge, expertise or experience beyond their actual level of knowledge, expertise or experience.
- Doctors and medical students should seek advice from a colleague or supervisor if they are unsure of the best course of action.
- Doctors and medical students should seek local solutions to problems that arise wherever possible and practicable.

You can get a full sense of the range of principles of medical professionalism that you may encounter in the Situational Judgement section on Test Day by reviewing the booklet *Good Medical Practice*.

Try to put the principles of medical professionalism into practice in the following Appropriateness scenario. Spend 30 seconds reading the scenario, then no more than 15 seconds assessing each response before reading the answer.

> As he is walking through the ward, a junior doctor, Bao, notices a patient waving him to come to her bedside. Bao approaches the patient, who says that no one will tell her what is wrong with her, and she wants to know if she can get treatment to help her stop feeling tired all the time and getting so many infections. Bao checks the patient's chart, and sees that she is 14 years old and has just been diagnosed with leukaemia.

How **appropriate** are each of the following responses by **Bao** in this situation?

6. Explain immediately to the patient that she has leukaemia, and answer any questions she has about her diagnosis

    A. A very appropriate thing to do
    B. Appropriate, but not ideal
    C. Inappropriate, but not awful
    D. A very inappropriate thing to do

Answer: From the patient's comments, it is very likely that she has not been informed of her diagnosis. Since Bao is not responsible for her care, it would be very inappropriate for him to share such a diagnosis with a patient who is a child in this way, in the absence of her parents and the doctor responsible for her care. The correct answer is **(D)**.

---

7.   Ask if there is anything in particular that he can do to help

     A.   A very appropriate thing to do
     B.   Appropriate, but not ideal
     C.   Inappropriate, but not awful
     D.   A very inappropriate thing to do

Answer: This is quite a neutral question, so it is not inappropriate. However, it is less than an ideal response, as the patient has already made a specific request for information about her diagnosis and recommended treatment, so Bao should already have a clear idea of what can be done to help the patient. Answer **(B)** is correct.

8.   Encourage the patient to discuss her concerns together with her parents and the doctor responsible for her care

     A.   A very appropriate thing to do
     B.   Appropriate, but not ideal
     C.   Inappropriate, but not awful
     D.   A very inappropriate thing to do

Answer: This response is highly appropriate, as it guides the patient to initiate this important and necessary conversation with the people who are best positioned to provide the emotional support she will need as she comes to terms with her diagnosis and begins treatment. The answer is **(A)**.

9.   Offer to speak to the patient's parents on her behalf

     A.   A very appropriate thing to do
     B.   Appropriate, but not ideal
     C.   Inappropriate, but not awful
     D.   A very inappropriate thing to do

Answer: Bao knows nothing about the patient's family situation; given that the patient is clearly unaware of her diagnosis, Bao should be careful not to do anything that implies that her parents have not told her something, or that there is a reason a discussion might need to be had with the patient's parents that does not involve the patient. It is likely, for example, that the patient's parents have just been told the diagnosis and need a short amount of time to process it themselves so they can be ready to support their daughter. Bao should not do anything that could imply to the patient that her parents are keeping something from her, or that they have done something wrong—so this option is highly inappropriate, answer **(D)**.

10.   Offer to speak to the doctor responsible for the patient's care on her behalf

     A.   A very appropriate thing to do
     B.   Appropriate, but not ideal
     C.   Inappropriate, but not awful
     D.   A very inappropriate thing to do

Answer: This is a very appropriate response, as it deflects the patient's concerns to the doctor responsible for her care. This doctor may not be aware of just how anxious the patient is; speaking to this doctor on the patient's behalf would address her concerns while also ensuring quality of care. Answer **(A)** is correct.

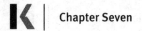

Kaplan Timed Practice Set—Appropriateness Scenarios

Set your timer for 90 seconds. Mark answers for all 5 questions before time is up!

> Imogen is a junior doctor at a large GP practice in a small city. One day, she has a consultation with a patient, Jade, who is in her final year of sixth form. Jade wants to discuss other options for birth control, since she sometimes forgets to take the pill. Looking over Jade's notes, Imogen sees that Jade has been treated twice for the same sexually transmitted infection. Due to her religious beliefs, Imogen is strongly opposed to the use of birth control and sex outside of marriage.

How **appropriate** are each of the following responses by **Imogen** in this situation?

11. Arrange for Jade to have a consultation with another doctor at the practice
    A. A very appropriate thing to do
    B. Appropriate, but not ideal
    C. Inappropriate, but not awful
    D. A very inappropriate thing to do

12. Advise Jade that she needs to start making better choices with regard to her sexual health
    A. A very appropriate thing to do
    B. Appropriate, but not ideal
    C. Inappropriate, but not awful
    D. A very inappropriate thing to do

13. Tell Jade that she is unable to provide any birth control options
    A. A very appropriate thing to do
    B. Appropriate, but not ideal
    C. Inappropriate, but not awful
    D. A very inappropriate thing to do

14. Call Jade's mum to discuss her concerns about Jade's sexual behaviour
    A. A very appropriate thing to do
    B. Appropriate, but not ideal
    C. Inappropriate, but not awful
    D. A very inappropriate thing to do

15. Ask Jade if there is anything else she would like to discuss with regard to her sexual health
    A. A very appropriate thing to do
    B. Appropriate, but not ideal
    C. Inappropriate, but not awful
    D. A very inappropriate thing to do

Kaplan Timed Practice Set—*Appropriateness Scenarios*: Answers and Explanations

In this scenario, there were two different issues to consider: the doctor's religious beliefs and the patient's sexual history, including her current request to switch to a different form of birth control. Notice that the scenario seems to set up a conflict between the two, but they are not necessarily in conflict. It's entirely possible for the doctor to behave ethically towards the patient, without passing judgement on her sexual history or her current request.

Also, note that it's not entirely clear that there is anything wrong with the patient's current choices with regard to her sexual health. She seems to have made some poor choices in the past, but she has decided to change to another form of birth control that will not rely on her remembering to take a pill every day, so this shows a degree of conscience and responsibility. Be careful not to infer a conflict between two different issues in a Situational Judgement scenario, unless the conflict is clearly stated in the scenario. If a possible response causes conflict, then assess it appropriately (as appropriate or inappropriate, depending on the nature of the conflict).

11. (A)

When a doctor has a religious objection to a particular procedure or treatment option, the General Medical Council requires that the doctor ensure that the patient can see another doctor. Thus, it would be entirely appropriate for Imogen to arrange for Jade to have a consultation with another doctor at the practice who can advise her on alternate birth control options and provide a suitable option.

12. (D)

It would be quite disrespectful for a doctor to make such a statement to a patient; in this case, Jade has been treated for STIs in the past, but she has acknowledged that she has trouble adhering to her birth control prescription, so she is actively seeking out an alternative form of birth control. She does not seem to have any other problems with her sexual health at the moment, and she seems to be in control of the choices she is making, so this comment is not at all appropriate.

13. (C)

This statement is factually correct, since Imogen has a religious objection to providing birth control to Jade or any patient. Thus, it is not awful. However, the response is inappropriate, since it does not make clear that the reason that birth control cannot be provided is due to a conscientious objection.

14. (D)

Jade's age is not clear, but the fact that she is in sixth form suggests that she is likely 17 or 18. Anyone aged 16 or older is legally allowed to consent to their own medical treatment, so it would be a grave violation of Jade's confidentiality for Imogen to call Jade's mother and disclose any information about Jade's sexual history from her medical records. This response is wholly inappropriate, and would likely result in severe professional consequences for Imogen.

15. (A)

This is quite a neutral question, and given that Jade is sexually active and has been treated previously for STIs, it would be very appropriate for Imogen to encourage Jade to share any other concerns or questions she might have. Imogen might not be comfortable with Jade's response, but this conversation could be very useful to Jade, and GPs are expected to discuss patients' needs and concerns regarding contraception and safer sex.

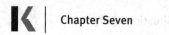

Importance Scenarios

The final few scenarios in the Situational Judgement section will ask you to assess the importance of a series of factors in deciding how to respond to the situation in the scenario. Just like with the possible responses to Appropriateness scenarios, you must assess these factors independently of each other. There may not necessarily be a 'best', or single 'very important', factor; there could be multiple very important factors, or multiple 'not at all important' factors.

In assessing the factors, you should only consider the implications to the person deciding how to respond if the factor is true. The principles of medical professionalism will help again here, with a few extra Kaplan top tips:

- Factors that mean the decider would be more aware of the principles of ethics or medical professionalism that have direct bearing on the scenario will generally be important or very important.

- Factors that are external pressures on the decider, with limited (or no) direct relevance to patients in the scenario, or to the principles of ethics or medical professionalism, will generally be of minor importance or not at all important.

- Factors that relate to the relationship (professional or otherwise) of the people directly involved in the scenario can sometimes be tricky to assess. Don't fret about these—they are tricky for everyone.

- Many of the Importance scenarios will involve doctors or medical students committing (or about to commit) gross misconduct, or other serious ethical or legal breaches. If you're a sixth-former, obviously you are unlikely to be aware of all of the nuances of issues that could be gross misconduct. Several of these (e.g. those that could get you struck off by the GMC) are detailed in *Good Medical Practice*, so it is well worth reviewing this booklet ahead of Test Day.

Put these Kaplan top tips into practice with the following Importance scenario. Be sure to read the scenario before assessing the factors, and be sure to mark an answer for each item before reading the answer. If you are unsure, try at least to choose a side (important or unimportant) and mark an answer on that side.

> A medical student, Ruchira, enters the supply cupboard at the university hospital to discover another medical student, Jake, sat there with a credit card in his hand, typing on his laptop. Ruchira can see that Jake is using a website notorious for selling essays to students. Jake closes the laptop quickly, and asks if Ruchira is spying on him.

How **important** to take into account are the following considerations for **Ruchira** when deciding how to respond to the situation?

16. There is no expectation of privacy in the supply cupboard

    A. Very important
    B. Important
    C. Of minor importance
    D. Not important at all

Answer: A supply cupboard is normally open to all staff at the hospital, and students have no expectation of privacy there. This factor undercuts Jake's claim that Ruchira is spying on him, as she has just as much right to be in the supply cupboard as he does. It is therefore a very important consideration. Answer **(A)** is correct.

17.   Jake and Ruchira dated for a few months, until he broke it off with her
    A.   Very important
    B.   Important
    C.   Of minor importance
    D.   Not important at all

Answer: Jake appears to be doing something that is highly unethical, and would likely be a breach of university policies about cheating, if he is buying an essay to submit as part of his coursework. Any personal relationship between Jake and Ruchira (current or former) would not mitigate his apparent guilt in any way; however, if Ruchira is Jake's ex-girlfriend, this would be a factor of minor importance in how she might decide how to respond to the situation, as it might explain his suspicion that she is spying on him, for instance. The answer is therefore **(C)**.

18.   Jake has a reputation for being honest and doing the right thing
    A.   Very important
    B.   Important
    C.   Of minor importance
    D.   Not important at all

Answer: Jake's reputation does not mitigate his current actions, which appear to be highly unethical, in any way. This factor is entirely unimportant. Answer **(D)** is correct.

19.   Ruchira thinks the website only sells essays for English and history modules
    A.   Very important
    B.   Important
    C.   Of minor importance
    D.   Not important at all

Answer: It would be unethical for a university student to buy an essay to be submitted as part of assessed coursework, whether it was his own coursework or he was buying the essay for someone else's. Ruchira could also be wrong in her impression about the website; if she is correct, however, that the essay could not be for Jake's coursework, it could point to a more complicated explanation for what exactly he is up to—so this factor is of minimal importance. Answer **(C)** is correct.

20.   Ruchira led a discussion on ethics at the most recent meeting of her tutor group
    A.   Very important
    B.   Important
    C.   Of minor importance
    D.   Not important at all

Answer: If Ruchira recently led a discussion on ethics, then that means that she should be well aware of the ethical responsibilities of doctors and students to behave with integrity at all times. This factor is thus very important. The answer is **(A)**.

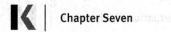

Kaplan Timed Practice Set—Importance Scenarios

Set your timer for 1 minute. Be sure to mark answers for all 4 questions before time runs out.

> Several staff from the hospital have been injured when a bus crashed into several cars in the city centre. The staff were on their way to a dinner honouring the hospital chairman, Mr Phillips. All the staff who had already arrived at the event have been called back to the hospital, as more than a dozen patients (including hospital staff) have been admitted with life-threatening injuries. A junior doctor working in the emergency department is treating a nurse who was injured in the accident. It is determined that she has bleeding on the brain and requires an operation immediately, or she is likely to suffer long-term brain damage or death. However, no neurosurgeons are available at the hospital, or at either of the nearby hospitals. Mr Phillips stops by, asking for an update on the nurse's condition. The junior doctor explains the situation, and Mr Phillips responds, 'All right then, I'll have to take her into theatre myself.' The junior doctor knows that Mr Phillips was once a highly regarded neurosurgeon, but he has not operated on a patient for several years.

How **important** to take into account are the following considerations for **the junior doctor** when deciding how to respond to the situation?

21. Mr Phillips has not operated on a patient for several years

    A. Very important
    B. Important
    C. Of minor importance
    D. Not important at all

22. Mr Phillips knows the nurse and is concerned about her condition

    A. Very important
    B. Important
    C. Of minor importance
    D. Not important at all

23. The junior doctor finds Mr Phillips very intimidating

    A. Very important
    B. Important
    C. Of minor importance
    D. Not important at all

24. Earlier in the evening, Mr Phillips mentioned to the junior doctor that he has not kept up with the latest developments in the field

    A. Very important
    B. Important
    C. Of minor importance
    D. Not important at all

Kaplan Timed Practice Set—*Importance Scenarios*: Answers and Explanations

In this timed set, you faced a more complicated scenario, with two difficult issues in conflict—the nurse's need for immediate, life-saving neurosurgery, balanced against the possibility that Mr Phillips, the only one who could perform the surgery, may not be sufficiently capable of doing so. Importance scenarios are more likely to put two issues in conflict, and the important thing in reading the scenario is to identify the issues, so you can keep them in mind in weighing the importance of the factors. Don't hesitate or deliberate too much on each option, though, or you will run out of time!

21. (B)

The nurse requires immediate brain surgery, but there are no neurosurgeons available to perform it. In this instance, not performing the surgery is likely to result in long-term brain damage or death. Thus, the risk to the patient in Mr Phillips performing the surgery is somewhat mitigated. The fact that he has not performed an operation on a patient in several years is still a significant concern, however. This factor is important to consider in responding to the situation. For example, the junior doctor might suggest that Mr Phillips should be assisted by junior doctors and nurses with recent neurosurgery experience. Note that in this case, it's somewhat of a grey area between being important and very important. However, it's clearly one of those two—so you would get partial marks if you chose the wrong answer. This highlights the importance of choosing a side first (important/not important), then trying to zero in on A or B. In this case, there are enough mitigating factors to justify answer **(B)**.

22. (C)

It is natural for Mr Phillips, as the hospital chairman, to be concerned about the welfare of all the staff who were injured in the accident, and even more so in the case of this nurse, whose life is at risk if she does not have immediate brain surgery. The guidance from the General Medical Council indicates that doctors must avoid providing medical to anyone with whom they have a close personal relationship, wherever it is possible to do so. In this case, the doctor and the nurse appear to have a purely professional relationship, and it is not possible for another neurosurgeon to operate on the nurse. Thus, the factor is of minor importance in responding to the situation. It is not entirely unimportant, since it is still a concern; the junior doctor might consider whether Mr Phillips is emotional or upset because of the accident, for example. But this is not an overriding concern.

23. (D)

It is not surprising that a junior doctor might find the hospital chairman intimidating. It's likely that many of the staff, even some of the consultants, feel the same way. This does not in any way mitigate the junior doctor's duty to ensure that the hospital chairman is confident and able to perform the surgery that the nurse requires. For this reason, this factor is not at all important.

24. (A)

The additional information here changes the situation significantly. We already know from the original scenario that Mr Phillips has not performed neurosurgery in several years, so it is possible that his skills are a bit rusty. However, if he also has not kept up with the latest developments in the field, then it is possible that he is unfamiliar with the equipment or techniques that are currently in use, which could cause considerable danger to the patient and confusion to the team assisting him, who would expect the surgeon to be familiar with the equipment and techniques used at the hospital. This factor is therefore of the utmost importance in responding to Mr Phillips.

Choosing Sides

The most important skill for Situational Judgement is the ability to choose sides quickly, as you read each response option or factor. The more confident your understanding of the principles of medical professionalism, the more secure you will feel in your ability to choose sides. This is very much a matter of making a 'snap judgement': Is the response appropriate or inappropriate? Is the factor important or not important?

Simply by making that snap judgement, you will eliminate two incorrect answers. In most cases, the 'strong' answer on the side you have chosen—**(A)** or **(D)**—will be correct; you will click it and move on to the next item. Thus, it is essential to force yourself to make a snap judgement quickly, as you read each of the remaining responses and factors in this chapter. It may feel awkward or uncertain at first, but your confidence (and your accuracy) will grow with practice.

Sometimes the correct answer will be **(B)** or **(C)**. Let's take a moment to consider, in the broadest possible terms, why each answer is usually correct:

- Select **(A)** if it is an ideal response for a medical professional in the same circumstances, with no negative consequences for patients or the profession, or if it is an essential factor for a medical professional to consider in responding to the scenario.

- Select **(B)** if the response is inferior for some reason (i.e. not ideal), but without any negative consequences for patients or the profession. For example, a response that does not address the underlying problem in the scenario but is not otherwise wrong would like be a **(B)**. A factor of some significance (but not overwhelming significance) would also tend to be a **(B)**.

- Select **(C)** if the response is negative in some way, but not terrible. For example, if the response is somewhat accurate/valid but adds a new problem, it's likely to be a **(C)**. A factor that is less relevant in responding to a scenario would also tend to be a **(C)**.

- Select **(D)** if the response has negative consequences for patient health, safety or dignity, or if it compromises the public's confidence in the medical profession, or if a factor should not be considered in responding to a scenario.

Note that there are some clear cases where something must be **(A)**, or must be **(D)**. Watch out for anything in a scenario that could risk patient health, safety or dignity, as these matters must be addressed with urgency. Often a response will be inferior or negative simply because it does not respond promptly or professionally to an issue of patient health, safety or dignity in the scenario.

Note as well that if you practise rigorously for this section, you shouldn't often find yourself choosing between **(B)** and **(C)**. First, choose a side; then, consider whether there is any mitigation that makes it **(B)** or **(C)**. If a response is not negative, for example, it must be **(A)** or **(B)**; if there's something seriously wrong with the response, then it's either **(C)** or **(D)**. Build your skill at choosing sides, and you will find it becomes much clearer to know when it's **(B)** or **(C)**.

Practise choosing sides in the following Appropriateness scenario. First, choose whether the response is generally good or bad. Next, decide whether it could be **(B)**—if you think the response is generally good—or if it could be **(C)**—if the response is generally bad. Bear in mind, however, that the majority of answers will be either ideal or awful—either **(A)** or **(D)**.

Do the same in the Importance scenario that follows. When assessing importance, the snap judgement is whether the factor is generally relevant or irrelevant. Next, decide whether it could be **(B)**—if you think the factor is generally relevant in responding to the scenario—or if it could be **(C)**—if the response is generally irrelevant in responding to the scenario. Don't hesitate to pick **(A)** or **(D)** if the factor is overwhelmingly relevant or utterly irrelevant.

> Luke, a junior doctor, notices that some of the staff on the psychiatry ward wear jeans for the night shift. Luke knows jeans are banned in the hospital dress code policy, but this is overlooked at night by most nurses, even the more senior nurses.

How **appropriate** are each of the following responses by **Luke** in this situation?

25. Talk to the ward manager who supervises the nurses the next morning about the relaxed dress code

   A. A very appropriate thing to do
   B. Appropriate, but not ideal
   C. Inappropriate, but not awful
   D. A very inappropriate thing to do

Answer: This response is appropriate, since the ward manager supervises the nurses and they are not following the hospital dress code. The ward manager may not be aware that nurses on the night shift are wearing jeans. This response is not ideal, however, because it is not a direct or immediate solution. If there were a hospital inspection during the night shift, for example, there could be trouble due to the nurses wearing jeans that Luke could have avoided by taking action sooner. Answer **(B)** is therefore correct.

26. Dress more casually on the night shift, in order to fit in with his colleagues

   A. A very appropriate thing to do
   B. Appropriate, but not ideal
   C. Inappropriate, but not awful
   D. A very inappropriate thing to do

Answer: An entirely awful response. The hospital dress code is clear; the fact that others are violating does not justify Luke doing the same. The correct answer is **(D)**.

27. Tell the nurses they shouldn't wear jeans the next time he sees them doing so

   A. A very appropriate thing to do
   B. Appropriate, but not ideal
   C. Inappropriate, but not awful
   D. A very inappropriate thing to do

Answer: This response is not ideal, since Luke is the nurses' colleague, not their supervisor; such a response could easily be misinterpreted or lead to problems. At the same time, the response is not awful, for the simple reason that the nurses are violating hospital policy by wearing jeans. Answer **(C)** is correct.

> A junior doctor, Scarlet, is leaving the ward for an important lunch with her department chair, who is known for placing a great emphasis on punctuality. In a corridor far from the main part of the ward, Scarlet sees an elderly patient lying on a trolley. There is no one else in the corridor. As Scarlet approaches, she notices the patient—who is wearing only a hospital gown—has been caught short and had an accident. The patient is crying quietly to herself.

How **important** to take into account are the following considerations for **Scarlet** when deciding how to respond to the situation?

28. The nurses on the ward are unlikely to walk down this corridor before the end of their shift
   A. Very important
   B. Important
   C. Of minor importance
   D. Not important at all

Answer: We are told the corridor is far from the main part of the ward. If it is also true that the nurses on the ward are unlikely to walk down the corridor anytime soon, then the patient will be left in discomfort and distress for some time if Scarlet does not help her. This factor is very important for Scarlet to consider. Answer **(A)** is correct.

29. The department chair's reputation for valuing punctuality
   A. Very important
   B. Important
   C. Of minor importance
   D. Not important at all

Answer: Patient dignity must take priority over other considerations. The ideal response would be for Scarlet to speak briefly with the patient, reassure the patient that she will get someone to help her straightaway, then go to the nurse's station to let them know of the urgent situation on the corridor. It sounds like this might make Scarlet late for lunch, but Scarlet should disregard this factor in responding to the scenario. The answer is **(D)**.

30. Scarlet does not know who is responsible for leaving the patient in the corridor
   A. Very important
   B. Important
   C. Of minor importance
   D. Not important at all

Answer: Scarlet must act urgently to help the patient. The question of who left the patient in the corridor is not especially relevant; Scarlet's overriding concern isn't placing blame, but restoring the patient's dignity. The correct answer is **(C)**.

Kaplan Timed Practice Set—*Choosing Sides*

Set your timer for 2 minutes. Be sure to mark answers for all 6 questions before time runs out.

> Dr McDowall has started work at a busy paediatric outpatient clinic with another, slightly more senior doctor, Dr Braidy. He notices that every afternoon Dr Braidy leaves half an hour early from clinic, leaving him to see the remaining patients alone. The result is that Dr McDowall often finishes work half an hour late. He has heard Dr Braidy discussing her child care difficulties with the clinic nurse on numerous occasions, and this this is why she leaves early.

How **appropriate** are each of the following responses by **Dr McDowall** in this situation?

31. Tell Dr Braidy that she needs to stay to help him finish clinic

    A. A very appropriate thing to do
    B. Appropriate, but not ideal
    C. Inappropriate, but not awful
    D. A very inappropriate thing to do

32. Suggest that Dr Braidy talks to their consultant if she is having difficulties with working hours

    A. A very appropriate thing to do
    B. Appropriate, but not ideal
    C. Inappropriate, but not awful
    D. A very inappropriate thing to do

33. Discuss the challenges of maintaining a work-life balance with Dr Braidy the next time they have lunch together

    A. A very appropriate thing to do
    B. Appropriate, but not ideal
    C. Inappropriate, but not awful
    D. A very inappropriate thing to do

Mrs Moore has been brought to a hospital appointment by her daughter. Mrs Moore has severe dementia and her daughter is her main carer. Ewa, the junior doctor responsible for Mrs Moore's care, starts to have severe concerns as the appointment proceeds. It seems that Mrs Moore is not being adequately cared for at home and that her daughter is not coping with her mother's complex physical health needs, although the daughter denies this. Ewa notes that Mrs Moore's other daughter died recently; the surviving daughter becomes tearful when talking about her sister's death.

How **important** to take into account are the following considerations for **Ewa** when deciding how to respond to the situation?

34.   Several patients are waiting to see Ewa once she finishes her appointment with Mrs Moore
    A.   Very important
    B.   Important
    C.   Of minor importance
    D.   Not important at all

35.   Mrs Moore states that she is also very upset about the recent death of her daughter
    A.   Very important
    B.   Important
    C.   Of minor importance
    D.   Not important at all

36.   Mrs Moore's daughter reports that she is doing a good job looking after her mother
    A.   Very important
    B.   Important
    C.   Of minor importance
    D.   Not important at all

Kaplan Timed Practice Set—*Choosing Sides*: Answers and Explanations

This timed set included two scenarios, so you had to work quickly to read both scenarios and answer all 6 questions before time ran out. Hopefully you managed to finish in time. If not, take a moment to reflect on what you can do differently in your next timed practice. For example, did you take too long to read the scenario? Did you fail to identify the conflict in the scenario before going on to the questions? If so, then you may have needed extra time to untangle it, and you may have had trouble answering the first question. Whenever you have problems in timed practice, be sure to make a note of what you did, and make a plan for next time.

31. (C)

This response is not awful because it is true; Dr Braidy should not be leaving him to finish the clinic by himself. Telling her what to do is not the best way to go about it, particularly because Dr Braidy is his senior.

32. (A)

This response would be highly appropriate, as it is a constructive suggestion to Dr Braidy that also implies that he is struggling with her leaving early.

33. (B)

There is nothing awful in this response. However, it is not ideal, since it may be some time before they next have lunch together; Dr McDowall would ideally address the issue more urgently.

34. (D)

Ewa seems to think something is not right with Mrs Moore's care. Ewa would do well to follow up on her concerns, regardless of whether other patients are waiting for their appointments with her. This factor is not at all important in deciding how to respond to the situation.

35. (B)

This factor is important to consider, since it would impact how Ewa responds to Mrs Moore, and how she addresses her concerns about Ewa's care. While the death of Mrs Moore's daughter has resulted in a change of carer, it is not really the central issue here—but Mrs Moore's feelings are important, as the patient must be treated with respect and dignity in this difficult situation.

36. (C)

Doctors should listen to patients and their relatives, but they must act in their patients' best interests in cases like this one. Ewa seems to feel that the surviving daughter is not taking adequate care of her mother, potentially putting her mother's health at risk. The daughter's views are not irrelevant, but they are minimally important.

Remember

Importance questions are a bit tougher to answer, since they are factors that the decider might consider in responding the scenario.

You have to infer the response based on the factor.

Focus on the key issue in the scenario—what is the main problem the decider is faced with? If there are multiple problems, which is most important?

Anything that directly affects patient safety or dignity would usually be of the highest importance—factors addressing these areas would almost always be of the highest importance.

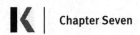

Keeping Perspective—Situational Judgement

You are about to complete a timed Situational Judgement quiz, consisting of 11 scenarios and a total of 34 responses/factors. If you pace yourself, and spend about a minute per scenario—and less than a minute on shorter scenarios, with fewer responses/factors—you should be able to attempt all the scenarios and answer all the items. Even if you find yourself running out of time near the end, do your best to choose a side for each item (appropriate/inappropriate or important/unimportant) and mark an answer on that side.

Before you start the quiz, let's consider some of the challenges in Situational Judgement that cause unprepared test-takers to waste time and earn a lower score:

You must understand the conflict in the scenario before assessing the responses/factors. This may seem a really obvious point, but we find that many students who struggle with Situational Judgement are skimming or glancing over the scenario without 'registering' the key conflict that must be understood in order to assess the possible responses or factors. You should always take 20–30 seconds to read the scenario in full, as you will be able to assess most responses/factors in 10–15 seconds each.

Don't waste time deliberating over any one response/factor. This is perhaps the most vital point. You have only 10–15 seconds for each individual response/factor, so you cannot spend any longer than that in deciding the appropriateness/importance. Always force yourself to choose a side straightaway, and then choose the stronger/weaker answer on that side.

Don't worry about full vs partial marks. The UKCAT Consortium has declined to disclose how the partial marks work. We know that you get full marks if you choose the correct answer; presumably, then, you would get partial marks for choosing an answer that is near (next to) the correct answer. Our best guess (based on years of analysing standardised tests at Kaplan) is that you get partial marks for the other answer on the same side. That is, if B is correct, you get partial marks for A (and vice versa); if C is correct, you get partial marks for D (and vice versa). If we get further information about partial marking from the test-maker, we'll post this in your Kaplan online companion—but it isn't worth worrying about. Do your best to choose a side, then narrow to B/C if appropriate. Simply choosing the correct side should be sufficient to get partial marks on most items that you do not answer correctly.

Take time to read through *Good Medical Practice*. We have mentioned this several times, as it is really the best guide to the principles of medical professionalism as practised by doctors in the UK. It is a relatively short and easy-to-read booklet, and you will have to read and get to know it very well in any case once you are a medical student—so it's worth putting in a bit of time now, so you can get more comfortable with the range of principles that could be tested in this section of the UKCAT.

Chapter 7 Kaplan UKCAT Quiz

Set your timer for 13 minutes. Try to assess all 34 items and mark an answer for each before time is up. If you have trouble with a particular scenario or response/factor, choose a side (appropriate/inappropriate or important/unimportant) and mark an answer on that side. Above all, do your best not to spend more than 15 seconds on any single item

> Janice, a patient with chronic cardiac problems and a very high body mass index (BMI), has been in the ward for a few weeks. Hideo, a first year medical student, asks Janice to spend 30 minutes talking to him about her medical history as practice for his exams. While discussing her family history of heart disease during the interview, Janice makes several unkind remarks about the junior doctor on the ward, who is rather overweight.

How **appropriate** are each of the following responses by **Hideo** in this situation?

37. Ask the doctor supervising his work on the ward what he should have done at their next meeting
    A. A very appropriate thing to do
    B. Appropriate, but not ideal
    C. Inappropriate, but not awful
    D. A very inappropriate thing to do

38. Ask Janice about her eating habits and whether she has made any effort to lose weight
    A. A very appropriate thing to do
    B. Appropriate, but not ideal
    C. Inappropriate, but not awful
    D. A very inappropriate thing to do

39. Tell Janice that she is being very rude
    A. A very appropriate thing to do
    B. Appropriate, but not ideal
    C. Inappropriate, but not awful
    D. A very inappropriate thing to do

> Colm and Vicki are junior doctors at a large GP practice. They are the only doctors working in the early evening hours, when Vicki receives a call from A&E at a nearby hospital. Her partner and their young son have been in a car crash and are very seriously injured. Vicki is shaken, and asks Colm if he could see her final two patients of the day, as she must go to the hospital. Vicki hands Colm the patients' records, and he sees that Vicki's handwriting is so impossible to read that he cannot make sense of either patient's notes.

How **appropriate** are each of the following responses by **Colm** in this situation?

40. Tell Vicki not to worry and that he will take good care of her patients

   A. A very appropriate thing to do
   B. Appropriate, but not ideal
   C. Inappropriate, but not awful
   D. A very inappropriate thing to do

41. Tell Vicki he doesn't feel right about trying to help, as her notes in the patient records are illegible

   A. A very appropriate thing to do
   B. Appropriate, but not ideal
   C. Inappropriate, but not awful
   D. A very inappropriate thing to do

42. Tell Vicki he can't read her handwriting

   A. A very appropriate thing to do
   B. Appropriate, but not ideal
   C. Inappropriate, but not awful
   D. A very inappropriate thing to do

43. Ask Vicki to brief him on the reasons for each patient's appointment, along with any underlying conditions or allergies, before she leaves

   A. A very appropriate thing to do
   B. Appropriate, but not ideal
   C. Inappropriate, but not awful
   D. A very inappropriate thing to do

44. Ask Vicki if there's anything else he can do to help

   A. A very appropriate thing to do
   B. Appropriate, but not ideal
   C. Inappropriate, but not awful
   D. A very inappropriate thing to do

A junior doctor, Greer, sees a new patient, Fiona, in her orthopaedic clinic. They end up talking about Fiona's home town, which it turns out is where Greer's family also originate, although they have never met before. Fiona makes frequent references to the fact that she expects better treatment from Greer, as they from the same town. Fiona jokes about being moved up the waiting list for her operation.

How **appropriate** are each of the following responses by **Greer** in this situation?

45. Explain patiently and politely how the waiting list system works

   A. A very appropriate thing to do
   B. Appropriate, but not ideal
   C. Inappropriate, but not awful
   D. A very inappropriate thing to do

46. Order the required blood tests for Fiona now, instead of following the standard protocol, as ordering the blood tests now will ensure that Fiona is booked in sooner for her operation

   A. A very appropriate thing to do
   B. Appropriate, but not ideal
   C. Inappropriate, but not awful
   D. A very inappropriate thing to do

47. Discuss a favourite memory of their home town

   A. A very appropriate thing to do
   B. Appropriate, but not ideal
   C. Inappropriate, but not awful
   D. A very inappropriate thing to do

A cardiothoracic consultant, Dr Sentongo, breaks the news to his patient that he likely has a terminal lung disease. The patient asks Dr Sentongo to pray with him. Dr Sentongo is not religious but has built up a good rapport with the patient over the last few years.

How **appropriate** are each of the following responses by **Dr Sentongo** in this situation?

48. Refuse, stating that praying is not going to help the patient now

    A. A very appropriate thing to do

    B. Appropriate, but not ideal

    C. Inappropriate, but not awful

    D. A very inappropriate thing to do

49. Offer for the patient to speak to the hospital faith leader instead

    A. A very appropriate thing to do

    B. Appropriate, but not ideal

    C. Inappropriate, but not awful

    D. A very inappropriate thing to do

50. Allow the patient to lead the prayer whilst remaining silent

    A. A very appropriate thing to do

    B. Appropriate, but not ideal

    C. Inappropriate, but not awful

    D. A very inappropriate thing to do

Aled is a medical student. His supervisor at the hospital instructs him to perform a certain procedure on a patient while his supervisor observes. Aled has seen the procedure demonstrated several times, and has practised the procedure a few times on an anatomical model, but he has never done the procedure on a living person. As Aled is about to start, the patient asks if he has done this before.

How **appropriate** are each of the following responses by **Aled** in this situation?

51. Ask if the patient would prefer for his supervisor to perform the procedure

    A. A very appropriate thing to do

    B. Appropriate, but not ideal

    C. Inappropriate, but not awful

    D. A very inappropriate thing to do

52. Explain that he has practised the procedure but has not performed it on a patient, and that his supervisor will observe and can intervene if there is a problem

    A. A very appropriate thing to do

    B. Appropriate, but not ideal

    C. Inappropriate, but not awful

    D. A very inappropriate thing to do

53. Tell the patient that he has performed the procedure before, and there has never been a problem

    A. A very appropriate thing to do

    B. Appropriate, but not ideal

    C. Inappropriate, but not awful

    D. A very inappropriate thing to do

Tasnia is a medical student currently undertaking her obstetrics placement. She is sitting in with her consultant, Miss Khan, when a patient comes in with her husband. Unbeknownst to Miss Khan, the patient does not speak much English, so her partner says he will act as a translator. However, Tasnia, who happens to understand a little of the language the couple speak, notices that the partner is not translating what the patient is actually saying, changing some vital facts which could potentially change the treatment required.

How **appropriate** are each of the following responses by **Tasnia** in this situation?

54. Stop the consultation and suggest to Miss Khan that they use a phone interpreter

   A. A very appropriate thing to do
   B. Appropriate, but not ideal
   C. Inappropriate, but not awful
   D. A very inappropriate thing to do

55. Offer to translate herself, as she understands a bit of the language

   A. A very appropriate thing to do
   B. Appropriate, but not ideal
   C. Inappropriate, but not awful
   D. A very inappropriate thing to do

56. Tell Miss Khan at their next one-to-one meeting next week what she thinks happened in this consultation

   A. A very appropriate thing to do
   B. Appropriate, but not ideal
   C. Inappropriate, but not awful
   D. A very inappropriate thing to do

Pritesh, a dentistry student, suspects that his friend and colleague, Lepina, has used an essay-writing website to write her essay for her. Pritesh strongly suspects Lepina has undiagnosed dyslexia (he has dyslexia himself) and that this causes Lepina to struggle with essay writing, although Lepina says things are fine.

How **important** to take into account are the following considerations for **Pritesh** when deciding how to respond to the situation?

57.   Lepina needs to pass the year, otherwise she will have to leave the course
      A.   Very important
      B.   Important
      C.   Of minor importance
      D.   Not important at all

58.   Lepina does not get on with the course supervisor
      A.   Very important
      B.   Important
      C.   Of minor importance
      D.   Not important at all

59.   He knows that the university uses anti-plagiarism software
      A.   Very important
      B.   Important
      C.   Of minor importance
      D.   Not important at all

> Fatima, a consultant at a large hospital, has been asked to help cover on a different ward where there is a staff shortage. Whilst covering on that ward, Fatima opens the door to the supply cupboard and sees a nurse take several bottles of painkillers and put them into her handbag. It looks like the nurse is taking the last bottles of that type of painkiller.

How **important** to take into account are the following considerations for **Fatima** when deciding how to respond to the situation?

60. Fatima's patient requires urgent treatment

    A. Very important
    B. Important
    C. Of minor importance
    D. Not important at all

61. Fatima is unlikely to work on this ward again in the near future

    A. Very important
    B. Important
    C. Of minor importance
    D. Not important at all

62. Fatima's patient needs the same painkiller that the nurse is putting in her bag

    A. Very important
    B. Important
    C. Of minor importance
    D. Not important at all

Finn and Albie are fifth year medical students on their paediatric rotation. The day before they start their placement, Albie realises he must have left his ID badge in his locker at their previous hospital, which he thinks he cannot collect until the weekend. Finn knows that the hospital has a strict policy about ID badges being worn, so Finn offers to lend Albie his ID badge for rest of the week, since he will be at a conference and will not need it.

How **important** to take into account are the following considerations for **Albie** when deciding how to respond to the situation?

63. Hospital policy states that name badges must be worn at all times

   A. Very important
   B. Important
   C. Of minor importance
   D. Not important at all

64. Albie and Finn are not meeting their consultant until next week

   A. Very important
   B. Important
   C. Of minor importance
   D. Not important at all

Diamond is a junior doctor responsible for supervising several newly qualified doctors in the gastroenterology outpatient clinic. One day, on the train to a mandatory training session, Diamond receives a phone call from Rob, a newly qualified doctor who is running the clinic for the day. Diamond told Rob to call her if he needed help, as there is no one else in the clinic. Rob sounds flustered; he asks Diamond how best to deal with a patient currently in the clinic. Diamond is aware the train is packed, and people might hear their potentially confidential conversation.

How **important** to take into account are the following considerations for **Diamond** when deciding how to respond to the situation?

65. Rob does not think the patient is acutely unwell

    A. Very important
    B. Important
    C. Of minor importance
    D. Not important at all

66. Rob is the only doctor in the clinic

    A. Very important
    B. Important
    C. Of minor importance
    D. Not important at all

67. Diamond has not met the patient in question

    A. Very important
    B. Important
    C. Of minor importance
    D. Not important at all

Olly and Simon attended the same medical school and are about to start working at the same London hospital as junior doctors. Before starting at the hospital, they take a weeklong trip to America. On their first night in Las Vegas, they are walking from their hotel to a nearby casino when they are stopped by police. Simon was carrying an open bottle of beer that he had not finished at the hotel; as a result, he is charged with violating the city's open container law. Simon appears in court the next day and is fined $250, as the offence is only a misdemeanour. On the flight back to London, Olly reminds Simon that he must disclose the incident to the General Medical Council, since he has been found guilty of a criminal offence. Simon responds that 'it's not a big deal,' points out that the same behaviour would be legal in the UK, and insists that 'what happens in Vegas, stays in Vegas.'

How **important** to take into account are the following considerations for **Olly** when deciding how to respond to the situation?

68. The General Medical Council have set out clear guidelines about what a doctor must do if he is found guilty of a criminal offence
    A. Very important
    B. Important
    C. Of minor importance
    D. Not important at all

69. Simon has never previously done anything illegal or unethical
    A. Very important
    B. Important
    C. Of minor importance
    D. Not important at all

70. Simon shared details about his arrest and court appearance on his social media accounts
    A. Very important
    B. Important
    C. Of minor importance
    D. Not important at all

STOP. IF YOU FINISH BEFORE TIME IS UP, CHECK ANY QUESTIONS YOU HAVE MARKED FOR REVIEW. YOU MAY GO BACK TO QUESTIONS IN THIS QUIZ ONLY.

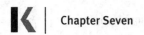

Chapter 7 Kaplan UKCAT Quiz: Answers and Explanations

37. (A)

As a medical student, it would be very appropriate for Hideo to ask the doctor supervising his work on the ward for advice at their next meeting. The situation with Janice is not serious enough to justify seeking advice more urgently.

38. (C)

It is not awful to ask Janice about her eating habits and whether she has attempted to lose weight, since she has a very high BMI and her weight issues could be a factor in her chronic cardiac problems. However, shifting to this topic now is not ideal, since it could be interpreted as a response to her comments about the junior doctor.

39. (D)

Whilst Janice is being rude, this response is not an appropriate way for a medical student to speak to a patient. There are more delicate ways of phrasing this sentiment.

40. (D)

Colm is right to help his colleague, as she is clearly upset by the news about her partner and son and should not be seeing patients in that state. However, there is a real problem in Colm covering for Vicki, as he cannot read her notes in the patient's records, so he has no idea why the patients are coming in for their appointments, or if they have any underlying conditions or allergies. This lack of information could seriously endanger the patients' health if Colm were to see them using Vicki's illegible notes, so this response is very inappropriate.

41. (C)

It is inappropriate for Colm to tell Vicki that he won't help in this situation, however it is not an awful response, as the reason he gives is the central problem here and puts patient safety at risk. All doctors are required to ensure that the notes they make in patient records are legible, and it is Vicki's failure to meet this fundamental professional obligation that makes it problematic for Colm to cover for her.

42. (A)

This is a very appropriate response, as it is true and is at the heart of the problem in this scenario.

43. (A)

This response is highly appropriate, as it is a quick and straightforward solution to the problem of Vicki's illegible notes, and will enable Colm to cover for her so she can join her family at the hospital.

44. (A)

This is a very appropriate thing to do, as Vicki may need some other support or help as a result of the emergency.

45. (A)

This response is ideal. Whilst it is possible that the patient is merely joking, Greer should take care not to mislead her in any way into thinking she is getting preferential treatment.

46. (D)

It would be wholly inappropriate for Greer to improve Fiona's position on the waiting list by modifying the standard protocol.

47. (B)

There are no negative consequences from this response, so it is not inappropriate. However, it is not ideal, since it does not really engage with any of the issues in the scenario. It is generally pleasant, inoffensive, and irrelevant; the answer is **(B)**.

48. (D)

This response is not appropriate. Although Dr Sentongo does not believe in the power of prayer, clearly the patient feels it is important and a source of comfort. Dr Sentongo should be sensitive to the patient's beliefs.

49. (A)

This response would be an appropriate way to provide for the patient's spiritual needs without involving the doctor in something that he is not comfortable with.

50. (A)

This response would allow the doctor to support the patient without having to share his own beliefs. It is a very appropriate thing to do.

51. (C)

Aled has been instructed to perform the procedure by his supervisor, so it is inappropriate for him to give the patient the option of having his supervisor take over before explaining his own level of experience with the procedure. Once he answers the patient's question, then this might be an appropriate course of action. However, this response is not awful, as it is clear that the patient doubts that Aled is qualified to undertake the procedure.

52. (A)

This response accurately describes Aled's experience with the procedure, whilst reassuring the patient of his supervisor's support, and it gives the patient the informed choice of whether to allow Aled to proceed. As such, it is a highly appropriate response.

53. (D)

It would be highly inappropriate for Aled to imply that he has performed the procedure on a patient, when in fact he has not practised it on a living person. It is serious violation of the principles of medical professionalism for a doctor or medical student to state or suggest that they have more experience or expertise than they actually do.

54. (A)

This response is very appropriate, because there is a real risk of a potentially incorrect treatment being given that could harm the patient. Tasnia must alert Miss Khan to her concerns about the translation errors as a matter of urgency.

55. (B)

This response is not ideal, since Tasnia only understands a little of the language. However, Tasnia would communicate this point clearly in this response, and it directly and urgently addresses the problem of the patient's partner translating inaccurately, reducing the potential for harm from an incorrect treatment.

56. (D)

There is a real risk to the patient of an incorrect treatment being given, which must be addressed urgently; waiting until next week to tell Miss Khan about the problem is very inappropriate, since it could result in harm to the patient.

57. (D)

This factor is not at all important. It might explain why Lepina is cheating, but it does not excuse her behaviour. Obviously all students want to pass the year.

58. (C)

This factor is of minor importance, because it might inform where Pritesh suggests that Lepina seeks help. For example, if she is struggling with the deadline or finding the topic difficult, Lepina might be able to discuss the problem with a lecturer instead of the course supervisor. The factor is not especially important, however, as it does not mitigate the fact that Lepina is cheating on her essay.

59. (D)

This factor is entirely irrelevant. The fact that Lepina is likely to get caught should not affect how she or Pritesh act. Pritesh is aware that his fellow student has cheated and, as her friend, he should address the issue.

60. (B)

This is an important factor to consider, as Fatima would want to be cautious not to take too long in dealing with the nurse's behaviour at the present moment. However, it does appear that a member of staff is stealing painkillers from the supply cupboard—this must be addressed immediately, and it is of more importance than the issue with her patient, which is why this factor is important but not of the greatest importance.

61. (D)

The serious nature of the nurse's transgression demands an immediate response. Fatima's responsibility to follow through on this is not diminished at all by the fact that she is unlikely to work on the ward again in the near future.

62. (A)

This is a very important factor, as Fatima will need to ensure that the painkiller is available for her patient. Thus, it will be all the more essential for her to respond to the nurse urgently and effectively.

63. (A)

This factor is very important to consider. Albie must wear his name badge at the hospital, so he must get it back as a matter of urgency. Albie would do well to ask for help from the hospital to resolve the issue; there might also be a facility to provide temporary name badges, for example.

64. (D)

It does not matter whether the consultant is on the ward this week; there are many other people who will meet Albie and Finn and need to know who they are. Medical students must comply with hospital policy at all times.

65. (B)

The fact that the patient is not in imminent danger might affect how urgently Diamond responds to Rob. For example, she could ask Rob to call her back in a few minutes when she is off the train. However, she told Rob she would help, so she should support him regardless of the urgency. This factor is therefore important, but not of the highest importance.

66. (A)

This factor is very important; it means that Rob is depending on Diamond, as there is no one else to help.

67. (D)

This factor is not at all important. Diamond told Rob she would help him remotely whilst he is working without any other doctors in the clinic. Since she is responsible for supervising Rob as a newly qualified doctor, Diamond should give him the support that he needs.

68. (A)

This factor is of the utmost importance. Since the GMC guidance on this issue is very clear, it would be irresponsible for Simon to claim that he was unaware or that he did not have a duty to disclose his offence from the visit to Las Vegas.

69. (D)

Simon's previous record of legal, ethical behaviour is entirely unimportant. He has been found guilty of a criminal offence, and he is required to disclose it to the GMC. Failure to do so is a breach of the GMC guidance, and would itself be an unethical act.

70. (B)

This factor is important to consider. If Simon has shared details about his arrest and court appearance on social media, then it is possible that some people in the UK who are aware that he is about to begin work as a junior doctor are now also aware that he is guilty of a criminal offence. If one such person were to inform the hospital or the GMC about his criminal offence before Simon does so, then there could be serious consequences to his medical career.

Kaplan UKCAT Mock Test

Mock Test General Instructions

You have 2 hours to complete the Kaplan UKCAT Mock Test. You will need the following items:

- This book
- A pen or pencil to record your answers
- Scrap paper for any scratch work and notations
- A timer (such as one on your watch, mobile or computer)
- A calculator with basic functions (i.e. not a scientific calculator or mobile phone)

- Time each section strictly, so you can practise under test-like conditions. Be sure to use the top tips wherever possible. You should also try to keep to the timing recommendations for each question or set of questions, but getting comfortable with the top tips is the primary goal of the Mock Test. Once you 'internalise' the top tips, you will find that your timing improves significantly.

- On Test Day, you will have an additional minute to read the directions for each section. That minute cannot be used to answer test questions, so it has not been included here. Time yourself using the timings given once you turn each instructions page and start work on each section.

- Answer the questions as quickly and accurately as possible. Now that you have a better understanding of how the UKCAT works, you have every incentive to ensure that you mark an answer for every question in each section.

- Record your answers on a sheet of paper, and check them against the explanations in Appendix C once you finish.

N.B. You cannot write on the test paper on Test Day, because the test is taken on a computer. Be careful not to get into the habit of writing on the practice questions in this book. Make any notations, eliminations or other markings entirely on scrap paper, and not directly on the questions themselves.

Your score on Test Day corresponds to the number of questions you answer correctly. You can find your equivalent score on the scoring table at the end of the test.

When you are ready to begin the Mock Test, turn the page and read the directions for the first section.

Section 1: Verbal Reasoning (22 Minutes)

This section contains 11 passages, each of which is followed by four items. Most items will be questions, each with four answer choices. Your task in a Verbal question is to select the best answer from the options given.

Other items will consist of a statement, with the answer choices True, False and Can't tell. You must assess the statement based on the passage. Select True if the information in the statement is stated explicitly in the passage or a valid inference from the passage. Select False if the information in the statement contradicts what is stated in the passage. Select Can't tell if there is not enough information to determine whether the statement is True or False.

Answer all 44 questions in Section 1, selecting one of the possible answers and circling the letter corresponding to the appropriate answer in your test paper.

When you are finished with this section, you may use any remaining time to review your work in this section only. Once you proceed to the next section, you may not return to this section.

You will have 22 minutes to answer the questions. It is in your best interest to select an answer for every item as there is no penalty for wrong answers.

Set your timer for 22 minutes, turn the page and begin the section.

Recently, scientists have observed surprising results in the population sizes of animals living within the irradiated exclusion zone of Chernobyl. The exclusion zone was created following the nuclear disaster in 1986, when the 116,000 inhabitants living within the 4,200 kilometre area worst affected by radiation were permanently evacuated from their homes. Shortly after the disaster, a team of researchers from the Polessye State Radioecological Reserve (PSRER) set out to discover the impact on the local wildlife of living on the radiated land in the decades following the disaster. Before collecting the data, researchers had predicted that the population growth of these animals would decline for the first 20 years following the disaster, and remain stalled at a lower level in the following decades.

As the researchers needed to examine the population of animals living within a hazardous radiation zone, data collection was particularly tricky. From 2008 to 2010, for instance, data was gained during winter by studying the tracks animals left in the snow when looking for prey after dark. This allowed researchers to discern both the size of individual packs of wolves, as well as the amount of different packs of wolves in a given area (which could be identified by the number of different track routes). This then allowed researchers to predict overall populations of individual species within the exclusion zone as a whole. As the researchers gathered this data from helicopters at a distance from the radiated land, they were able to avoid exposure to the extreme radiation present at ground level. Overall, the research showed that animal populations had flourished compared not only to the researchers predicted results, but also compared to animals living outside of the exclusion zone, on healthy land without radiation damage. In one instance, research found that the population of wolves was seven times greater inside the exclusion zone than it was in nearby, uncontaminated land.

Of course, though the data shows an increase in animal populations, this does not mean that radiation is beneficial for animals. Many humans exposed to radiation from the initial nuclear explosion died from acute radiation syndrome, and the population of most animal breeds within the exclusion zone initially showed a severe decrease. Though serious mutations in animals were documented only in the immediate aftermath of the accident, lingering problems persist. Voles living within the area have shown a higher susceptibility to developing cataracts than voles living on uncontaminated land; and partial albinism (a lack of pigment in the skin and feathers) is higher among swallows living within the exclusion zone. What the study appears to show, instead, is that despite the significant impact the polluted land has on the population size of animals, living on extremely irradiated land has a less harmful impact than humans do on the animals' ability to grow in population size. The findings of the study have shown that despite the terrible effects Chernobyl has had on the environment, it has at least not deterred the local animals' determination to survive.

1. Which of the following is not mentioned in the passage as a result of radiation?

   A. Acute radiation syndrome in humans affected by the nuclear explosion.
   B. Infertility in some animals directly affected by the nuclear explosion.
   C. An initial decline in population numbers of animals living within the exclusion zone.
   D. An increased risk of developing cataracts in some animals.

2. The author would most likely agree that the results of the PSRER study suggest:

   A. radiation only affects wildlife in the immediate aftermath of nuclear explosions.
   B. animals need to be closely observed in order to gauge population size.
   C. the detrimental impact of living on irradiated land outweighs the population increase.
   D. proximity to humans can be more detrimental to wildlife populations than exposure to radiation.

Recently, scientists have observed surprising results in the population sizes of animals living within the irradiated exclusion zone of Chernobyl. The exclusion zone was created following the nuclear disaster in 1986, when the 116,000 inhabitants living within the 4,200 kilometre area worst affected by radiation were permanently evacuated from their homes. Shortly after the disaster, a team of researchers from the Polessye State Radioecological Reserve (PSRER) set out to discover the impact on the local wildlife of living on the radiated land in the decades following the disaster. Before collecting the data, researchers had predicted that the population growth of these animals would decline for the first 20 years following the disaster, and remain stalled at a lower level in the following decades.

As the researchers needed to examine the population of animals living within a hazardous radiation zone, data collection was particularly tricky. From 2008 to 2010, for instance, data was gained during winter by studying the tracks animals left in the snow when looking for prey after dark. This allowed researchers to discern both the size of individual packs of wolves, as well as the amount of different packs of wolves in a given area (which could be identified by the number of different track routes). This then allowed researchers to predict overall populations of individual species within the exclusion zone as a whole. As the researchers gathered this data from helicopters at a distance from the radiated land, they were able to avoid exposure to the extreme radiation present at ground level. Overall, the research showed that animal populations had flourished compared not only to the researchers predicted results, but also compared to animals living outside of the exclusion zone, on healthy land without radiation damage. In one instance, research found that the population of wolves was seven times greater inside the exclusion zone than it was in nearby, uncontaminated land.

Of course, though the data shows an increase in animal populations, this does not mean that radiation is beneficial for animals. Many humans exposed to radiation from the initial nuclear explosion died from acute radiation syndrome, and the population of most animal breeds within the exclusion zone initially showed a severe decrease. Though serious mutations in animals were documented only in the immediate aftermath of the accident, lingering problems persist. Voles living within the area have shown a higher susceptibility to developing cataracts than voles living on uncontaminated land; and partial albinism (a lack of pigment in the skin and feathers) is higher among swallows living within the exclusion zone. What the study appears to show, instead, is that despite the significant impact the polluted land has on the population size of animals, living on extremely irradiated land has a less harmful impact than humans do on the animals' ability to grow in population size. The findings of the study have shown that despite the terrible effects Chernobyl has had on the environment, it has at least not deterred the local animals' determination to survive.

3.　Based on the passage, it must be true that wolves living within the exclusion zone:

A. grew in population size by a factor of seven in the decades following the nuclear disaster.
B. hunt in packs after dark.
C. are more likely to develop cataracts than wolves living on uncontaminated land.
D. have developed a method to avoid exposure to harmful radiation.

4.　Which of the following can be inferred from the passage?

A. All civilians living with the 4,200km exclusion zone left their homes.
B. The researchers found the low population levels surprising.
C. The exclusion zone offers some health benefits to animals.
D. Since the nuclear disaster in Chernobyl, the local wildlife has become more determined to survive.

The colour black is created when a surface absorbs all wavelengths of light. The more light the surface absorbs than it reflects, the darker the black appears to the human eye. In 2014, the darkest man-made substance, called the blackest black, was developed by British scientists. It is structurally similar to other light absorbing materials, such as those created by NASA, in that it is made up of carbon nanotubes.

Carbon nanotubes are formed when single-atom thick sheets of carbon, called graphene, are rolled into long hollow tubes with a diameter measuring on the nanometre scale. A nanometre is 10,000 times smaller than the diameter of a human hair. This process gives them high tensile or conductive properties, depending on how the sheet is rolled and the radius of the tube. In order to create this new black material, millions of these nanotubes were "grown" onto an aluminium foil surface using a variation of the chemical vapour deposition process. The surface structure created was highly unique in that all the carbon nanotubes aligned vertically, forming a tightly-packed array of tubes, like a clump of drinking straws standing up on end.

This structure causes the surface to appear so incredibly black by absorbing 99.965% of all the visible light that hits it. Light cannot travel through the nanotubes itself, but instead passes into the spaces between them, where it becomes trapped. Once inside these spaces, the light is repeatedly deflected until it is eventually absorbed and dissipates as heat. When the surface is looked at by human eyes, no reflections can be seen, meaning no topographical information on the surface can be picked out by the brain. This creates what is described as an odd sensation of looking into a void; the experience is thought to be the closest that humans can come to staring into a black hole.

The material itself has promise for several possible applications. For example, telescopes are calibrated against black in order to detect light from distant stars. Using this nanotube material, they would be able to pick out even fainter light sources from deep space, greatly increasing their sensitivity. It could also be used as an insulating material, increasing the performance and accuracy of the telescope by preventing stray light from entering the array. Other potential uses exist in the form of Infra-Red cameras and solar power technology, where it could increase the absorption of heat, as well as military applications such as thermal camouflage. However it could not yet be used for clothing, as despite having low outgassing and particle fallout properties, the surface remains brittle. Damage to the material would lead to the release of carbon nanotubes into the atmosphere, and these tiny particles have already been linked to respiratory illnesses in humans.

5. Carbon nanotubes have an average diameter of one nanometre.

   A. True
   B. False
   C. Can't tell

6. The darkest man-made substance is comprised of carbon nanotubes.

   A. True
   B. False
   C. Can't tell

7. Carbon nanotubes can be used in military uniforms to camouflage soldiers.

   A. True
   B. False
   C. Can't tell

8. Carbon nanotubes are not a naturally occurring material.

   A. True
   B. False
   C. Can't tell

The zoo, or zoological garden, is one of the most ancient institutions of leisure still utilized in modern society. The earliest origins of this institution lie in the world of antiquity, where kings and emperors would showcase the vastness of their territories by bringing together exotic species from the farthest reaches of the lands they ruled over. The oldest such space to be uncovered, at the ancient city of Hierakonpolis in Egypt, dates from 3500 BC. Menageries were also built throughout the following millennia by the rulers of Assyria, Babylonia and China, being filled with animals that served for decoration, as meals on special feast occasions, and, infrequently, as trained performers in parades and circus-type events. The idea of using captured animals as fighting champions was largely novel to the Roman Empire: the cost and difficulty of transporting exotic beasts back to Italy tended to militate against such a wasteful slaughter.

In Britain, the earliest zoos were cultivated by monarchs and were intended to impress the power and opulence of these patrons upon visitors. After the fall of the Roman Empire and the commencement of the Dark Ages, with the concomitant severing of communicative and commercial links between far-flung parts of the world, Europe was not to see large-scale menageries again for several centuries. Following the Renaissance and the era of exploration and discovery, European monarchs in the 16th and 17th centuries began assembling large menageries as a means to demonstrate, not only their power and riches, but also the globe-straddling culture and scholarly advancement of their ruling houses. It was in this period that Elizabeth I opened the Tower of London, which was then home to a group of majestic lions, to the public, making it Britain's first open menagerie. In contrast with the strict prohibition on feeding the animals at most modern zoos, visitors were invited to feed a cat or a dog to the lions by way of an entrance fee! Thereafter, the royal selection of animals was steadily enlarged to include the new specimens that English explorers came into contact with over time, and was spread across several locations in London. In many cases, new animals were acquired by the Crown as diplomatic gifts—in 1664, for example, St James's Park became home to a group of white pelicans gifted to England by the Russian Tsar; the descendants of the very same birds still inhabit the area today. By the late 18th century, most of the major European powers had opened their own menageries; the oldest zoo still in existence, the Tiergarten Schönbrunn, was founded in Vienna in 1752.

These menageries, growing out of royal patronage, were the immediate forerunners of modern or scientific zoos, the first of which was established in 1828 at Regent's Park by the Zoological Society of London, absorbing most of the collection of the closing Tower of London menagerie throughout the 1830s. The initial intention of this new zoo was that it would be used solely by scholars, for the purpose of dispassionate research. However, funding proved hard to come by, and in 1847 London Zoo ended up opening its doors to an eager public. Over the next half-century, catering to popular demand and abiding by government directives, the Zoo became a focal point for displays of the unprecedented geographical scope and scientific prowess of the British Empire. Somehow—for the time being at least—the attempt to take zoos away from their role as flashy political status symbols had come full circle.

9. Which of these statements must be false?

    A. Menageries were used in Europe to demonstrate advances in learning.
    B. Vienna is the home of the world's first zoo.
    C. Animals in ancient Babylonia were sometimes trained to perform in parades.
    D. Britain's first open menagerie housed only native British animals.

10. The passage suggests that the zoo in Regent's Park:

    A. was established in order to display the wealth and prowess of the British Empire.
    B. continues to house a rare breed of white pelican.
    C. was not initially open to the public.
    D. continues to be used for scientific research.

The zoo, or zoological garden, is one of the most ancient institutions of leisure still utilized in modern society. The earliest origins of this institution lie in the world of antiquity, where kings and emperors would showcase the vastness of their territories by bringing together exotic species from the farthest reaches of the lands they ruled over. The oldest such space to be uncovered, at the ancient city of Hierakonpolis in Egypt, dates from 3500 BC. Menageries were also built throughout the following millennia by the rulers of Assyria, Babylonia and China, being filled with animals that served for decoration, as meals on special feast occasions, and, infrequently, as trained performers in parades and circus-type events. The idea of using captured animals as fighting champions was largely novel to the Roman Empire: the cost and difficulty of transporting exotic beasts back to Italy tended to militate against such a wasteful slaughter.

In Britain, the earliest zoos were cultivated by monarchs and were intended to impress the power and opulence of these patrons upon visitors. After the fall of the Roman Empire and the commencement of the Dark Ages, with the concomitant severing of communicative and commercial links between far-flung parts of the world, Europe was not to see large-scale menageries again for several centuries. Following the Renaissance and the era of exploration and discovery, European monarchs in the 16th and 17th centuries began assembling large menageries as a means to demonstrate, not only their power and riches, but also the globe-straddling culture and scholarly advancement of their ruling houses. It was in this period that Elizabeth I opened the Tower of London, which was then home to a group of majestic lions, to the public, making it Britain's first open menagerie. In contrast with the strict prohibition on feeding the animals at most modern zoos, visitors were invited to feed a cat or a dog to the lions by way of an entrance fee! Thereafter, the royal selection of animals was steadily enlarged to include the new specimens that English explorers came into contact with over time, and was spread across several locations in London. In many cases, new animals were acquired by the Crown as diplomatic gifts—in 1664, for example, St James's Park became home to a group of white pelicans gifted to England by the Russian Tsar; the descendants of the very same birds still inhabit the area today. By the late 18th century, most of the major European powers had opened their own menageries; the oldest zoo still in existence, the Tiergarten Schönbrunn, was founded in Vienna in 1752.

These menageries, growing out of royal patronage, were the immediate forerunners of modern or scientific zoos, the first of which was established in 1828 at Regent's Park by the Zoological Society of London, absorbing most of the collection of the closing Tower of London menagerie throughout the 1830s. The initial intention of this new zoo was that it would be used solely by scholars, for the purpose of dispassionate research. However, funding proved hard to come by, and in 1847 London Zoo ended up opening its doors to an eager public. Over the next half-century, catering to popular demand and abiding by government directives, the Zoo became a focal point for displays of the unprecedented geographical scope and scientific prowess of the British Empire. Somehow—for the time being at least—the attempt to take zoos away from their role as flashy political status symbols had come full circle.

11. Which of the following must be true of zoos and menageries in Britain?

A. The public gained access to Britain's first scientific zoo in the first half of the 19th century.
B. They generally require visitors to pay an entrance fee.
C. None existed in Britain prior to the Dark Ages.
D. They were initially furnished solely with animals brought home by English explorers.

12. The author would most likely agree with the assertion that:

A. modern zoos share more similarities with menageries of the 16th century than with scientific zoos of the 19th century.
B. in the early Roman menageries, animals were frequently made to fight each other.
C. public zoos geared towards making money should focus more energy on research.
D. Elizabeth I brought lions to the Tower of London after opening the menagerie to the public.

Founded in 1838 as Spring Hill College in Birmingham, Mansfield College was not fully integrated into the University of Oxford until 1995. Today the college, which is home to 210 undergraduates, 130 graduate students, and 35 visiting scholars, is Oxford's smallest, except for Harris Manchester, the university's college for mature students. Mansfield has a reputation for friendliness and informality.

Spring Hill College was founded as a Nonconformist college for those who could not attend major national universities such as Oxford or Cambridge, which required allegiance to the Church of England. The college stood in Birmingham for almost 50 years, moving to Oxford after the 1871 Universities Test Act, which abolished religious tests for admission of non-theological students at Oxford, Cambridge and Durham. With the move, the college also renamed in recognition of its greatest donors, George and Elizabeth Mansfield. Though Mansfield was Oxford's first Nonconformist college, it lost much of its religious character over time, becoming increasingly secular.

Still, signs of the college's religious heritage still stand. A prominent portrait of Oliver Cromwell, the ultimate English dissenter who was killed in 1658, hangs in the Senior Common Room, and in the halls and library of Mansfield hang portraits of the 1662 dissenters who separated from the Church of England after the Act of Uniformity required Anglican ordination for all clergy. Chapel services continue to be performed in the nonconformist tradition, and the College Chaplain is always from a Nonconformist denomination. The college's religious past has also historically strengthened its ties to universities in the United States, from which the college still carries a long tradition of accepting a number of American junior year abroad students each year.

13. Durham University once required a religious admissions test.

    A. True
    B. False
    C. Can't tell

14. Mansfield is Oxford's smallest college.

    A. True
    B. False
    C. Can't tell

15. The Mansfield College Chapel is not consecrated.

    A. True
    B. False
    C. Can't tell

16. Oliver Cromwell was one of the 1662 dissenters.

    A. True
    B. False
    C. Can't tell

The UK has less usable water per person than most European countries. Despite the insatiable rainfall in Britain, research suggests that the Sudan and Syria have more available water than the South East of England. In the last few years, the UK has launched a campaign to conserve water, asking citizens to find small ways to reduce the amount of water they use on a daily basis. The average person in England and Wales currently uses 150 litres of water per day, the equivalent of 264 pints of milk. Most of this water is expended in washing and toilet flushing; in fact, water use has increased by almost 50% in the last 50 years due to new technological developments. Those numbers are on the rise; the need for fresh water is expected to increase by 30% when the population exceeds 8 billion, which is projected to happen in the next 20 years. The government's goal is to decrease per capita water usage by 20 litres per day. This is easier than most people imagine. For example, turning off the tap while brushing your teeth and cutting down shower time by one minute saves 15 litres of water a day.

Still, the problem is much bigger than these smaller conservation efforts. New studies estimate that UK consumers only see about 3% of the water usage they are responsible for. This is because of what environmental scientists term embedded water, the total amount of water necessary to produce the things we use on a daily basis. For example, a pint of beer contains 74 litres of embedded water, expended in growing the ingredients and running the processes that make the beer. A cup of coffee is worse; its embedded water content is about 140 litres. A cotton t-shirt embeds about 2,000 litres. Many developing countries currently use a large portion of their limited water resources for crops that they export to developed nations. Thus, the problem of embedded water raises many additional questions about how to really impact water conservation, both at home and abroad.

17. The author would least likely agree with which of these conclusion?
    A. The UK's water conservation schemes are inadequate.
    B. Conserving water is not as difficult as people might think.
    C. Current efforts to conserve water in the UK are sufficient.
    D. More effective water conservation will require further measures.

18. Most water in England and Wales is used in:
    A. toilets, baths and showers.
    B. milk production.
    C. making food and drink.
    D. gardens, lawns and farms.

19. The passage includes examples of embedded water that involve all of the following except:
    A. alcoholic and non-alcoholic drinks
    B. agricultural exports
    C. livestock
    D. clothing

20. Which of the following statements is true of embedded water?
    A. In the UK, it accounts for 3% of the total water supply.
    B. A cup of coffee embeds almost twice as much water as a pint of beer.
    C. The majority of embedded water is used for crops in developing countries.
    D. Leaving the tap running longer than necessary is an example of embedded water.

The International Table Tennis Federation (ITTF) has recently changed some of the key rules of competitive table tennis, also known as ping-pong. Starting in 2000, the ITTF increased the diameter of table tennis balls from 38 mm to 40 mm. While this difference in diameter may seem a minor issue, the resulting reduction in speed and spin gave an advantage to players who favoured a slower style of play. The change in ball size was challenged unsuccessfully by the Chinese National Team, whose players led the world table tennis rankings before the change, and who were known at the time for a playing style marked by smashes and quick attacks. ITTF-sanctioned balls must be white or orange, and are printed with three stars, which indicate the quality of the ball; lesser quality balls might be printed with only one or two stars. The stars on ITTF-approved balls may be printed in certain possible colours: most balls have black or blue stars, though the stars on some will feature a second colour (red, green or purple). Balls of these colours are thought to be easiest to see on tables with a green or blue surface, the only two colours of table surface that are approved for ITTF competition.

A year after their decision changing the size of table tennis balls, the ITTF adjusted the scoring system for competitive table tennis, so that the first player to score 11 points wins a game, unless both are tied on 10, in which case the first player to score a 2-point lead is the winner. Prior to this, a game was won by the first player to reach 21 points. The ITTF felt the change in scoring was necessary to make games more exciting, and to shorten the length of matches, so these would be more engaging to television audiences. (A match consists of an odd number of games, and a player must win a majority of games to win the match; matches in competitive table tennis consist of five or seven games.) Whether the scoring change succeeded in meeting this goal is an open question, but matches finish much more quickly, since nearly half as many points are now required to win most games (except, of course, in the case of a 10-10 tie). In spite of this, amateur players often play a game until someone scores 21 (or wins by at least 2 points), either because they are nostalgic for the old scoring system, or because they are unaware of the ITTF's decision.

21. The author would most likely agree that non-professional players:

    A. do not always know of rule changes in professional sport.
    B. always abide by the current rules of sporting associations.
    C. do not have an opinion on the actions of sporting associations.
    D. always prefer to play a sport under the rules they first learned.

22. Under current ITTF rules, a table tennis game could be won by a score of:

    A. 11-10
    B. 12-11
    C. 13-11
    D. 21-20

23. It must be false that the Chinese National Team:

    A. were known for a faster style of play.
    B. campaigned against the increase in ball size.
    C. did better with smaller balls, as they had more spin.
    D. prefer the larger ball size.

24. The stars on table tennis balls sanctioned for ITTF play may include any of the following combinations except:

    A. a white ball with blue stars.
    B. an orange ball with black stars
    C. a white ball with black and purple stars
    D. an orange ball with green and white stars.

In the mid-nineteenth century, the French novelist Emile Zola announced to his publisher that he was embarking on a cycle of novels in the style of Balzac that would explore various aspects of life in France during the Second Empire. Unlike *La Comedie Humaine*, though, Zola's cycle would focus its attentions on one family, allowing Zola to explore his strong interests in heredity, evolution, and genealogy at the same as he offered a literary account of the Second Empire. What resulted was Zola's twenty novel cycle, collectively known as *Les Rougon-Macquart* and subtitled *Histoire naturelle et sociale d'une famille sons le Second Empire* (Natural and social history of a family during the second empire). Zola's work in these novels established his reputation as a preeminent proponent of naturalism, a literary movement that emphasised the harsh realities of life through a frank, if pessimistic, depiction of subject matter such as sexuality, corruption and disease that had previously been considered too sordid to be included in literature.

Almost all of the protagonists of the Rougon-Macquart family are introduced in Zola's first novel, *La Fortune des Rougon*. The family centres on Adelaide Fouque, a middle-class French woman from Provence with a slight mental deficiency, and her three children: Pierre Rougon, the legitimate child from her marriage to Rougon, and Antoine and Ursule Macquart, illegitimate children by her lover, the smuggler Macquart. With Adelaide at the centre-point, the novel explores the three strands of her family: the Rougons, who are upper-class and well-educated; the Macquarts, who are mostly blue-collar workers or soldiers; and the Mourets (the family of Adelaide's illegitimate daughter Ursule Macquart), who live a more middle-class and balanced life.

Zola traced each of his more than 300 characters carefully. Before even beginning to write *La Fortune des Rougon*, he set about creating an elaborate family tree that included each character's name, date of birth, properties of heredity (including their mental proclivities and physical likeness), details of their biography, and death date. In each character, Zola traces the competing influences of blood and environment, set against the political, economic, cultural, and artistic backdrop of France (and Paris, particularly) from 1852 to 1870. Even in closing this cycle of novels, Zola accounts for the fate of all of his characters. In his final novel *Le Docteur Pascal*, Zola includes a long chapter that reconnects with all of his living characters, tying up loose ends in their narratives and finishing each of their stories. In this respect, Zola succeeded where Balzac failed; Balzac never finished *La Comedie Humaine*, consisting at the time of his death of more than 90 novels, short stories and essays that represented his only cycle of novels—and, indeed, the entire literary output of his adult life.

25. The Second Empire occurred in the 19th century.

    A. True
    B. False
    C. Can't tell

26. Zola was a notable naturalist.

    A. True
    B. False
    C. Can't tell

27. Zola's novels are set in Paris.

    A. True
    B. False
    C. Can't tell

28. Balzac wrote a cycle of twenty novels, featuring a number of different families.

    A. True
    B. False
    C. Can't tell

Single-sex education for both men and women is declining in the UK. Today, only about 11% of all boys and girls graduate from a single-sex secondary school, and the number of all-women's secondary schools is down to 400, from an historical UK high of about 2,500 in the 1960s. Nevertheless, a debate about the necessity, quality, and advantages of single-sex education continues among academics and public officials.

The 1944 Education Act guaranteed free education for all students, regardless of gender, from primary to secondary school. Full access to all levels of education, however, was not fully instituted until the late 1980s, until which point many universities and grammar schools maintained strict quotas on the number of female students they would admit. The increased access women enjoy to all levels of education may explain some of the reasons why the country has seen a decline in the number of women's-only institutions; in fact, women now outnumber men in higher education in the UK. However, there still seem to be some benefits to single-sex education. All-girls schools regularly report highly competitive GCSEs and low dropout rates. Studies suggest that those pupils who are most struggling when they enter the single-sex educational environment are often the students most likely to benefit. Other studies, targeted at adults in their 40s, indicate that graduates of single-sex schools of either gender are less likely to have studied gender-stereotyped subjects in school. Women from this group who graduated from all-girls schools also have higher earnings on average than women who attended school with boys.

Some researchers suggest that the results from these studies, particularly test scores and graduation rates, may be skewed by the economic and class differences at work. Alan Smithers, Professor of Education at Buckingham University, argues that pupils in these schools succeed because of their ability and social background, and not the particular environment of the schools.

29. Women in the UK first had full and equal access to education at all levels in the:

   A. 1940s
   B. 1960s
   C. 1980s
   D. 1990s

30. The author seems open to the possibility that:

   A. no students would benefit from a single-sex school.
   B. single-sex schools do not benefit women students.
   C. student success depends only on student ability.
   D. student success is tied to socioeconomic factors.

31. Which of the following cannot be inferred from the information in the passage?

   A. Prior to 1944, not all students in the UK were entitled to free education.
   B. Students who attend single-sex schools often come from affluent families.
   C. In the 1960s, the number of all-girls schools was at its peak.
   D. Graduates of all-girls schools earn, on average, more than graduates of mixed schools.

32. At their peak, secondary schools in the UK that enrolled only women students numbered:

   A. fewer than two thousand.
   B. more than two thousand.
   C. more than three thousand.
   D. fewer than five hundred.

From 2007 to 2013, at least 10 million domestic beehives were lost. The sudden, sharp decline in bee populations, caused by a mysterious phenomenon known as colony collapse disorder (CCD), posed a substantial threat, due to the significant share of the world's diet that depends on pollination by bees. More than four-fifths of food crops worldwide that require pollination are pollinated by honey bees; thus, colony collapse disorder—which rapidly spread throughout Europe, Asia and South America—represented a serious threat to the food supply

What, exactly, caused this outbreak of CCD? Pesticides were the original suspect, and were known to have exterminated the entire population of bees in one Chinese province in the 1980s. Other research suggested that a combination of two infections—a virus and a fungus—were far deadlier for bees than either would be on its own. One hundred percent of collapsed hives in the study were found to have traces of invertebrate iridescent viruses (IIV); however, since these were also found in many strong colonies, IIV could not have been responsible for colony collapse. A variety of microbes that attacked invertebrates were found in most of the collapsed colonies, but most could be eliminated as possible culprits, as they occurred in only a few collapsed hives. However, one fungus called Nosema, which consists of a single cell and targets bees specifically, was found in most of the collapsed colonies in the study. Scientists determined that, though Nosema was unlikely to predict the likelihood of collapse when found in an otherwise healthy hive, absent any traces of IIV; the presence of both Nosema and IIV was a strong indicator of the likelihood of collapse, given the high correlation of the two in collapsed colonies in the study.

In recent years, reported cases of CCD have declined. In the winter of 2007-2008, 28.7% of bee hives worldwide did not survive over winter, this level dropped to 23.1% for the winter of 2014-2015. In 2017, the number of honeybees in the US rose from the previous year. Despite these figures, the population level of bees worldwide remains troubling. Tests that had earlier proven that pesticides commonly used on flowers and crops in the USA and Europe are not significantly harmful to bees, were shown to be flawed. The USA's Environmental Protection Agency confirmed in a confidential report that was subsequently leaked to the press that clothianidin, a pesticide widely used on corn, can be 'highly toxic' and present a 'long-term risk' to bee colonies. Studies in 2017, funded in part by the makers of clothianidin, linked the use of neonicotinoids with decreased reproduction and shorter life expectancy in bees in Europe and Canada. We're still a long way from fully understanding how our actions impact bee populations, but until we understand the cause, we will not be able to fully address the impact.

33. Which of the following statements about the world's food supply is best supported by the passage?

   A. Most of the world's crops depend on bees for pollination.
   B. Nosema infections posed the greatest threat to the world's food supply in 2007.
   C. Pesticides are now the greatest threat to the world's food supply.
   D. Most of the world's pollinated food crops depend on bees for pollination.

34. Which of the following is true of bee populations in the US?

   A. The number of hive deaths was greater in the winter of 2007-2008 than that of 2014-2015.
   B. The number of beehives decreased by four fifths.
   C. The population size was greater in 2017 than 2016.
   D. 10 million bees died between 2007 and 2013.

From 2007 to 2013, at least 10 million domestic beehives were lost. The sudden, sharp decline in bee populations, caused by a mysterious phenomenon known as colony collapse disorder (CCD), posed a substantial threat, due to the significant share of the world's diet that depends on pollination by bees. More than four-fifths of food crops worldwide that require pollination are pollinated by honey bees; thus, colony collapse disorder—which rapidly spread throughout Europe, Asia and South America—represented a serious threat to the food supply

What, exactly, caused this outbreak of CCD? Pesticides were the original suspect, and were known to have exterminated the entire population of bees in one Chinese province in the 1980s. Other research suggested that a combination of two infections—a virus and a fungus—were far deadlier for bees than either would be on its own. One hundred percent of collapsed hives in the study were found to have traces of invertebrate iridescent viruses (IIV); however, since these were also found in many strong colonies, IIV could not have been responsible for colony collapse. A variety of microbes that attacked invertebrates were found in most of the collapsed colonies, but most could be eliminated as possible culprits, as they occurred in only a few collapsed hives. However, one fungus called Nosema, which consists of a single cell and targets bees specifically, was found in most of the collapsed colonies in the study. Scientists determined that, though Nosema was unlikely to predict the likelihood of collapse when found in an otherwise healthy hive, absent any traces of IIV; the presence of both Nosema and IIV was a strong indicator of the likelihood of collapse, given the high correlation of the two in collapsed colonies in the study.

In recent years, reported cases of CCD have declined. In the winter of 2007-2008, 28.7% of bee hives worldwide did not survive over winter, this level dropped to 23.1% for the winter of 2014-2015. In 2017, the number of honeybees in the US rose from the previous year. Despite these figures, the population level of bees worldwide remains troubling. Tests that had earlier proven that pesticides commonly used on flowers and crops in the USA and Europe are not significantly harmful to bees, were shown to be flawed. The USA's Environmental Protection Agency confirmed in a confidential report that was subsequently leaked to the press that clothianidin, a pesticide widely used on corn, can be 'highly toxic' and present a 'long-term risk' to bee colonies. Studies in 2017, funded in part by the makers of clothianidin, linked the use of neonicotinoids with decreased reproduction and shorter life expectancy in bees in Europe and Canada. We're still a long way from fully understanding how our actions impact bee populations, but until we understand the cause, we will not be able to fully address the impact.

35. According to the information in the passage, what led scientists to believe that IIVs are not the sole cause of colony collapse disorder?

A. IIVs were found in 100% of collapsed colonies.
B. IIVs occurred in strong colonies as well as collapsed colonies.
C. IIVs are not found in colonies that are infected with Nosema.
D. IIVs are more likely to be found in hives that have been sprayed with clothianidin.

36. According to the passage, recent studies into the effect of pesticides suggest:

A. a pesticide used on corn can decrease reproduction in bees.
B. research may not always be funded by impartial parties.
C. neonicotinoids are highly toxic to bee populations
D. pesticides are not significantly harmful to bees.

In November 1936, Crystal Palace, relocated since the Great Exhibition of 1851 to Sydenham Hill, burned to the ground. The enormous glass and cast iron construction had by that time fallen into disrepair, though in recent years it had seen a revival under the leadership of Sir Henry Buckland and his board of trustees. What started as a small office fire took off quickly, and 89 fire engines and 400 firemen could not stop the blaze. 10,000 people came out to Sydenham Hill to watch the palace as it burned to the ground.

The building that was destroyed in 1936 was very different from that erected in Hyde Park for the Great Exhibition over eighty years earlier. Though all the construction materials had been moved south of London after the six months of the exhibition, what was erected on Sydenham Hill was really a Beaux Arts form, and not the greenhouse-like construction designed by Chatsworth House gardener Joseph Paxton. This new building has some of the same features—public toilets, for example, which had debuted at Crystal Palace during the Great Exhibition, were installed in the new site as well. But, the structure had been modified and enlarged, so much so that it exceeded the bounds of the new park designed for its construction.

The relocation of Crystal Palace was an expensive feat, costing £1.3 million (£96.5 million today), over a £1 million more than it had taken to build the original structure. The relocation put Crystal Palace in debt from which it never recovered. Although two separate train stations were built to serve the permanent exhibition, by the 1890s the structure had seriously deteriorated. The palace was used in World War I as a naval training establishment and was later the site of the first Imperial War Museum. Buckland's leadership in the 1920s and 30s improved the gardens and brought visitors back to the palace for the exhibitions and regular fireworks shows, but the 1936 fire prevented him from fully realising the palace's old glory. Nevertheless, as Buckland predicted, Crystal Palace is not forgotten today. In fact, the area of Penge Common and Sydenham Hill, where the structure was relocated over 150 years ago, is now known as Crystal Palace.

37. The Imperial War Museum is located at Crystal Palace.
    A. True
    B. False
    C. Can't tell

38. The Great Exhibition of 1851 featured the first public toilets.
    A. True
    B. False
    C. Can't tell

39. Crystal Palace was originally in Hyde Park.
    A. True
    B. False
    C. Can't tell

40. A fireworks display started the fire that destroyed Crystal Palace.
    A. True
    B. False
    C. Can't tell

A charity is an organisation that is run on a not-for-profit basis: rather than being beholden to share-holders seeking financial returns, any revenue a charitable organisation raises must be used towards further fulfilling its mission, defined in its Memorandum of Understanding. This may include contributions towards overheads, recruitment costs and salaries for valuable employees, building capacity to scale up operations, or else contributing towards a reserve, through savings or investments.

The definition and subsequent regulation of charitable trusts has been a relatively longstanding feature of English law. The Charitable Uses Act of 1601 outlines the scope of what constitutes a charitable purpose, al-though as is the nature of English law, the workable definition is derived from case law. Lord Macnaghten stated that charitable trusts must work to relieve poverty; advance education; advance religion or else benefit the wider public. The public aspect to this is key: while there exist a number of benevolent funds that seek to alleviate poverty or hardship amongst professions and vocations including musicians, doctors and service personnel, the *Oppenheim v Tobacco Securities Trust* decision made it clear that the beneficiaries of a trust may not be related to one another by links to a single company alone. The scope of charities to undertake political campaigning to make changes to the law is prohibited: as regulation of charities is a responsibility shared between the Charity Commission and the High Court of Justice, the assumption is that the law in its current state must be upheld. Moreover, advocacy of this nature may contravene the stipulation for charities to act within the public benefit.

With respect to governance, charities are overseen by trustees, who may not take a salary from the organi-sation but have a responsibility and duty to uphold the charity's mission and ensure no funds are misap-propriated. Trustees may be removed from their position by the Charity Commission, should they not be fulfilling their duties, be this due to diminished mental capacity, bankruptcy, absence from the country or any such other reason. As charities are exempt from paying VAT and their donations are not subject to the basic rate of tax (through a scheme known as 'Gift Aid,' initially established through the 1990 Finance Act), they receive financial benefits profit-making companies are not party to. However, charities are subject to enhanced scrutiny of their accounts; alongside the statutory filing of annual accounts with both Companies House and HMRC they have enhanced audit procedures.

41. Which of the following can be inferred from the passage?

    A. Charities must not align themselves with any specific religion.

    B. Those who work for charitable organisations do not get paid.

    C. If a charity is not benefitting the wider public or relieving poverty, it must advance education.

    D. If a charity sought to change the law, it might not be acting with the intention of benefitting the public.

42. It must be false that:

    A. Gift Aid enables donations to charities to be exempt from tax.

    B. if a charity's revenue is not used towards fulfilling its mission, a trustee may be removed from their position.

    C. the trustees of a charity are solely responsible for its regulation.

    D. employees of a single company may not be the sole beneficiaries of a charity.

43. Which of the following is true of the Charitable Uses Act?

    A. It states that charities must not take part in political campaigning.

    B. It has been heavily revised since its initial creation in 1601.

    C. It conforms to the traditions of English law.

    D. It outlines that the beneficiaries of a trust may not be doctors or service personnel.

44. According to the passage, trustees of a charity:

    A. must ascertain that the charity's Memorandum of Understanding is followed.

    B. are often compensated for their work.

    C. are exempt from tax, as a result of the 1990 Finance Act.

    D. must remain in the same country as the charity they oversee.

STOP. IF YOU FINISH BEFORE TIME IS CALLED, CHECK ANY QUESTIONS YOU HAVE MARKED FOR REVIEW. YOU MAY GO BACK TO QUESTIONS IN THIS SECTION ONLY.

Section 2: Decision Making (31 Minutes)

This section contains 29 questions. Each question is a standalone item. Some questions may include information in the form of charts, graphs, tables or diagrams. Most questions will have five answer choices. Your task is to select the best option based on the data provided.

Some questions will include five parts, instead of five answer choices. You must drag and drop the correct answer (Yes or No) for each of the five parts. These questions are worth 2 marks each. You only get 2 marks if you answer all five parts correctly. If you answer mostly correctly, you will get 1 mark.

Answer all 29 questions in Section 2, selecting one of the possible answers and circling the letter corresponding to the appropriate answer in your test paper. For drag-and-drop questions, write YES or NO in the grey box beside each of the five parts.

When you are finished with this section, you may use any remaining time to review your work in this section only. Once you proceed to the next section, you may not return to this section.

You will have 31 minutes to answer the questions. It is in your best interest to select an answer for every item as there is no penalty for wrong answers.

Set your timer for 31 minutes, turn the page and begin the section.

1. Not all the rides at the fair were deemed unsafe, except for those visited by the health inspector. Place 'Yes' if the conclusion does follow. Place 'No' if the conclusion does not follow.

Some of the rides at the fair were not deemed unsafe.	
All the rides at the fair were deemed unsafe.	
All the rides at the fair that were visited by the health inspector were deemed unsafe.	
All the rides at the fair that were deemed unsafe were visited by the health inspector.	
The health inspector visited all the rides at the fair.	

2. The leaving students at a UK sixth form college are all either going to university or into full-time employment next year. Fewer than half of the students going to university will study abroad. 70% of the leaving students are going to university.

Place 'Yes' if the conclusion does follow. Place 'No' if the conclusion does not follow.

None of the students are going into full-time employment abroad.	
Some of the students at the sixth form college will study in the UK.	
All of the students are leaving the college next year.	
There are fewer students going into full-time employment than going to university in the UK.	
Some of the students are taking a gap year.	

3. DTP is a business conglomerate consisting of three corporations: Dizon, Transmet and Pearton. All employees of Transmet work in the service sector, compared to only 35% of Dizon's. All Pearton employees work in either the manufacturing or the service sector.

    Place 'Yes' if the conclusion does follow. Place 'No' if the conclusion does not follow.

Sheila is a Pearton employee but does not work in the service sector. Sheila works in the manufacturing sector.	
Dizon employees who do not work in the service sector are employed in the manufacturing sector.	
Beatrice works in the service sector, so she must be employed by Transmet.	
Mahmood does not work in the service sector, so he must not be employed by Transmet.	
Anyone who works in the service sector must be employed by Dizon, Transmet or Pearton.	

4.   A shopping centre food court has both restaurants and takeaway food outlets. Some of the takeaway food outlets sell Chinese food. The majority of the restaurants sell Italian food. The remainder of establishments in the food court only offer Indian food.

Place 'Yes' if the conclusion does follow. Place 'No' if the conclusion does not follow.

There are more Italian restaurants than Indian takeaways in the food court.	
Any shop selling Chinese food must be a takeaway.	
A person buying Italian food must be in a restaurant.	
There are more places to buy Indian food than either other cuisine.	
Indian food could be sold at both takeaways and restaurants in the food court.	

5. All clowns are unhappy. All morticians are happy. Happy people always attend funerals. This person is either a mortician or a clown.

    Place 'Yes' if the conclusion does follow. Place 'No' if the conclusion does not follow.

This person is either happy or a mortician.	
If this person never attends funerals, then they are a clown.	
If this person is a mortician, then they do not attend funerals.	
If this person always attends funerals, then they are a mortician.	
People who never attend funerals are unhappy.	

The table below shows the length of three types of steel tubes. Barry has constructed three flagpoles, labelled I, II, and III. Each flagpole is made from four steel tubes.

Steel Tubes	
Type	**Height (cm)**
P	120
Q	80
R	160

Flagpole I has been constructed with all three types of steel tube.

Flagpole II has been constructed with only P-type and R-type tubes.

Flagpole III has been constructed with four steel tubes of the same length.

No flagpole has been constructed with more than two R-type tubes.

6. Which of the following statements must be true?

A. Flagpole I is the longest flagpole.
B. Flagpole III is the shortest flagpole.
C. Flagpole I and Flagpole II are the same length.
D. Flagpole II is longer than Flagpole III.

A publisher of science fiction and historical novels is releasing one book per financial quarter (Q1, Q2, Q3 and Q4). Each book is by a different author but the publisher never releases novels of the same genre in successive quarters.

Levi's novel will be published after Wilkins's novel.

Neither Prandesh nor Gordell writes historical novels.

The publisher is releasing a work of science fiction in Q2.

7. Which of the following MUST be true?

A. Wilkins's novel will be released in Q1.
B. Gordell's novel will be released in Q2.
C. Prandesh's novel will be released in Q3.
D. Levi's novel will be released in Q4.

Five friends—Artemis, Charlie, Deandre, Frank and Roxie—are seated together at the back of a bus.

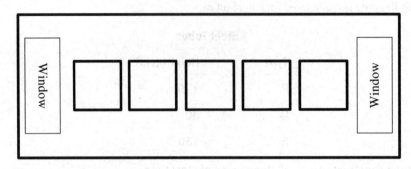

Artemis is not sat in the middle seat.

Deandre has a window seat.

There are two people between Roxie and Charlie.

8.   Which of the following must be true?

   A.   Roxie is sat next to Frank.
   B.   Frank is sat next to Artemis.
   C.   Artemis is sat next to Charlie.
   D.   Charlie is sat next to Deandre.

Five sales reps attending a conference notice that their shirts and socks are each a different combination of colours. All the colours mentioned describe their shirts and socks only.

Their shirts are white, blue, pink, purple and grey.

Their socks are white, blue, pink, black and green.

No one is wearing a shirt and socks of the same colour.

No one is wearing a shirt and socks of colours that start with the same letter.

The sales rep wearing blue socks is sitting between two sales reps wearing pink.

The sales reps wearing white are not sitting next to the sales rep wearing green, nor next to each other.

One sales rep is wearing blue and pink.

9.   Which of the following must be worn by one of the sales reps?

   A.   A blue shirt and white socks.
   B.   A grey shirt and pink socks.
   C.   A pink shirt and black socks.
   D.   A purple shirt and blue socks.

10. Should tourists be denied access to cultural sites such as Machu Picchu and the Great Wall of China, in order to protect these sites for future generations?

Select the strongest argument from the statements below.

A. Yes, current unsustainable levels of tourism will result in irreparable damage to these sites within 20 years.
B. Yes, some of these sites have cultural or religious significance which is not appreciated by tourists.
C. No, revenue generated by tourism already helps to maintain these sites, providing the main source of income to local communities.
D. No, everyone should be able to appreciate these sites of interest.

11. Should schools with gardens and fields use some of this land for student allotments to grow vegetables, in order to improve the health of their students?

Select the strongest argument from the statements below.

A. Yes, because eating vegetables is part of a balanced diet lifestyle.
B. Yes, research shows that students who grow their own food are more likely to choose healthy meals.
C. No, because most schools use these fields to allow students to play sports, which is equally important for student health.
D. No, because some students will not like to eat the vegetables that could be grown at school.

12. Should the NHS no longer prescribe gluten-free foods because they are now available in most supermarkets?

Select the strongest argument from the statements below.

A. Yes, the NHS needs to save money so that it can prescribe more drugs for serious illnesses.
B. Yes, conditions such as gluten intolerance are not life-threatening and do not need to be treated by the NHS.
C. No, because gluten-free foods are more expensive and not everyone can afford them.
D. No, because there are some areas of the country where gluten-free foods are not widely available in supermarkets.

13. Should it be compulsory for all students taking GCSEs in the UK to study at least one modern foreign language?

    Select the strongest argument from the statements below.

    A. Yes, learning a foreign language has been shown to improve cognitive skills and extend attention spans so it would help these students in other subjects.
    B. Yes, having studied an additional language will make students more desirable when they apply for full-time jobs after finishing their studies.
    C. No, many students can already speak another modern foreign language.
    D. No, the use of technology to translate foreign languages makes the need to learn them obsolete.

14. Should customers be made to pay a small charge for disposable cups in order to encourage people to bring their own mugs to coffee shops?

    Select the strongest argument from the statements below.

    A. Yes, 2.5 billion disposable coffee cups are thrown away each year and they are bad for the environment.
    B. Yes, this would reward people for bringing their own mug to coffee shops with a small saving.
    C. No, disposable coffee cups should just be made from environmentally friendly materials instead.
    D. No, this would mean coffee shops would have to raise their prices.

15. The vitamin content of various fruit and vegetables from one grower were analysed and ten results shown in the following table (in mg per 100 g).

	Vitamin B1 (mg)	Vitamin B2 (mg)	Vitamin B6 (mg)	Vitamin C (mg)
Grapefruit	0.07	0.02	0.03	40
Artichoke	0.14	0.01	0.03	15
Lychee	0.09	0.04	0.04	23
Asparagus	0.04	0.04	0.03	12
Avocado	0.06	0.12	0.36	17
Kiwi	0.01	0.02	0.1	30

Place 'Yes' if the conclusion does follow. Place 'No' if the conclusion does not follow.

Weight for weight, asparagus contains more vitamin B6 than grapefruit.	
Avocado contains less than 50% of the vitamin C of grapefruit per 100g.	
No vegetable grown in the UK contains more Vitamin B1 than artichoke.	
A kilogram of grapefruit contains the same amount of vitamin B1 as 7 kg of kiwi.	
A person wanting to increase their intake of Vitamin B2 should be encouraged to eat kiwi rather than avocado.	

16. Coelacanths are an order of fish long considered to have gone extinct at around the same time as the dinosaurs, some 65 million years ago. Experts received a pleasant surprise, however, in 1938, when a living specimen was discovered off the coast of South Africa. Today, it is thought that there are two living species of coelacanths in existence, both of which are endangered. The first species is found primarily in the western Indian Ocean, particularly around the Comoros Islands, while a second, discovered in the late 1990s, lives thousands of miles away in Indonesian waters. Typically, coelacanths are found in volcanic caves between 150 m to 250 m underwater, where they feed on octopuses, squids and other fishes.

A large fish which can grow up to 2 m in length and can live for as long as sixty years, the coelacanth also has certain unique features which have led some researchers to believe they mark a crucial step in the evolution from water-based to land-based animals. Most prominent among these are the coelacanth's limb-like fins, which when in motion have been compared to the movement of a trotting horse. Other distinctive characteristics include a joint in the skull that allows the creature to greatly expand its mouth to swallow larger prey, and thick scales that are found only in ancient species of fish.

Place 'Yes' if the conclusion does follow. Place 'No' if the conclusion does not follow.

There are likely more living species of coelacanth yet to be discovered.	
Squid are not normally found more than 250 metres underwater.	
The unique anatomical features of the coelacanth suggest that it could represent a stage in the evolution from aquatic to terrestrial animals.	
Coelacanths did not go extinct at the time of the dinosaurs offspring.	
Coelacanths are most commonly found more than 100 metres underwater.	

17. Sixty-one per cent of adults in England visit their dentist regularly, compared to an average of 65% across Northern Ireland, Wales and Scotland, although 25% of adults in the United Kingdom say they have not seen a dentist in at least two years. This is certainly an improvement since 30 years ago, when dentist visits were less frequent. In those days, 37% of adults would eventually lose all of their natural teeth, compared to just 6% of people nowadays. Whilst visiting a dentist regularly means you are a 25% less likely to suffer from tooth decay, brushing your teeth twice daily is even more vital, as this simple twice-daily activity reduces tooth decay by a third compared to brushing your teeth once a day.

Place 'Yes' if the conclusion does follow. Place 'No' if the conclusion does not follow.

Brushing your teeth once a day is not the most effective way to reduce tooth decay.	
English people are more likely to visit the dentist frequently than people from the rest of the UK.	
The public should be told that visiting the dentist more frequently is the best way to prevent tooth decay.	
British people today are 31% more likely to have all of their own teeth.	
Three-quarters of people in the UK have seen a dentist in the last two years.	

18. Fruit flies can either be wild type, which means they have red eyes, or they can have white eyes. Following a genetic cross, flies were grown on either Medium A or Medium B. The number of wild type and white eye flies was recorded, along with the number of males and females on the different mediums.

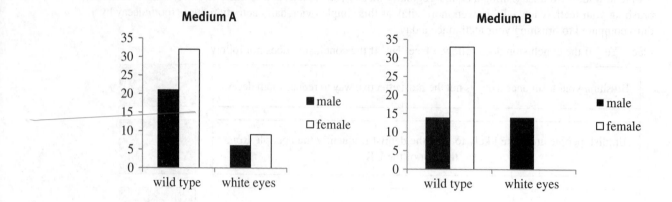

Place 'Yes' if the conclusion does follow. Place 'No' if the conclusion does not follow.

The proportion of male flies with white eyes grown on Medium B is more than twice the proportion of male flies grown on Medium A.	
Medium A produced twice as many red-eyed male flies as Medium B.	
Medium B produced more female wild type flies than all males combined.	
The difference in medium had most effect on females with red eyes.	
Medium A produced more males than females.	

A class of female school children were asked what they wanted to be when they grow up. Some children gave more than one answer.

The hexagon represents happy.

The circle represents rich.

The trapezium represents married.

The triangle represents a doctor.

The star represents famous.

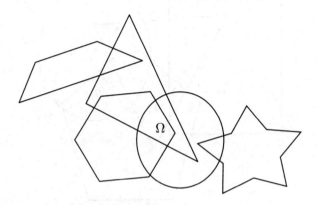

19. Which of the following is represented by the letter omega?

   A. Rich, a doctor, not famous, married, not happy.
   B. Rich, famous, not happy, a doctor, not married.
   C. Rich, a doctor, not married, not famous, not happy.
   D. Rich, not famous, happy, a doctor, not married.

The diagram shows the different events in which members of an athletics club compete.

The circle represents those who compete in the 100 metres.
The square represents those who compete in the 1500 metres.
The triangle represents those who compete in the javelin.
The pentagon represents those who compete in the discus.

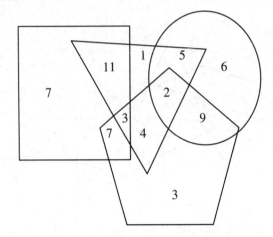

20. Which of the following statements is true?

   A. Of the members who compete, more than half compete in the javelin.
   B. There are the same number of discus competitors as 1500 metres competitors.
   C. The number of competitors in the discus is exactly half of the total number of competitors.
   D. The number of people competing in exactly two events is six times the number of people competing in exactly three events.

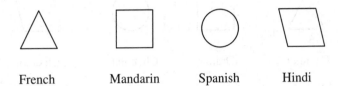

The diagram shows the various numbers of teachers at an international school that speak languages other than English.

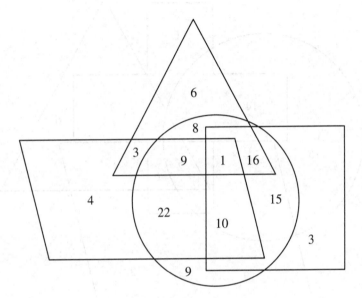

French   Mandarin   Spanish   Hindi

21. Which of the following must be true?

A. More than half of the teachers who speak both French and Spanish also speak Hindi.

B. The number of teachers whose non-English languages are Hindi and Spanish is fewer than the number of those whose non-English languages are Mandarin and Spanish.

C. There are twice as many Spanish speakers as Mandarin speakers.

D. Of the teachers who can speak at least three of these languages, one-third cannot speak Mandarin.

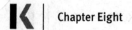
The diagram shows the ingredients used in dishes prepared by contestants on a cookery show.

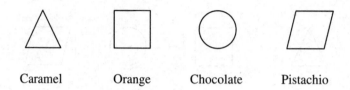

Caramel   Orange   Chocolate   Pistachio

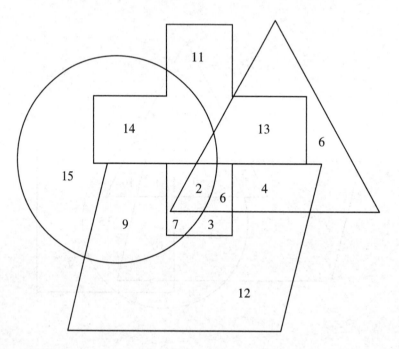

22. Which of the following must be true?

    A. Of the dishes represented in this diagram, more than half used orange.

    B. The number of dishes that used caramel and at least two other ingredients was fewer than the number of dishes that only used caramel.

    C. Of the dishes containing three or more of these ingredients, the majority contained chocolate.

    D. There were more dishes containing pistachio than dishes containing chocolate

A community orchestra struggles with recruitment, so they often hires musicians who play more than one instrument. The diagram below shows the instrument playing skills of the musicians.

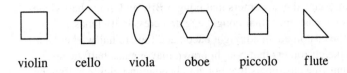

violin   cello   viola   oboe   piccolo   flute

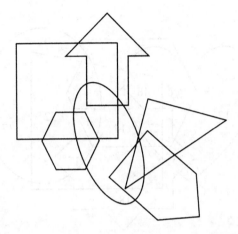

23.   Which of the following combinations of instruments is **not** played by any of the musicians?

A.   Viola, violin and oboe.
B.   Flute and piccolo.
C.   Viola, violin and flute.
D.   Cello and violin.

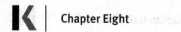

A sandwich shop known for its cheese sandwiches (Brie and cheddar) sells 'halfwiches'—half sandwiches—so customers may mix and match different fillings. The shop records the number of customers that buy each type of half sandwich over the course of a single day. These customer figures are given in the diagram.

The quadrilateral represents the customers that bought Brie and grape halfwiches.
The heart represents the customers that bought egg and cress halfwiches.
The star represents the customers that bought bacon and tomato halfwiches.
The oval represents the customers that bought prawn mayonnaise halfwiches.
The hexagon represents the customers that bought cheddar and pickle halfwiches.

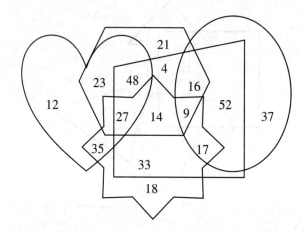

24. How many customers bought halfwiches containing cheese or bacon?

    A. 264
    B. 285
    C. 308
    D. 317

25. Which of the following diagrams best represents the statements 'all coyotes are dogs', 'all dogs are mammals', 'some dogs are pets' and 'some, but not all, pets are mammals'?

A.

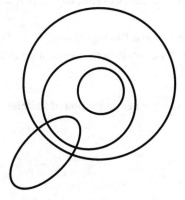

B.

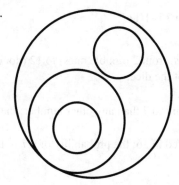

C.

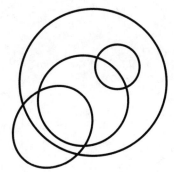

D.

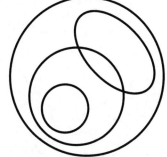

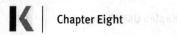

26. Two classes take their end-of-year exams. In Class A, 95% of the students passed the Biology exam, whilst 10% of students failed the Chemistry exam. In Class B, 7% of students failed the Biology exam, and 90% passed the Chemistry exam.

Based **only** on the percentage of students who passed the Biology and Chemistry exams, did Class B achieve better exam results?

A. Yes, a greater proportion of students in Class B passed the Chemistry and Biology exams.
B. Yes, although the same percentage of students passed the Chemistry exam in both classes, a greater proportion of Class B passed the Biology exam.
C. No, both classes had equal proportions passing each exam.
D. No, the two classes performed equally in the Chemistry exam, but a greater proportion of students in Class A passed the Biology exam.

27. Stefan rolls two fair 6-sided dice simultaneously.

Stefan states: 'The probability that the upward faces on the dice add to 7 is 1/11.'

Is Stefan correct?

A. Yes, because there are 11 possibilities for the sum of the two faces, from 2 (double ones) to 12 (double sixes); only one of the 11 possibilities will result in a single roll of the dice.
B. Yes, because the number on each dice is independent of the other.
C. No, because there are more possible combinations of faces that sum to 7 than any other number; the probability would be greater than 1/11.
D. No, because there are 6 possible values for each dice, and 6 squared in 36; the probability of a 7 is 1/36.

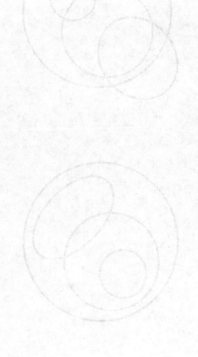

28. Two new medications for a certain condition are currently being trialled.

    Medication I is effective at treating the condition in all but 36% of patients.
    Only 12.5% of patients successfully treated with Medication I experience a relapse of the condition.
    Medication II is effective at treating the condition in 76% of patients.
    Of patients successfully treated with Medication II, 75% do not experience a relapse of the condition.

    Judging only on effectiveness at treating the condition without relapse, is Medication I the better treatment?

    A. Yes, because it treats the condition successfully in a greater proportion of patients.
    B. Yes, because it treats the condition successfully without relapse in a greater proportion of patients.
    C. No, because patients treated with Medication II are less likely to experience a relapse of the condition.
    D. No, because Medication II treats 1% more patients successfully without a relapse of the condition.

29. At the start, a bag contains an equal number of white and black counters.

    Jasmine randomly selects two counters from the bag, one at a time, without replacing them.

    Has the probability of a white counter being selected now decreased from the start?

    A. Yes, if both counters selected on the first and second draw are white.
    B. Yes, if at least one of the counters selected on the first or second draw is white.
    C. No, unless both counters selected on the first and second draw are black.
    D. No, unless there were four white counters in the bag at the start.

STOP. IF YOU FINISH BEFORE TIME IS CALLED, CHECK ANY QUESTIONS YOU HAVE MARKED FOR REVIEW. YOU MAY GO BACK TO QUESTIONS IN THIS SECTION ONLY.

Section 3: Quantitative Reasoning (24 Minutes)

This section contains 9 sets of data, each of which is followed by four questions. Each question will have five answer choices. Your task is to select the best option based on the data provided. Some sets may consist of four individual questions, each with its own data.

You may use a calculator to answer the questions in this section. On Test Day, you will be provided with an onscreen calculator that can perform the four basic operations (addition, subtraction, multiplication and division) along with only a few extra features (percentage, reciprocal, square root and memory buttons). You should not use any functions beyond these on the calculator used for this Mock Test.

Answer all 36 questions in Section 3, selecting one of the possible answers and circling the letter corresponding to the appropriate answer in your test paper.

When you are finished with this section, you may use any remaining time to review your work in this section only. Once you proceed to the next section, you may not return to this section.

You will have 24 minutes to answer the questions. It is in your best interest to select an answer for every item as there is no penalty for wrong answers.

Set your timer for 24 minutes, turn the page and begin the section.

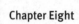

Below is John and Sandra's weekly work schedule:

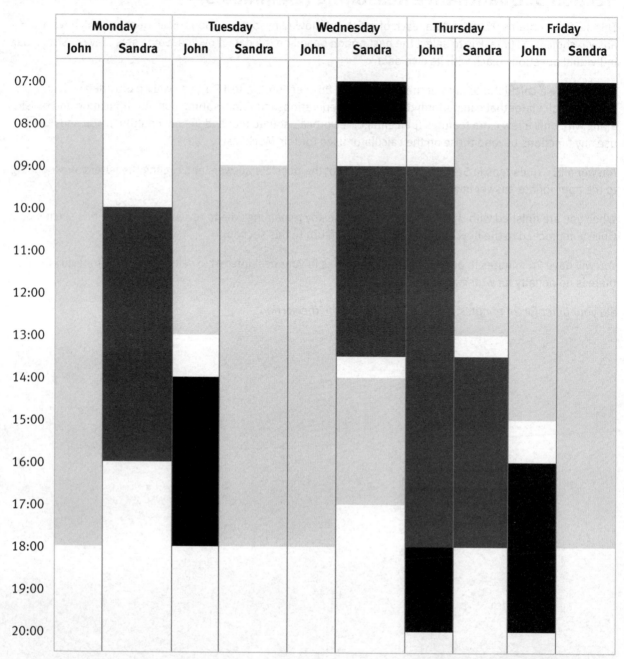

	Monday		Tuesday		Wednesday		Thursday		Friday	
	John	Sandra	John	Sandra	John	Sandra	John	Sandra	John	Sandra

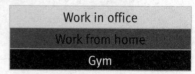

Work in office
Work from home
Gym

- John pays 21% tax on his income
- Sandra pays 24% tax on her income
- John pays £8.99 per week for gym membership
- Sandra pays £7.50 per week for gym membership
- Sandra's office is 16.2 km from the gym

1. Sandra decides to do all her work from home on days where she goes to the gym. What is the per cent increase in hours worked from home, for the couple?

   A. 39.1%
   B. 46.2%
   C. 52.4%
   D. 58.8%
   E. 61.2%

2. John makes £15.17 an hour before tax when he works from home. How much does he make per week after tax, working from home?

   A. £115.92
   B. £125.48
   C. £131.78
   D. £139.98
   E. £166.87

3. How much do John and Sandra pay per hour of use for their gym memberships?

   A. £1.65
   B. £1.80
   C. £2.25
   D. £2.50
   E. £2.75

4. On Friday morning, Sandra leaves the gym immediately and arrives at her workplace 22 minutes early. What was her mean driving speed that morning?

   A. 17.97 km/h
   B. 18.86 km/h
   C. 21.40 km/h
   D. 23.25 km/h
   E. 25.58 km/h

The diagram below shows the floor plan of a new suite of offices for a small company.

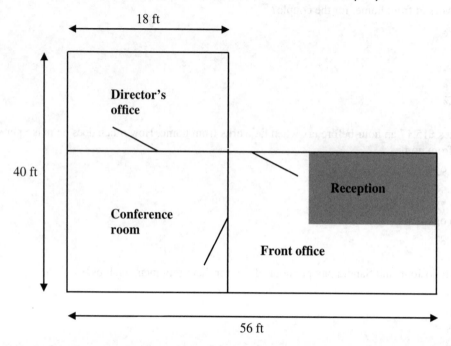

- The reception area (shaded in the diagram above) is 35% of the area of the combined reception/front office room. This is shown as an approximation, and is not to scale.
- The floors of the offices can be covered with carpeting, at a cost of £2.99 per square foot, or with laminate flooring, at a cost of £4.45 per square foot.

5.   The director's office is 108 square feet smaller than the conference room. What is the area of the conference room, in square feet?

   A.   306
   B.   414
   C.   684
   D.   720
   E.   874

6.   What is the total area of the reception/front office room?

   A.   306 ft²
   B.   484 ft²
   C.   568 ft²
   D.   874 ft²
   E.   Can't tell

The diagram below shows the floor plan of a new suite of offices for a small company.

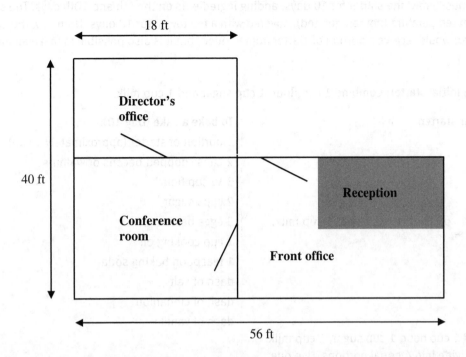

- The reception area (shaded in the diagram above) is 35% of the area of the combined reception/front office room. This is shown as an approximation, and is not to scale.
- The width of the reception area is 12 ft.
- The floors of the offices can be covered with carpeting, at a cost of £2.99 per square foot, or with laminate flooring, at a cost of £4.45 per square foot.

7. What are the dimensions of the reception area?

    A. 12 ft x 13.5 ft
    B. 12 ft x 15.4 ft
    C. 12 ft x 18.3 ft
    D. 12 ft x 24.2 ft
    E. 12 ft x 25.5 ft

8. What is the total cost of carpeting the entire suite of offices, except for the reception area?

    A. £3,851.42
    B. £4,766.06
    C. £5,732.05
    D. £6,120.50
    E. £7,093.30

Jeremy's distant cousin living in the USA has shared a recipe for an Amish friendship cake with him. To make the cake, he must 'grow' the starter for 10 days, adding ingredients on the 5th and 10th days. The starter must be left at room temperature (not refrigerated), covered with a tea towel, for 10 days. Normally, the baker of a friendship cake would receive a portion of starter from a friend, but it is also possible to make an initial starter.

To make the initial starter: Combine 1 cup flour, 1 cup sugar and 1 cup milk.

To grow your starter:	To bake a cake (Day 10):
Day 1: Stir.	1 portion of starter (approximately 1 cup)
Day 2: Stir.	2 cups chopped pecans or walnuts
Day 3: Stir.	3 ½ cup flour
Day 4: Stir.	2 cups sugar
Day 5: Add 1 cup flour, 1 cup sugar, 1 cup milk. Stir.	3 eggs beaten
Day 6: Stir.	1 cup cooking oil
Day 7: Stir.	1 teaspoon baking soda
Day 8: Stir.	dash of salt
Day 9: Stir.	dash of cinnamon
Day 10: Add 1 cup flour, 1 cup sugar, 1 cup milk. Stir. Then, divide into 4 equal portions. Use one portion to bake a cake; give the other three to friends.	dash of vanilla
Alternatively, you might give two portions to friends, use one portion to bake a cake and use the fourth portion to begin the cycle again.	1. Preheat oven to 325°F
	2. Mix eggs, sugar and oil; then, add the starter.
	3. Sitr in half of the flour, followed by salt, bking soda, cinnamon and vanilla. Stir well.
	4. Add nuts and the rest of the flour. Mix well. Dough will be stiff.
	5. Bake in a greased cake pan at 325°F for 90 minutes.

325°F = 170°C = Gas Mark 3.
1 cup = 240 ml = 240 g
1 teaspoon = 4.9 ml

9.   If Jeremy makes the initial starter and completes the cycle 3 times, baking one cake with each cycle and giving the extra portions to his friends, how much sugar will he have used?

   A.   1.44 kg
   B.   1.68 kg
   C.   2.16 kg
   D.   2.88 kg
   E.   3.12 kg

In 2011, a total of 39.7 billion text messages were sent over mobile phone networks in the UK.

However, this number had fallen to 21 billion by 2014, due to the rise in popularity of data-based messaging apps, which allowed users to send texts via WiFi or their data plans instead of the phone network, thereby avoiding the charges levied on text messages by mobile companies.

A total of 50 billion messages were sent on these data-based apps in the UK in 2014; this figure is predicted to rise in future years, whilst the amount of text messages sent through over the phone network will continue to drop.

10. The total amount of text messages sent over mobile phone networks in the UK dropped by what percentage from 2011 to 2014?

   A. 42.0%
   B. 47.1%
   C. 52.9%
   D. 79.4%
   E. 89.0%

A pig farmer weighs her prize pigs (in kg) once a month throughout the spring and summer.

Pig	Sex	March	April	May	June	July	August
Anastasia	F	67.9	68.5	70.2	71.6	73.4	74.7
Horatio	M	46.1	49.5	53.3	56.0	59.8	62.4
Otto	M	25.4	27.3	28.9	31.2	34.5	36.8
Queenie	F	53.3	53.7	53.9	54.6	55.3	59.1
Sebastian	M	38.1	42.9	44.6	48.3	51.8	54.5

11. The average weight of the male pigs has increased by how much from March to August?

   A. 10.4%
   B. 24.6%
   C. 38.7%
   D. 40.2%
   E. 43.0%

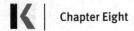
The table shows the ratio of milk to espresso for four different drinks.

Drink	Size (ml)	Milk : Espresso
Cappuccino	200 ml	4:2
Latte	250 ml	10:2
Espresso	40 ml	0:1
Macchiato	80 ml	1:8
Breve	180 ml	9:6

12. If all of the drinks are made from only milk and espresso, which drink contains the largest amount of espresso?

    A. Cappuccino

    B. Latte

    C. Espresso

    D. Macchiato

    E. Breve

Below are the profits Equinox Holdings made from their different businesses across sectors including Retail, Leisure, Commercial and Industrial across three years.

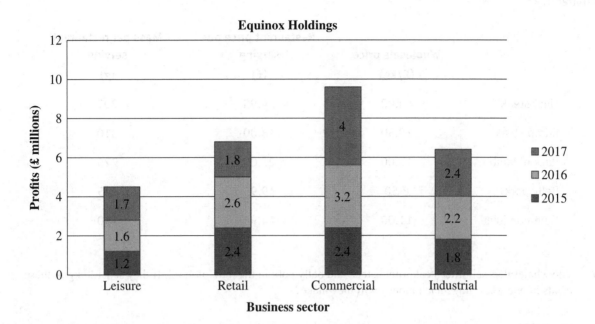

Profit figures above are given in millions of pounds, eg 2.2 refers to £2,200,000.

13. How much profit did businesses in the Retail sector make in 2016?

    A. 2,400,000
    B. 2,600,000
    C. 2,800,000
    D. 24,000,000
    E. 26,000,000

14. How much profit did businesses in the Leisure sector make in 2017?

    A. 1,200,000
    B. 1,600,000
    C. 1,700,000
    D. 16,000,000
    E. 17,000,000

15. The profits of the Commercial sector increased by what percentage from 2015 to 2016?

    A. 20%
    B. 25%
    C. 30%
    D. 33%
    E. 37%

16. What was the total profit across all business sectors in 2016?

    A. 7.8 million
    B. 8.6 million
    C. 9.6 million
    D. 9.9 million
    E. 10.3 million

A restaurant purchases meat from a local wholesaler. The amount that they pay for each type of meat and the price that they charge for each meal is shown below. The quantity of meat varies according to the meal that is prepared.

	Wholesale price (£/kg)	Restaurant price per serving (£)	Mass per restaurant serving (g)
Fillet steak	44.00	24.95	200
Rump steak	19.50	18.00	310
Rack of lamb	17.00	21.00	225
Belly pork	8.50	19.95	325
Gammon joint	11.00	14.95	250

17. The wholesalers sell fillet steak, rump steak and belly pork in the ratio of 4:3:2. If they sell 120 kg of these meats in one week, how much money will they make?

    A. £3343
    B. £3353
    C. £3580
    D. £3610
    E. £3627

18. On average the restaurant sells 55 servings of fillet steak, 47 servings of belly pork and 42 servings of gammon joint per week. How much does the restaurant spend at the wholesalers?

    A. £702
    B. £714
    C. £721
    D. £730
    E. £736

19. What is the total profit that the restaurant makes when they sell one serving of each of the five meats?

    A. £62
    B. £70
    C. £75
    D. £79
    E. £83

20. The wholesale prices of rump steak and belly pork increase by 3% and 5% respectively. What is the percentage reduction in profit when one serving of each is sold?

    A. 1.1%
    B. 1.3%
    C. 1.5%
    D. 1.6%
    E. 1.8%

Whilst holidaying in Majorca, Christos and Vasilis enjoy spending time on the water, riding in a motorboat and on jet skis with a top speed of 60 miles per hour.

21. Christos rides a jet ski for 1 hour, 12 minutes, at an average speed of 45 miles per hour. How far does Christos travel on his jet ski?

   A. 48 miles
   B. 50 miles
   C. 52 miles
   D. 54 miles
   E. 56 miles

22. Vasilis starts out on his jet ski at the same time as Christos, but Vasilis travels 16 miles further than Christos, in a total time of 75 minutes. What is Vasilis's average speed, in miles per hour?

   A. 46
   B. 47
   C. 56
   D. 57
   E. 58

23. How many minutes will it take Christos to catch up to Vasilis, if he travels at top speed?

   A. 16
   B. 21
   C. 23
   D. 25
   E. 26

24. The next day, Vasilis covers the same distance at a more leisurely pace, completing his jet ski ride in 2 hours. By what percentage has his journey time increased?

   A. 40%
   B. 60%
   C. 64%
   D. 67%
   E. 167%

Mr Singh has circular area in his garden that he wishes to renovate. The radius of this area is 5 metres. He has two options for the ground work in the garden and the cost of purchasing the materials for these is listed in the table below.

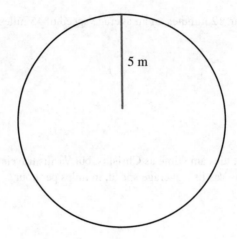

5 m

	Materials cost (£/m²)	Labour cost (£/m²)
Lawn turf	£2.00	£3.00
Paving slabs	£6.00	£2.00

25. If Mr Singh uses lawn turf on the entire circular garden, how much will the materials cost?

    A. £78.50
    B. £95.50
    C. £157.00
    D. £314.00
    E. £412.50

26. If Mr Singh uses paving slabs on the entire circular garden, how much will the materials cost?

    A. £235.50
    B. £471.00
    C. £612.00
    D. £720.50
    E. £760.00

27. Mr Singh has a budget of £750 for the renovation project. If he uses paving slabs across the entire garden, how much money will he have left in his budget after considering material and labour costs?

    A. £14.00
    B. £43.50
    C. £122.00
    D. £174.50
    E. £279.00

28. Mr Singh decides to put a new circular garden fountain with a diameter of 2 m in the middle of the garden. What is the area of the garden that is not covered by the new fountain?

    A. 56.2 m
    B. 65.9 m
    C. 67.2 m
    D. 68.4 m
    E. 75.4 m

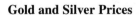

The trend in gold and silver prices per ounce for an entire decade is shown below. Gold and silver are both traded in US Dollars.

Gold and Silver Prices

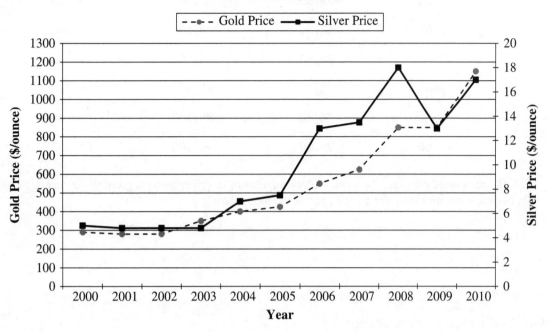

29. Approximately what was the price of gold in dollars per ounce in 2007?

   A. 550
   B. 590
   C. 610
   D. 850
   E. 890

30. Which year recorded the greatest difference between gold and silver, in price per ounce?

   A. 2002
   B. 2003
   C. 2006
   D. 2008
   E. 2010

31. By what percentage did silver increase in price per ounce from 2000 to 2010?

   A. 183%
   B. 240%
   C. 260%
   D. 325%
   E. 350%

32. At 2010 prices, how many ounces of silver could you buy for the value of 100 ounces of gold?

   A. 104
   B. 620
   C. 6,197
   D. 6,765
   E. 7,500

Below is a table showing the exam scores for a group of friends.

	English	Maths	Science	French
Tyron	44/60	39/80	84/100	80/100
Zack	48/60	64/80	78/100	65/100
Amna	29/60	74/80	54/100	42/100
David	4/60	75/80	47/100	18/100
Emily	58/60	76/80	89/100	100/100
Joel	41/60	28/80	96/100	74/100

33. What is the percentage difference between the total number of incorrect answers given by Amna and the total number of incorrect answers given by Joel, across the four exams?

    A. 28.9%
    B. 31.6%
    C. 34.5%
    D. 37.8%
    E. 39.6%

34. Who scored the best across all subjects?

    A. Amna
    B. Tyron
    C. Emily
    D. Joel
    E. Zack

35. David resits his English exam, and scores 36/60. What is the percentage rise in his English score?

    A. 60%
    B. 80%
    C. 600%
    D. 800%
    E. Can't tell

36. What is the mean score of all the Science marks of all six friends to the nearest integer?

    A. 69/100
    B. 75/100
    C. 79/100
    D. 84/100
    E. 88/100

STOP. IF YOU FINISH BEFORE TIME IS UP, CHECK ANY QUESTIONS YOU HAVE MARKED FOR REVIEW. YOU MAY GO BACK TO QUESTIONS IN THIS SECTION ONLY.

Section 4: Abstract Reasoning (13 Minutes)

This section contains 11 sets of five items each. There are four different question types:

Type 1: These items appear in sets of 5 test shapes, along with Set A and Set B. All the items in Set A are similar to each other, and all the items in Set B are similar to each other. Your task is determine in what way the shapes in each set are similar and to decide whether each test shape fits into Set A, Set B or neither set.

Type 2: These items appear as individual questions. You will see a progression of four boxes in a single row. Your task is to select the test shape that comes next in the progression.

Type 3: These items appear as individual questions. You will see a statement, with two boxes in the top row and two boxes in the bottom row. There will be some progression from the first box to the second box in the top row; the second box in the bottom row will be blank. Your task is to select the test shape that fills the blank box, so that the progression in the bottom row is the same as the progression in the top row.

Type 4: These items appear in sets of 5 questions, along with Set A and Set B. All the items in Set A are similar to each other, and all the items in Set B are similar to each other. Your task is to choose the test shape that belongs to the set mentioned in the question.

Answer all 55 questions in Section 4, selecting one of the possible answers and circling the letter corresponding to the appropriate answer in your test paper.

When you are finished with this section, you may use any remaining time to review your work in this section only. Once you proceed to the next section, you may not return to this section.

You will have 13 minutes to answer the questions. It is in your best interest to select an answer for every item as there is no penalty for wrong answers.

Set your timer for 13 minutes, turn the page and begin the section.

Set A

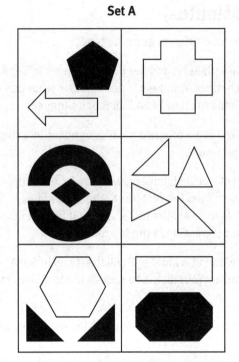

Set B

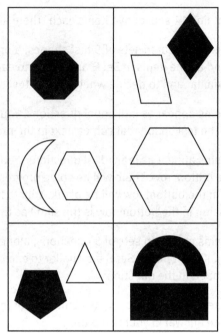

Test Shapes

1	2	3	4	5

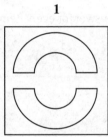
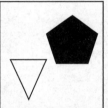

A. Set A
B. Set B
C. Neither

A. Set A
B. Set B
C. Neither

A. Set A
B. Set B
C. Neither

A. Set A
B. Set B
C. Neither

A. Set A
B. Set B
C. Neither

Set A

Set B

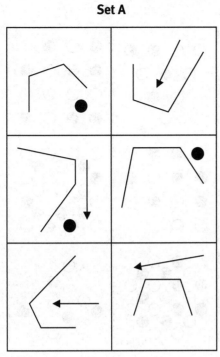
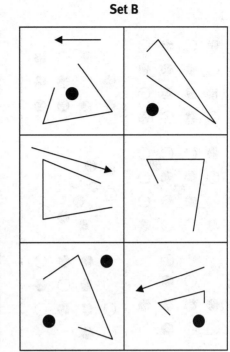

Test Shapes

| 6 | 7 | 8 | 9 | 10 |

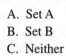

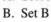
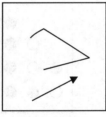
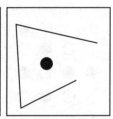

A. Set A
B. Set B
C. Neither

A. Set A
B. Set B
C. Neither

A. Set A
B. Set B
C. Neither

A. Set A
B. Set B
C. Neither

A. Set A
B. Set B
C. Neither

Set A   **Set B**

11. Which of the following test shapes belongs in Set A?

A.   B.   C.   D.

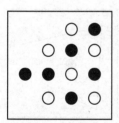 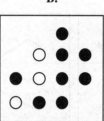 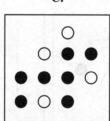 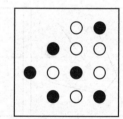

12. Which of the following test shapes belongs in Set A?

A.   B.   C.   D.

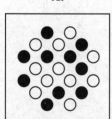 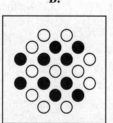 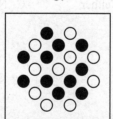 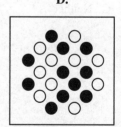

13. Which of the following test shapes belongs in Set B?

A.   B.   C.   D.

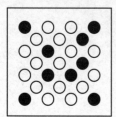 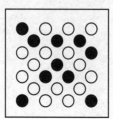 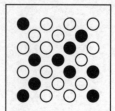 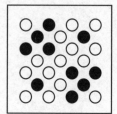

14. Which of the following test shapes belongs in Set A?

A. 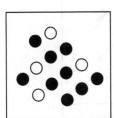 B. 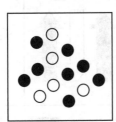 C. 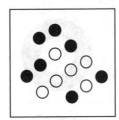 D.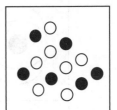

15. Which of the following test shapes belongs in Set B?

A. 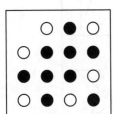 B. 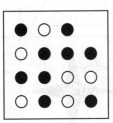 C. 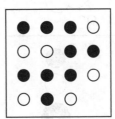 D.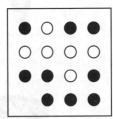

Set A

Set B

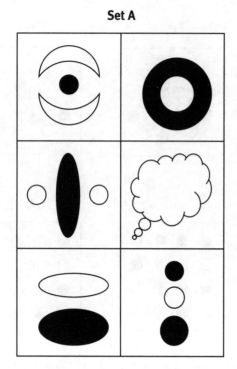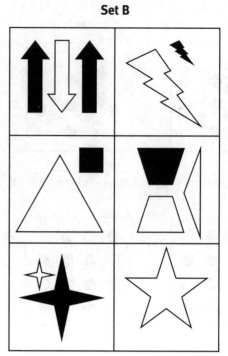

Test Shapes

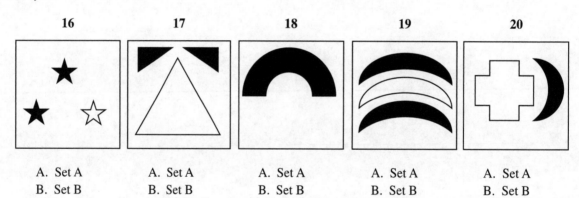

16	17	18	19	20

A. Set A
B. Set B
C. Neither

A. Set A
B. Set B
C. Neither

A. Set A
B. Set B
C. Neither

A. Set A
B. Set B
C. Neither

A. Set A
B. Set B
C. Neither

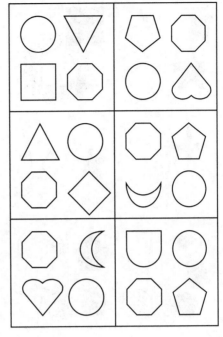

Set A

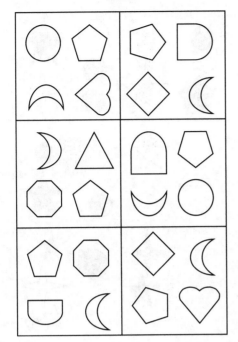

Set B

Test Shapes

21	22	23	24	25

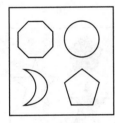
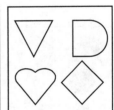

A. Set A
B. Set B
C. Neither

A. Set A
B. Set B
C. Neither

A. Set A
B. Set B
C. Neither

A. Set A
B. Set B
C. Neither

A. Set A
B. Set B
C. Neither

Set A

Set B

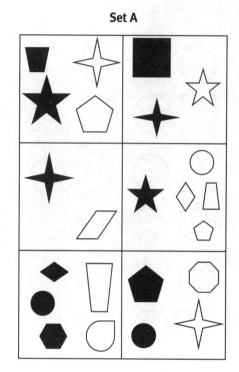
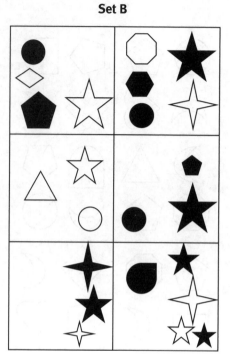

Test Shapes

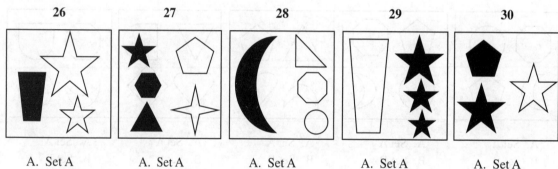

26	27	28	29	30
A. Set A	A. Set A	A. Set A	A. Set A	A. Set A
B. Set B	B. Set B	B. Set B	B. Set B	B. Set B
C. Neither	C. Neither	C. Neither	C. Neither	C. Neither

Set A

Set B

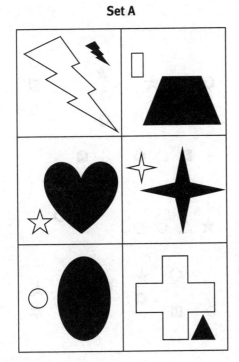
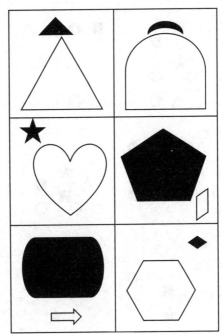

Test Shapes

31	32	33	34	35

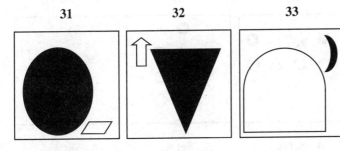
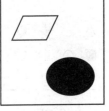

A. Set A   A. Set A   A. Set A   A. Set A   A. Set A
B. Set B   B. Set B   B. Set B   B. Set B   B. Set B
C. Neither C. Neither C. Neither C. Neither C. Neither

Set A

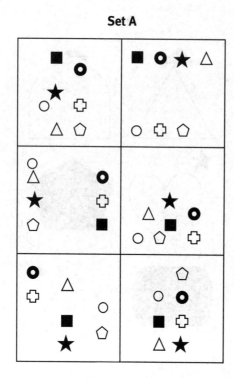

Set B

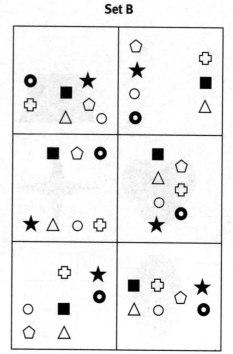

Test Shapes

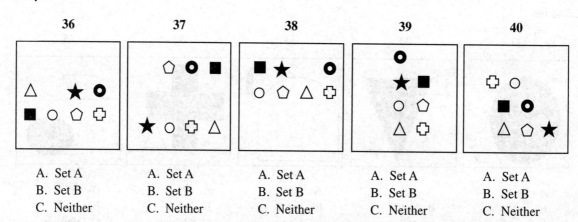

36	37	38	39	40
A. Set A	A. Set A	A. Set A	A. Set A	A. Set A
B. Set B	B. Set B	B. Set B	B. Set B	B. Set B
C. Neither	C. Neither	C. Neither	C. Neither	C. Neither

Set A

Set B

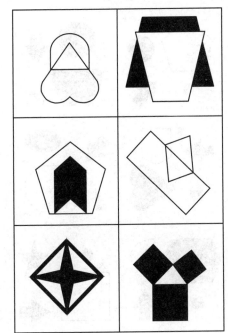

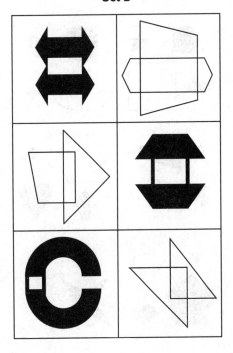

Test Shapes

41	42	43	44	45

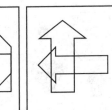
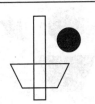
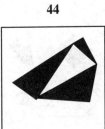
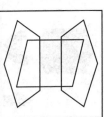

A. Set A
B. Set B
C. Neither

A. Set A
B. Set B
C. Neither

A. Set A
B. Set B
C. Neither

A. Set A
B. Set B
C. Neither

A. Set A
B. Set B
C. Neither

Set A   **Set B**

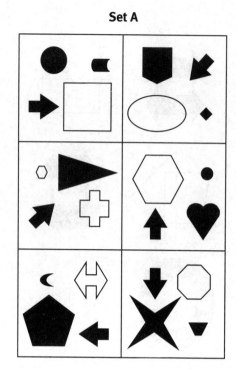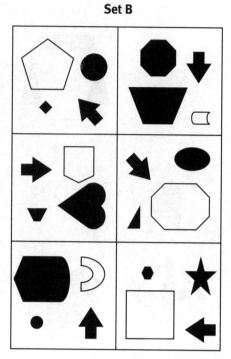

Test Shapes

46	47	48	49	50

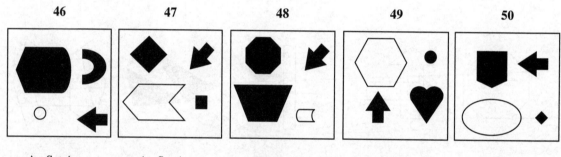

A. Set A   A. Set A   A. Set A   A. Set A   A. Set A
B. Set B   B. Set B   B. Set B   B. Set B   B. Set B
C. Neither C. Neither C. Neither C. Neither C. Neither

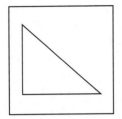  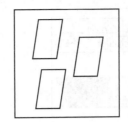 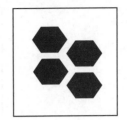

51. Which figure completes the series?

A.   B.   C.   D.

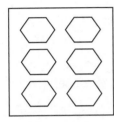 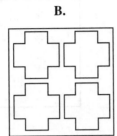 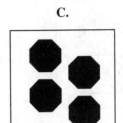 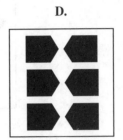

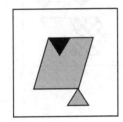  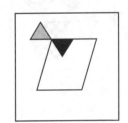

52. Which figure completes the series?

A.   B.   C.   D.

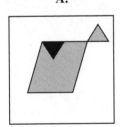 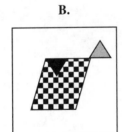 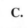 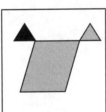 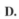 

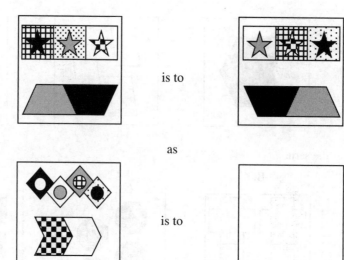

is to

as

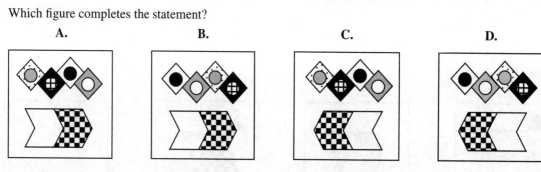

is to

53. Which figure completes the statement?

A.   B.   C.   D.

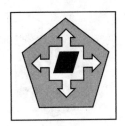 is to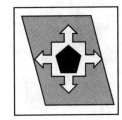

as

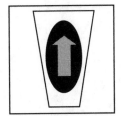 is to

54. Which figure completes the statement?

A. 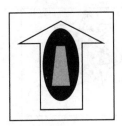 B.  C.  D.

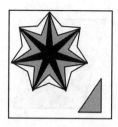

is to

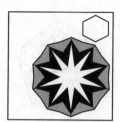

as

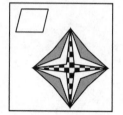

is to

55. Which figure completes the statement?

A.   B.   C.   D.

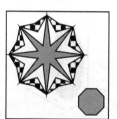 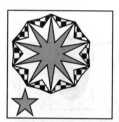 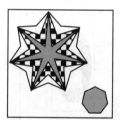

STOP. IF YOU FINISH BEFORE TIME IS UP, CHECK ANY QUESTIONS YOU HAVE MARKED FOR REVIEW. YOU MAY GO BACK TO QUESTIONS IN THIS SECTION ONLY.

Section 5: Situational Judgement (26 Minutes)

This section contains 21 theoretical scenarios, each involving a medical or dental professional, or a student preparing for a career in medicine or dentistry. Your task is to read the scenario carefully, and then make a series of judgements about possible options for responding to the situation in the scenario. There are two types of scenarios in this section:

Appropriateness: These scenarios will ask you to rate whether possible responses to the scenario are appropriate or inappropriate.

Importance: These scenarios will ask you to rate whether certain factors are important or not important to consider when responding to the scenario.

The first part of the section will contain Appropriateness scenarios; the final part of the section will contain Importance scenarios. Be sure to answer based on the appropriateness or importance of the response/factor to the person who is named in the question under the scenario. Evaluate the responses/factors independently of each other; do not assume that there will be a response/factor corresponding to each answer choice for each scenario.

Answer all 68 questions in Section 5, selecting one of the possible answers and circling the letter corresponding to the appropriate answer in your test paper.

When you are finished with this section, you may use any remaining time to review your work in this section only. Once you complete this section, you are finished with the Diagnostic Test. You may then assess your results using the scoring tables that follow.

You will have 26 minutes to answer the questions. It is in your best interest to select an answer for every item as there is no penalty for wrong answers.

Set your timer for 26 minutes, turn the page and begin the section.

> Adam is a second year medical student who must attend anatomy and dissection classes as part of his preclinical training. During his first session he felt very queasy, but manages to make it through the class without vomiting. He is thus very nervous about his second session. He decides to attend; however, before even starting the dissection, he began to feel very sick. His friend, Bella, says that he looks very pale.

How **appropriate** are each of the following responses by **Adam** in this situation?

1. Tell Bella he feels sick, ask her to inform the tutor, and leave the class

    A. A very appropriate thing to do
    B. Appropriate, but not ideal
    C. Inappropriate, but not awful
    D. A very inappropriate thing to do

2. Walk out immediately so as not to disrupt his peers and avoid being sick in the classroom

    A. A very appropriate thing to do
    B. Appropriate, but not ideal
    C. Inappropriate, but not awful
    D. A very inappropriate thing to do

3. Tell the instructor he feels unwell, leave the class and catch up on what has been missed later

    A. A very appropriate thing to do
    B. Appropriate, but not ideal
    C. Inappropriate, but not awful
    D. A very inappropriate thing to do

4. Finish this session, and in future pretend to be ill during anatomy sessions

    A. A very appropriate thing to do
    B. Appropriate, but not ideal
    C. Inappropriate, but not awful
    D. A very inappropriate thing to do

Umar is a junior doctor working on a busy hospital ward. He enters the supply cupboard, turns on the light and discovers another junior doctor, Darryl, sat on the floor, crying and drinking from a bottle of whisky. Darryl says that his wife has just left him for another man, and there is no point in going on.

How **appropriate** are each of the following responses by <u>Umar</u> in this situation?

5. Ask Darryl if he would like to chat about what is going on
   - A. A very appropriate thing to do
   - B. Appropriate, but not ideal
   - C. Inappropriate, but not awful
   - D. A very inappropriate thing to do

6. Ask Darryl if he is seeing patients today
   - A. A very appropriate thing to do
   - B. Appropriate, but not ideal
   - C. Inappropriate, but not awful
   - D. A very inappropriate thing to do

7. Contact the hospital anonymously through their website to report that a doctor has a drinking problem
   - A. A very appropriate thing to do
   - B. Appropriate, but not ideal
   - C. Inappropriate, but not awful
   - D. A very inappropriate thing to do

8. Encourage Darryl to let his consultant know that he is having a hard time
   - A. A very appropriate thing to do
   - B. Appropriate, but not ideal
   - C. Inappropriate, but not awful
   - D. A very inappropriate thing to do

> Saba is a junior doctor on the surgical ward. She is well liked by the patients who say she is always friendly and cheerful. One morning Saba receives a message from a social networking site from a man who she recognises as being a former patient. The patient has requested to add Saba as a contact on the social networking site; Saba can accept, deny or ignore his request.

How **appropriate** are each of the following responses by <u>Saba</u> in this situation?

9. Accept the man's request temporarily, so that she can email him to explain why they cannot socialise

   A. A very appropriate thing to do
   B. Appropriate, but not ideal
   C. Inappropriate, but not awful
   D. A very inappropriate thing to do

10. Ignore the man's request

   A. A very appropriate thing to do
   B. Appropriate, but not ideal
   C. Inappropriate, but not awful
   D. A very inappropriate thing to do

Dr Davies approaches the nurse's station to make an urgent enquiry regarding a patient. The two nurses at the nurse's station continue to gossip about whether or not an attractive doctor has a girlfriend, without acknowledging Dr Davies.

How **appropriate** are each of the following responses by **Dr Davies** in this situation?

11. Instruct the nurses that they are behaving unprofessionally

    A. A very appropriate thing to do
    B. Appropriate, but not ideal
    C. Inappropriate, but not awful
    D. A very inappropriate thing to do

12. Clear her throat several times

    A. A very appropriate thing to do
    B. Appropriate, but not ideal
    C. Inappropriate, but not awful
    D. A very inappropriate thing to do

13. Ask the nurses if one of them could assist with her urgent enquiry regarding a patient

    A. A very appropriate thing to do
    B. Appropriate, but not ideal
    C. Inappropriate, but not awful
    D. A very inappropriate thing to do

Anwen is a junior doctor currently working in the outpatient clinic at the county hospital. Anwen receives an email with dates for three mandatory training courses, all in the next month. Anwen checks the clinic diary and sees that she already has several patients booked in on all three dates.

How **appropriate** are each of the following responses by **Anwen** in this situation?

14. Call all of the patients to reschedule their appointments for dates that do not conflict with her training courses

    A. A very appropriate thing to do
    B. Appropriate, but not ideal
    C. Inappropriate, but not awful
    D. A very inappropriate thing to do

15. Ask her consultant for advice on how best to proceed

    A. A very appropriate thing to do
    B. Appropriate, but not ideal
    C. Inappropriate, but not awful
    D. A very inappropriate thing to do

16. Reply to the email to request alternative dates for the training courses

    A. A very appropriate thing to do
    B. Appropriate, but not ideal
    C. Inappropriate, but not awful
    D. A very inappropriate thing to do

Ian is seated directly behind his best friend, Ben, in a written examination. During the examination, Ian notices that Ben has notes written on his arm, hidden by the sleeve of his hoodie, and Ben keeps referring to them. Ian has never witnessed Ben cheating before and knows he would not normally do so, but Ian knows that recently Ben has been very upset over the divorce of his parents, and so may not have had time to prepare adequately for this exam.

How **appropriate** are each of the following responses by **Ian** in this situation?

17. Raise his hand and discreetly tell an invigilator about Ben
    A. A very appropriate thing to do
    B. Appropriate, but not ideal
    C. Inappropriate, but not awful
    D. A very inappropriate thing to do

18. Wait until the end of the examination to tell an invigilator
    A. A very appropriate thing to do
    B. Appropriate, but not ideal
    C. Inappropriate, but not awful
    D. A very inappropriate thing to do

19. Contact the medical school anonymously explaining what has been witnessed in the exam
    A. A very appropriate thing to do
    B. Appropriate, but not ideal
    C. Inappropriate, but not awful
    D. A very inappropriate thing to do

A junior doctor, Arissa, is attempting to obtain consent for treatment from a patient, but the patient does not respond to any of her questions. The patient appears to listen to what Arissa is saying, but says nothing in response.

How **appropriate** are each of the following responses by **Arissa** in this situation?

20. Check the patient's name to see if she is foreign
    A. A very appropriate thing to do
    B. Appropriate, but not ideal
    C. Inappropriate, but not awful
    D. A very inappropriate thing to do

21. Proceed with the treatment, explaining each step calmly and clearly
    A. A very appropriate thing to do
    B. Appropriate, but not ideal
    C. Inappropriate, but not awful
    D. A very inappropriate thing to do

22. Seek advice from a senior colleague
    A. A very appropriate thing to do
    B. Appropriate, but not ideal
    C. Inappropriate, but not awful
    D. A very inappropriate thing to do

Joanna and Freddie are the two new junior doctors on the wards. Joanna decides to spend most afternoons teaching the medical students, leaving Freddie to do the boring paperwork.

How **appropriate** are each of the following responses by **Freddie** in this situation?

23. Tell their consultant that Joanna is not doing her fair share of the work
    A. A very appropriate thing to do
    B. Appropriate, but not ideal
    C. Inappropriate, but not awful
    D. A very inappropriate thing to do

24. Talk to Joanna about taking it in turns to teach the medical students
    A. A very appropriate thing to do
    B. Appropriate, but not ideal
    C. Inappropriate, but not awful
    D. A very inappropriate thing to do

25. Tell Joanna he does not want to do all the paperwork himself
    A. A very appropriate thing to do
    B. Appropriate, but not ideal
    C. Inappropriate, but not awful
    D. A very inappropriate thing to do

Olubayo is a dentist who is about to perform a procedure on a patient that requires the use of several different electrical instruments that must be plugged into the mains. There have been severe storms throughout the day, and the power to the dentist's surgery has gone out twice. The backup generator failed the second time the power went out. Olubayo hears thunder in the distance, and is certain that another severe storm is approaching. The lights in the surgery begin to flicker.

How **appropriate** are each of the following responses by **Olubayo** in this situation?

26. Ask if the patient is comfortable with going ahead with the procedure

    A. A very appropriate thing to do
    B. Appropriate, but not ideal
    C. Inappropriate, but not awful
    D. A very inappropriate thing to do

27. Notify the patient that it is unsafe to proceed due to inclement weather

    A. A very appropriate thing to do
    B. Appropriate, but not ideal
    C. Inappropriate, but not awful
    D. A very inappropriate thing to do

28. Close the surgery for the rest of the day, and reschedule patients for the earliest available appointments

    A. A very appropriate thing to do
    B. Appropriate, but not ideal
    C. Inappropriate, but not awful
    D. A very inappropriate thing to do

Two junior doctors, Emmanuel and Simone, are working in a busy A&E department. Emmanuel comes out of an examination room and tells Simone that the patient inside is a leader of an extreme right-wing political group known for its anti-immigrant policies. Emmanuel's parents are from Nigeria, and he does not feel comfortable treating this patient. Emmanuel asks Simone if she will take the patient instead.

How **appropriate** are each of the following responses by **Simone** in this situation?

29.　Ask Emmanuel if the patient has said anything to make him uncomfortable

　　A.　A very appropriate thing to do
　　B.　Appropriate, but not ideal
　　C.　Inappropriate, but not awful
　　D.　A very inappropriate thing to do

30.　Ask the patient if Emmanuel said anything to make him uncomfortable

　　A.　A very appropriate thing to do
　　B.　Appropriate, but not ideal
　　C.　Inappropriate, but not awful
　　D.　A very inappropriate thing to do

31.　Remind Emmanuel of his duty to treat all patients, regardless of their beliefs

　　A.　A very appropriate thing to do
　　B.　Appropriate, but not ideal
　　C.　Inappropriate, but not awful
　　D.　A very inappropriate thing to do

Hannah, a paediatrician, is examining a patient, Alfie, who is aged seven and has a headache and a sore throat. Whilst listening to Alfie's breathing, Hannah notices several bruises in various stages of healing on Alfie's chest, all of which are concealed by his shirt. Alfie's carer is not in the examination room; she has stepped outside to have a cigarette. Alfie seems shy and withdrawn, and tries to pull away when he sees that Hannah has noticed the bruises on his chest.

How **appropriate** are each of the following responses by **Hannah** in this situation?

32. Ask Alfie what happened

   A. A very appropriate thing to do
   B. Appropriate, but not ideal
   C. Inappropriate, but not awful
   D. A very inappropriate thing to do

33. Step outside and ask Alfie's carer for consent to examine the bruises on his chest

   A. A very appropriate thing to do
   B. Appropriate, but not ideal
   C. Inappropriate, but not awful
   D. A very inappropriate thing to do

34. Reassure Alfie that she wants to help him feel better

   A. A very appropriate thing to do
   B. Appropriate, but not ideal
   C. Inappropriate, but not awful
   D. A very inappropriate thing to do

35. Phone children's services at the local council immediately to report a suspected case of child abuse

   A. A very appropriate thing to do
   B. Appropriate, but not ideal
   C. Inappropriate, but not awful
   D. A very inappropriate thing to do

Dr Miller, a junior doctor, has just finished ward rounds when a woman approaches him in the corridor. She says that she is the niece of a patient that Dr Miller is looking after in the Intensive Care Unit. She wants to know everything about her uncle and how long it will be until he is well enough to go home. Dr Miller's consultant will be busy in clinic all day, and Dr Miller knows that the patient is very sick, with only days to live; the patient asked the consultant to inform the family of this himself.

How **appropriate** are each of the following responses by **Dr Miller** in this situation?

36. Tell the woman that he is too busy to talk to her

  A. A very appropriate thing to do
  B. Appropriate, but not ideal
  C. Inappropriate, but not awful
  D. A very inappropriate thing to do

37. Tell the woman that he cannot tell her anything regarding a patient

  A. A very appropriate thing to do
  B. Appropriate, but not ideal
  C. Inappropriate, but not awful
  D. A very inappropriate thing to do

38. Suggest that the woman wait for the consultant in the relatives' room

  A. A very appropriate thing to do
  B. Appropriate, but not ideal
  C. Inappropriate, but not awful
  D. A very inappropriate thing to do

Two consultants at the hospital, Dr Zaghari and Dr Khavari, agree to jointly supervise a junior doctor. Each consultant is expected to meet regularly with the junior doctor and complete several assessments over the course of the year. Halfway through the year, however, Dr Zaghari notes that Dr Khavari has never met with the junior doctor and has not completed any assessments for him.

How **important** to take into account are the following considerations for **Dr Zaghari** when deciding how to respond to the situation?

39.   Dr Zaghari knows that the junior doctor has tried to schedule meetings with Dr Khavari, but Dr Khavari always cancels at the last minute

    A. Very important
    B. Important
    C. Of minor importance
    D. Not important at all

40.   Dr Khavari also supervises another junior doctor

    A. Very important
    B. Important
    C. Of minor importance
    D. Not important at all

Jackson and Zakariyah are medical students. Upon walking into the supply cupboard one day, Zakariyah sees Jackson filling a rucksack with bags of intravenous fluid and equipment for inserting drips. He asks Zakariyah not to tell the nurse in charge or their consultant.

How **important** to take into account are the following considerations for **Zakariyah** when deciding how to respond to the situation?

41. Jackson says that he is sending the supplies to a charity hospital in Cambodia

    A. Very important
    B. Important
    C. Of minor importance
    D. Not important at all

42. Zakariyah has heard Jackson discussing putting up drips on himself and his friends when they have been out drinking

    A. Very important
    B. Important
    C. Of minor importance
    D. Not important at all

43. The intravenous fluid bags are past their expiry dates

    A. Very important
    B. Important
    C. Of minor importance
    D. Not important at all

44. Zakariyah knows that Jackson is on his final warning in terms of appropriate behaviour whilst at medical school

    A. Very important
    B. Important
    C. Of minor importance
    D. Not important at all

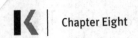

> Liam, a junior doctor, approaches Conor, another junior doctor, and asks Conor to take over the case of a patient he has just been assigned, Mr Abdul. Conor asks why, and Liam explains he cannot deal with 'another one of those people.' Conor asks Liam to explain himself, and Liam says Conor knows all about 'all these outsiders' coming to the UK so they can 'go on benefits' and 'impose their religion' on this country.

How **important** to take into account are the following considerations for **Conor** when deciding how to respond to the situation?

45.   Liam's brother was injured in the war in Afghanistan

    A.   Very important
    B.   Important
    C.   Of minor importance
    D.   Not important at all

46.   Whether there are any patients or staff nearby

    A.   Very important
    B.   Important
    C.   Of minor importance
    D.   Not important at all

47.   Liam has not made comments of this nature to Conor before

    A.   Very important
    B.   Important
    C.   Of minor importance
    D.   Not important at all

48.   Conor and Liam are supervised by the same consultant

    A.   Very important
    B.   Important
    C.   Of minor importance
    D.   Not important at all

49.   Liam recently helped Conor when his mother was seriously ill

    A.   Very important
    B.   Important
    C.   Of minor importance
    D.   Not important at all

The medical team decides that a patient should have a non-urgent chest x-ray before he goes home, but that this would not alter his treatment whilst in hospital. A junior doctor, Dr O'Keefe, is asked by the team to organise the x-ray. The next day, however, Dr O'Keefe admits to Dr Bates, a senior doctor on the medical team, that she has forgotten to organize the x-ray.

How **important** to take into account are the following considerations for **<u>Dr Bates</u>** when deciding how to respond to the situation?

50.   The consultant had specifically asked for the x-ray to be completed in the next 24 hours

    A.   Very important
    B.   Important
    C.   Of minor importance
    D.   Not important at all

51.   Dr O'Keefe was dealing with a very sick patient all of the previous afternoon

    A.   Very important
    B.   Important
    C.   Of minor importance
    D.   Not important at all

52.   The patient is not scheduled to go home until next week

    A.   Very important
    B.   Important
    C.   Of minor importance
    D.   Not important at all

53.   Dr O'Keefe had some bad news about her grandmother's cancer diagnosis a few days ago

    A.   Very important
    B.   Important
    C.   Of minor importance
    D.   Not important at all

A group of medical students have been assigned to prepare and give a presentation; they will be assessed jointly for their work. At the first group meeting, they select Maisie as group leader. A few minutes before the second group meeting, Maisie receives a text message from Catriona, another group member, stating that she has car trouble and cannot come to the meeting; Catriona asks Maisie to cover for her.

How **important** to take into account are the following considerations for **Maisie** when deciding how to respond to the situation?

54. There is a private spot near the meeting room, where Maisie could ring Catriona

    A. Very important
    B. Important
    C. Of minor importance
    D. Not important at all

55. Whether Catriona lives near enough to the meeting venue that she could walk or take public transport

    A. Very important
    B. Important
    C. Of minor importance
    D. Not important at all

56. The assignment clearly requires them to prepare and give the presentation as a group

    A. Very important
    B. Important
    C. Of minor importance
    D. Not important at all

Two junior doctors, Addison and Petra, are called to a meeting with a hospital administrator to discuss what happened during a procedure that caused serious health problems for the patient, leading to a formal complaint from the patient and the threat of a lawsuit. When asked to explain what she did during the procedure, Petra omits to mention a minor error she made that Addison remembers noticing at the time.

How **important** to take into account are the following considerations for **Addison** when deciding how to respond to the situation?

57. Petra's error may be directly responsible for the patient's health problems that resulted form the procedure

    A. Very important
    B. Important
    C. Of minor importance
    D. Not important at all

58. The administrator does not ask Addison directly about the error made by Petra

    A. Very important
    B. Important
    C. Of minor importance
    D. Not important at all

59. Other staff present at the time may have noticed Petra's error

    A. Very important
    B. Important
    C. Of minor importance
    D. Not important at all

Rhiannon is a junior doctor on a busy hospital ward. Rhiannon pops into the staff lounge for a quick cup of tea on her mid-morning break and discovers a group of medical students sitting round the table. Rhiannon does not know them well, but was introduced when they started their placements the week before. The medical students tell Rhiannon that they have barely spoken to the consultant who is responsible for their placement; the consultant told them to 'just get stuck in' but they don't know what they are meant to be doing. Rhiannon finds the consultant in the corridor and asks to have a quick word. Rhiannon explains that the medical students need guidance as to what they should be doing for their placement work. The consultant says he is 'too busy to be bothered' and tells Rhiannon to 'just come up with something' and mentor the students herself.

How **important** to take into account are the following considerations for **Rhiannon** when deciding how to respond to the situation?

60. The medical students are meant to be assessed on clear criteria set out by their university

  A. Very important
  B. Important
  C. Of minor importance
  D. Not important at all

61. The hospital requires a doctor to supervise the medical students in all their interactions with patients

  A. Very important
  B. Important
  C. Of minor importance
  D. Not important at all

62. The consultant is the only consultant on their ward at the moment, as several other consultants are on annual leave or medical leave

  A. Very important
  B. Important
  C. Of minor importance
  D. Not important at all

Holly is a medical student completing a placement in the emergency department at a local hospital. A patient is brought in with a serious leg injury. The consultant that Holly is shadowing tries to explain the course of treatment to the patient, only to discover that she does not speak any English. The consultant tells Holly that the patient 'looks to be Latin American,' so he will try to speak to her in Spanish, 'seeing as I got an A in GCSE Spanish.' Holly does not speak Spanish, but she observes that the consultant is speaking it very badly, struggling to remember words. The patient is confused, then becomes agitated as the doctor continues in broken Spanish; the patient clearly does not understand a word that the doctor is saying.

How **important** to take into account are the following considerations for **Holly** when deciding how to respond to the situation?

63. The consultant does not speak Spanish very well

   A. Very important
   B. Important
   C. Of minor importance
   D. Not important at all

64. The patient's injury is not life-threatening

   A. Very important
   B. Important
   C. Of minor importance
   D. Not important at all

65. The consultant has not made an effort to determine what language the patient speaks

   A. Very important
   B. Important
   C. Of minor importance
   D. Not important at all

> A consultant paediatrician is finishing a busy shift on the children's ward when she notices that one of her patients, Alice, aged 7, is curled up on her bed, clutching a teddy bear and crying.

How **important** to take into account are the following considerations for **the consultant paediatrician** when deciding how to respond to the situation?

66. She has already stayed on the ward an hour after her shift was supposed to end, and she is extremely tired

   A. Very important
   B. Important
   C. Of minor importance
   D. Not important at all

67. Alice's father is travelling on business, and Alice's mother has not been in to see her today

   A. Very important
   B. Important
   C. Of minor importance
   D. Not important at all

68. Alice is recovering well from her latest operation and is due to be discharged the next day

   A. Very important
   B. Important
   C. Of minor importance
   D. Not important at all

STOP. IF YOU FINISH BEFORE TIME IS CALLED, CHECK ANY QUESTIONS YOU HAVE MARKED FOR REVIEW. YOU MAY GO BACK TO QUESTIONS IN THIS SECTION ONLY.

Kaplan UKCAT Mock Test Answer Key: Sections 1–4

Verbal Reasoning

1. B
2. D
3. B
4. A
5. C
6. A
7. B
8. C
9. D
10. C
11. A
12. A
13. A
14. B
15. C
16. B
17. C
18. A
19. C
20. A
21. A
22. C
23. D
24. D
25. A
26. A
27. C
28. B
29. C
30. D
31. D
32. B
33. D
34. C
35. B
36. B
37. C
38. A
39. A
40. B
41. D
42. C
43. C
44. A

Decision Making

1. YES; NO; YES; NO; NO
2. NO; YES; NO; YES; NO
3. YES; NO; NO; YES; NO
4. NO; NO; YES; NO; YES
5. NO; YES; NO; NO; YES
6. D
7. A
8. B
9. C
10. C
11. B
12. D
13. A
14. B
15. NO; YES; NO; YES; NO
16. NO; NO; YES; YES; YES
17. YES; NO; NO; NO; YES
18. YES; NO; YES; NO; NO
19. D
20. B
21. C
22. A
23. C
24. D
25. A
26. D
27. C
28. D
29. A

Quantitative Reasoning

1. B
2. C
3. A
4. E
5. B
6. D
7. E
8. A
9. E
10. B
11. D
12. E
13. B
14. C
15. D
16. C
17. B
18. D
19. C
20. A
21. D
22. C
23. A
24. B
25. C
26. B
27. C
28. E
29. C
30. E
31. B
32. D
33. E
34. C
35. D
36. B

Abstract Reasoning

1. B
2. B
3. C
4. C
5. A
6. A
7. B
8. C
9. C
10. B
11. C
12. D
13. C
14. A
15. D
16. B
17. B
18. C
19. A
20. C
21. C
22. C
23. A
24. C
25. B
26. C
27. A
28. A
29. B
30. A
31. B
32. A
33. C
34. B
35. C
36. A
37. C
38. A
39. C
40. B
41. A
42. C
43. B
44. A
45. B
46. B
47. C
48. A
49. C
50. C
51. B
52. C
53. A
54. D
55. A

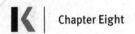

Kaplan UKCAT Mock Test Scoring Table: Sections 1–4

1. Count up your number of correct answers in each scored section. For Decision Making, count multiple choice questions as 1 mark each. For each five-part question, give yourself 2 marks if you answered all five parts correctly; if you answered three or four parts correctly, give yourself 1 mark.

2. Find your approximate score for each section in the table below.

	NUMBER CORRECT	APPROXIMATE UKCAT SCORE
Verbal Reasoning	_____	_____
Decision Making	_____	_____
Quantitative Reasoning	_____	_____
Abstract Reasoning	_____	_____

3. Add your section scores to find your total score: _____

Approximate UKCAT Score	Number of Questions Answered Correctly			
	Verbal Reasoning	**Decision Making**	**Quantitative Reasoning**	**Abstract Reasoning**
300	0–5	0–4	0–3	0–6
330	6	5	4–5	7–8
350	7	6	6	9–10
370	8	7	7	11–12
400	9–10	8	8	13–14
430	11–12	9	9	15–16
450	13–14	10	10	17–18
470	15	11	11	19–20
500	16	12–13	12	21–22
530	17–18	14–15	13	23–24
550	19–20	16–17	14–15	25–26
570	21–22	18–19	16–17	27–29
600	23–24	20–21	18–19	30–32
630	25–26	22–23	20–21	33–34
650	27–28	24–25	22–23	35–36
670	29–30	26–27	24	37
700	31	28–29	25	38–39
730	32	30	26	40–41
750	33	31	27	42–43
770	34	32	28	44–45
800	35–36	33	29	46–47
830	37–38	34	30	48–49
850	39–40	35	31–32	50–51
890	41–42	36	33–34	52–53
900	43–44	37–38	35–36	54–55

N.B. These scores are for approximation purposes only. Scores on the UKCAT are given in 10-point intervals; actual scores will vary slightly from this scheme. This table is designed to err on the side of caution. In most cases, a similar performance on the UKCAT would result in a slightly higher score.

Kaplan UKCAT Mock Test Answer Key: Section 5

1. C	18. C	35. D	52. B
2. C	19. D	36. D	53. D
3. A	20. D	37. D	54. A
4. D	21. D	38. A	55. B
5. A	22. A	39. A	56. A
6. A	23. D	40. D	57. A
7. D	24. A	41. D	58. D
8. A	25. C	42. B	59. C
9. D	26. D	43. D	60. A
10. A	27. A	44. D	61. A
11. C	28. A	45. D	62. B
12. C	29. A	46. A	63. C
13. A	30. D	47. D	64. D
14. D	31. B	48. A	65. A
15. A	32. A	49. C	66. D
16. A	33. A	50. A	67. A
17. A	34. A	51. A	68. C

Kaplan UKCAT Mock Test Scoring Table: Section 5

1. Count up your number of correct answers in this section: _____

2. Count up your number of partially correct answers in this section: _____

   Your answers are partially correct if:

   - you chose A, but the correct answer was B.

   - you chose B, but the correct answer was A.

   - you chose C, but the correct answer was D.

   - you chose D, but the correct answer was C.

3. Multiply the number of partially correct answers by 0.5, and add to your number of correct answers for your total marks:

Partially correct answers	Correct answers	Total marks
0.5(_____) +	_____ =	_____

4. Find your approximate scoring band for this section in the table below.

Approximate UKCAT Scoring Band	Total Marks in Situational Judgement
Band 4	0–16.5
Band 3	17–33.5
Band 2	34–50.5
Band 1	51–68

Getting Ready for Test Day

You are nearly ready for Test Day. You have completed two full-length Kaplan UKCAT practice tests, and learned and practised Kaplan's top tips for each section of the UKCAT. Hopefully, the top tips helped you improve your performance from the Kaplan UKCAT Diagnostic Test to the Kaplan UKCAT Mock Test. You will most likely have made some mistakes on the Mock Test, and these mistakes are to your advantage: any mistake you make while practising is one you can learn from, and avoid on Test Day. Be sure to review the worked answers for the Mock Test in full, so you can learn from your mistakes. You should also review the explanations for the questions you got right, to ensure that you got them right for the right reasons.

When athletes prepare for a major match or competition, they visualise success: a boxer imagines the series of punches and jabs that will defeat his opponent; a runner sees herself breaking away and crossing the finish line ahead of her rivals. When faced with an important and challenging exam such as the UKCAT, you must also get ready for success by visualising it. Imagine yourself working through each section of the test, applying the Kaplan top tips, keeping an eye on the clock while you work at a good pace, eliminating answers and moving on rather than fretting about a difficult question, maximising your marks section by section, and then the moment when you finish and are handed your result: it will be a happy moment indeed!

The remaining tips in this chapter are designed to help you get ready for Test Day, so you can get ready for success. Some of these tips may seem a bit obvious, or a bit unusual, but they have been tried and tested by thousands of students. Getting ready for Test Day is not simply about revising and practising, but also about preparing yourself, in body, mind and spirit.

Kaplan Top Tips for Getting Ready for Test Day

1. Make a study plan for the final days/weeks, and stick to it

Count up the number of weeks and days from now to Test Day, and work out exactly what you are going to do in that time to finish getting ready. If you have only a few days from now until Test Day, then keep it simple: review the Kaplan top tips and practice questions (and explanations) in this book. You should sit one of the free practice tests on the UKCAT website (www.ukcat.ac.uk). If you have a week until Test Day, then you should complete the online practice questions, and be sure to allow time afterwards for a full review of the worked answers. If you have more than a week, then you should try and take one or two practice tests per week. These could include the free practice tests from the UKCAT website, and also the free Mock Online test in your Kaplan Online Centre. If you have taken the Kaplan UKCAT preparation course and thus have access to further Kaplan practice tests, then you would do well to plan to take one or two of these a week, always reviewing the full worked answers very soon after completing a practice test. Be cautious about using any practice tests from other sources, as these are likely to diverge significantly from the format, timing or style of the UKCAT. Don't negate all your hard work by studying with flawed materials.

Allow time to use your Score Higher Question Bank, which may help to build mastery of individual question types, or to improve pacing in one or more sections. If you have the time, you may want to complete all 400 questions in the Score Higher Question Bank. More practice builds higher scores.

Be sure to check your Kaplan Online Centre, along with the UKCAT website, so that you are aware of any changes to the test format (including number of questions and timing for each section) in the year that you sit the UKCAT. The UKCAT website is normally updated in late April with the basic details of the exam format for the current year; the practice tests on this website may be updated again in late June or early July, just before testing begins, to reflect the proportion of question types in each section in the current year. We will post any related updates in your Kaplan Online Centre, once the information on the UKCAT website has changed—so be sure to plan to check online in the weeks ahead of Test Day.

2. Stress is normal—expect it, and manage it

Everyone feels anxious and pressurised about doing well on the UKCAT. Feelings of stress are to be expected when an exam is so important to your future. The best way to deal with stress is to understand it, acknowledge it, and limit its impact on your Test Day performance. By 'stress', we mean any factor that can keep you from doing your best on Test Day. Stress can include your own anxieties, comments from family and friends, and any problems that arise on Test Day. Feeling stress does not mean that you are unprepared, or stupid, or weak, or any other negative thing that might come to mind; feeling stress means that you're human. By acknowledging stress, you can then proceed to manage it, depending on its source:

Stress about the test itself. As we've seen through the course of this book, the UKCAT is a challenging and very tightly timed exam. This is its very nature, so the UKCAT is objectively stressful for everyone. However, consider the fact that most test-takers do very little to prepare for the UKCAT. Some even believe that it is impossible to prepare, so they do nothing at all. Most test-takers will look over a few practice questions, and perhaps try a full mock test. But relatively few among the UKCAT cohort will take the time to learn the Kaplan top tips, practise them so they become second nature, and practise as well for pacing. You are among the select few who are very well positioned for success on Test Day. Sure, the UKCAT is challenging and fast-paced; but you're prepared to work fast, and to meet its challenges. This gives you a huge advantage, and should also give you confidence.

Stress from family and friends. It is natural for family and friends to ask about how you're getting on with your UKCAT revision, and for them to want you to do well on the exam. Sometimes, though, comments from parents or friends that are meant to be supportive and encouraging have the unintended result of increasing stress. Such added pressure is more likely to result when comments are frequent—for instance, if your parents check in on your progress at least once a day. To limit stress from such friendly sources, you might mention to your parents (or friends, or whoever's the source) that you are getting on very well with your UKCAT preparation, and that it will help you do even better on Test Day if you can clear your head when you're not revising. They can help you succeed by keeping your mind on other things when you're not revising—even the most talented and brilliant among us need a break!

Stress about Test Day. The procedures on Test Day can be a source of anxiety and uncertainty. You should read through the information about what to expect on Test Day on the UKCAT website, and review their simulation of the Pearson testing centre. Sitting the official UKCAT practice tests will also help you to familiarise yourself with the format of the test interface that you will use on Test Day. You will also want to ensure you review the route from home to the test centre a day or two before the test. Be sure to plan for an alternate route to the test centre, whether you're driving or taking public transport; this will ensure that transport problems do not keep you from making it to the test centre in time.

3. Wind down your preparations in the last day or two before Test Day

Many students assume that it's best to keep on revising right up until the minute they walk into the exam room. In fact, such last-minute preparations are unhelpful for the UKCAT, because it's not a content-based exam. The skills you need for UKCAT success are developed through practice; they can't be 'crammed' for. Following the guidance in this book, and coming up with a study plan to incorporate any practice tests you can reasonably fit in between now and Test Day, is the best way to revise for the UKCAT.

In the last day or two before the UKCAT, however, you need to finish your revision efforts and make more time to relax in a 'test-free zone'. It is okay to finish looking over the worked answers from your final practice test, but don't assume that cramming in one more practice test will make you more prepared. You would do better to look back over the Kaplan top tips from each chapter of this book, to make sure that these are 'fresh', but otherwise to spend time taking your mind off the UKCAT. Returning to basics and relaxing in a 'test-free zone' is the best way to build confidence, reduce stress and make the most of your time just before Test Day.

You will also want to ensure that you get a good night's sleep each night in the week before Test Day. Don't stay up very late studying and then sleep late, as you will be sitting the exam during the day, and will want to be rested and fully awake. Getting into a regular sleep cycle will ensure that you do not feel tired while sitting the UKCAT.

Once you get ready for Test Day, the only thing that remains is to sit the UKCAT. Our final set of Kaplan top tips will help you make the most of the Test Day experience.

Kaplan Top Tips for Test Day

1. Warm up your brain and body before the test

Allow yourself plenty of time for a pre-test ritual, and ensure that you wake up early enough to do so. Eat a decent breakfast, with servings of protein and carbohydrates, so you are fully energised and don't get hungry during the test. Spend some time before the test reading something stimulating, to 'activate' your brain for the level of thinking and speed required on the UKCAT. You could read during breakfast or on the journey to the test centre. Just be sure not to go into the exam with an empty stomach, or without 'jump-starting' your brain. Students who do so usually have difficulty with the first section, which usually results in a far lower than expected Verbal Reasoning score. Warm up properly, so you can attack the Verbal section with the full force of your awesome UKCAT skills arsenal!

2. Make sure everything's in your bag

Before you leave home, check (and then double-check) that you have a copy of your UKCAT registration and an approved photo ID. You will also want to be prepared to put everything else except your clothes and your photo ID into your bag, which you will have to put in a locker before entering the exam room. You will only be allowed to take your photo ID and the locker key (and whatever clothes you didn't leave in the locker) into the exam room. Any jewellery and anything in your pockets—including your phone, wallet, watch and tissues—must be left in the locker. This is a rule that cannot be waived, so make sure everything is in your bag.

3. Ask for an extra noteboard

Just before you enter the exam room, the invigilator will give you a wet-erase pen and a 'noteboard', which is a plasticised sheet of A4 paper. You can write on both sides of the noteboard, but you can't rub it out without a moist cloth. You are welcome to ask for an additional noteboard during the exam—and should do so by raising your hand, ideally just before the end of a section, so you'll have a new noteboard at the start of the next section. However, there's no harm in asking for an extra noteboard before starting the exam. The invigilator may say no—but they may just as well say yes.

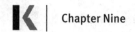

4. Take control of your testing station

Once you enter the exam room, you will be assigned to a testing station, consisting of a desktop computer, with mouse and keyboard, and a chair. Most testing stations will be separated by partitions; you must ensure that you do not get out of the chair without first getting the invigilator's permission, and you must take special care to make sure your eyes do not look anywhere other than inside your testing station during the exam. Even so, you can take control of your testing station before starting the exam. If the chair is a swivel chair, adjust the seat to an appropriate and comfortable height.

You might also move the keyboard out of the way, and set up your noteboard and mouse so you can use them easily and quickly. Just be sure to bring the keyboard out for the Decision and Quantitative sections, as you'll work much more quickly by typing the figures into the onscreen calculator than by using the mouse. If you take the test in a centre with touchscreen monitors, we strongly advise that you do not touch the screen to operate the calculator. Our experience is that these screens can be quite desensitised, so you may struggle to get all the numbers and signs to function correctly with a single touch. Students who have attempted the touchscreen have almost universally found it slower and less satisfying than using the keyboard number pad or the mouse.

If something is wrong in the testing room, raise your hand immediately and notify the invigilator. If a problem can be fixed, it's better to address it straightaway so you can return your full focus to the exam. If a problem can't be fixed, then notify the UKCAT Consortium as soon as possible after the test.

5. Take 'mini-breaks' between the sections

Remember, you have one minute to read the instructions for each section. However, the instructions are always the same. At Kaplan, we find that many of our students like to take a 'mini-break' during the minute for instructions. A mini-break might involve stretching in your seat—extending your arms and legs, and shaking them a bit to get the blood flowing; you might do the same with your head, neck and shoulders, but just be careful not to look outside your partition! You might also try blinking rapidly for several seconds, or closing and opening your eyes at 10-second intervals, to alleviate any eyestrain and freshen your eyes for the next section. You should not take a toilet break during the exam, as this will cost valuable time for answering questions. Most students find it helpful to use the toilet just before entering the exam room, as this will minimise the likelihood of any disruptive emergencies—so you can focus on building a great UKCAT score.

6. One question at a time

This is the simplest tip, and perhaps the most important. On Test Day, keep your focus on the question at hand. You will get through each section by answering the questions one at a time; great results are built on success in individual questions. Remember to follow the tips about maximising marks, and don't waste time on questions that are especially difficult or time-consuming. There won't be very many of these questions, and they will be difficult or time-consuming for all test-takers. Only the prepared test-taker will have the foresight and confidence to expect such questions, and to deal with them quickly and efficiently, marking an answer, marking for review, and moving on to quicker, easier marks.

7. Don't think about your score during the exam

You will get your result as soon as you finish. So don't think about how well you're doing, or whether the questions seem generally easy or difficult. Just focus on answering the questions one by one, and keep an eye on the clock so that you pace yourself and mark an answer for all the questions in each section.

8. Answer every question

There's no negative marking, so there is no reason not to mark an answer for every question. The computer cannot tell whether you got a question correct because you worked it out, because you eliminated the wrong answers, or because you guessed blindly. The computer only knows that you got the question correct, and so you get the mark. You do have to work very quickly on the UKCAT, and will almost certainly have to make your best guess after partial elimination on at least a few questions in each section. Expect this, embrace it, mark your best answers confidently, and keep moving. Students who don't understand how to pace themselves on the UKCAT and how to eliminate and guess strategically leave lots of questions unanswered—ensuring they get low scores. Answering all the questions will help you secure a top score.

Now that you have learned the Kaplan top tips for UKCAT success, all that remains is to follow through on your study plan, and put the top tips into practice on Test Day. We at Kaplan are honoured to have helped you prepare for the UKCAT, and wish you all the very best, on Test Day and in your future medical practice. Hard work makes great doctors—you are on your way!

Score Higher Online

Many students do not use all the available practice questions.

Make time to work through the resources in your Kaplan Online Centre, including all the items in your UKCAT Score Higher Question Bank.

Unless you are consistently scoring 100% correct, you can improve your speed and accuracy with further practice.

Kaplan Top Tips for Test-Takers with Learning Difficulties

The UKCAT Consortium offers a second standardised version of the exam, UKCATSEN, or UKCAT Special Educational Needs, for candidates with learning difficulties. You can sign up for UKCATSEN through the UKCAT website, and this version of the exam allows approximately 25% extra time in each section. This extra time is intended to help candidates with common learning difficulties, such as dyslexia, dysgraphia or working memory deficit.

Candidates should only register for UKCATSEN if they normally receive extra time on exams, and should ensure that they will be able to provide clinical evidence of the relevant learning difficulty, in the form of a written diagnosis in an approved format. This evidence is not required until later in the admissions process, and must be given directly to the universities; candidates who sit the UKCATSEN and are subsequently unable to furnish the required evidence will have their test results voided. So you should only sit UKCATSEN if you have a diagnosed learning difficulty. Check the UKCAT website for the latest details on timing for UKCATSEN, and follow up directly with the UKCAT Consortium with any questions about required evidence, as this can vary from country to country.

If you require test accommodations for other reasons—for example, if you need wheelchair access or an adjustable height desk—check the UKCAT website for a list of available accommodations and current procedures well in advance of Test Day. You will likely need to contact Pearson VUE customer services to ensure that the accommodation can be provided; you may be required to take the test at certain test centres, as not all locations can provide all accommodations. Note that the same procedure applies for access accommodations if you are taking UKCAT or UKCATSEN.

Kaplan Top Tips for Test-Takers with Learning Difficulties

1. Determine which sections require a different approach

Depending on the exact nature of your learning difficulty, you may need to take a slightly different approach in one or more sections. Some common adjustments include:

Verbal Reasoning: If you have trouble scanning for keywords, try reading the first statement, then reading through the passage quickly, in about a minute. Then, use your knowledge of the passage to evaluate the statements. If you find the answer to the first statement while reading the passage, mark it, read the next statement, and continue reading the passage. This is a slower approach overall, but dyslexic test-takers may find it more useful than scanning for keywords.

Decision Making: These question types require a mix of verbal and quantitative skills, so the challenges may be similar to the sections that come before and after Decision Making. As you practise, keep track of your progress with the different question types. If you are stronger in some than others, you might prioritise your strengths on Test Day, so you can build up marks on those questions as quickly as possible; come to more challenging question types on a second pass through the section, and work through these as efficiently as you can.

Quantitative Reasoning: If you have trouble thinking through how to solve the questions quickly, try skipping to the end of each question, rather than reading through from the beginning. Most of the time, the last few words of the question will describe what you must solve for—reading this first can help you to focus, and can save time and limit confusion as you set up and solve.

Abstract Reasoning: If you have trouble keeping the patterns in Set A and Set B distinct in your mind, then jot down a few notes on each on your noteboard. This can be especially helpful when there are multiple features, but test-takers with working memory deficit might want to make brief notes on the patterns in each set, to save time and avoid frustration.

Situational Judgement: The challenges in this section are very similar to those in Verbal Reasoning. Test-takers with dyslexia will want to allow a bit of extra time to read through each scenario before evaluating the related responses; if you read quickly, it is very easy to miss out a word or two that could be the key to the central issue in the scenario. Practise for this as you revise, to build your confidence and work out the best balance of time between scenario vs responses for you. You may find that it works better to spend more like 45 seconds or a minute per scenario, rather than the standard 30 seconds, so you can be certain of identifying the key issues.

2. Understand exactly how much extra time you have

Whilst it is true that UKCATSEN gives you 25% extra time per section, note that this is 25% more than the total time, which includes the 1 minute to read instructions in each section in the standard UKCAT—which cannot be used to answer questions. Furthermore, there is an increase in the time to read instructions in UKCATSEN—to 1 minute, 15 seconds per section—which, again, cannot be used to answer questions. As a result, the actual extra time to answer questions in each section is slightly less than 25%.

Section	UKCAT timing	UKCATSEN timing	Time for questions in UKCATSEN	Time per question in UKCATSEN
Verbal Reasoning	22 minutes	27.5 minutes	26.25 minutes	35 seconds
Decision Making	32 minutes	40 minutes	38.75 minutes	1 minute, 20 seconds
Quantitative Reasoning	25 minutes	31.25 minutes	30 minutes	50 seconds
Abstract Reasoning	14 minutes	17.5 minutes	16.25 minutes	17.7 seconds
Situational Judgement	27 minutes	33.75 minutes	32.5 minutes	28.6 seconds

It's true that this difference may vary slightly from the 25% advertised by the test-maker, but the time that really matters is the time to answer questions. Note that for each Abstract set, you have about a minute and a half (88.5 seconds). Note as well that the table indicates the average time per question in UKCATSEN If you need to adjust your pacing in a section, work out how much time you should expect to spend per question (or per set). Keep a note of your progress as you finish each timed set, quiz or practice test, so you can congratulate yourself when you do well and track your success in the days and weeks leading up to Test Day.

3. Practise your different approach, for speed and accuracy as well as for timing

While you will be able to spend 25% more time in each section of the UKCAT, this is not a huge amount of extra time. You will still want to ensure you can answer the questions as efficiently as possible, and should practise for this through your remaining UKCAT practice tests, and in any questions in this book you have not yet attempted. Practising your different approach for any sections requiring one will build your speed, accuracy and confidence, and will help you to answer the most possible questions correctly in the time allotted. You will also need to think about how many minutes/seconds to spend per set and per question. Your ability to pace yourself, even in sections that are especially challenging, is essential.

When you take an online practice test, be sure to select the option that includes the extra timing. The official practice tests on the UKCAT website include a UKCATSEN version; you can also take all the Kaplan UKCAT practice tests in our Online Study Plan (including the Mock Online Test in your Kaplan Online Centre provided with this book) with UKCATSEN timing.

4. Prepare for all sections of the test

Due to the varied nature of the sections on the UKCAT, your learning difficulty may affect your approach to one or more sections, but may not affect your approach to all sections. For example, a test-taker with dyslexia will not experience any extra challenges in Abstract Reasoning. Such a test-taker should follow the Kaplan top tips for Abstract Reasoning, and should see that section as a special opportunity to maximise marks. If you put in extra effort in a section that does not present extra challenges, and earn a score that is well above average, then you will make yourself truly stand out from the competition. An especially high result in such a section will also counterbalance a less than stellar performance in a section that is more challenging. So you should use the varied nature of the test to your advantage.

5. Remember—the UKCAT is objectively difficult for everyone

The final tip may seem a bit obvious, and perhaps not so helpful. But it's essential to remember that the UKCAT is designed to be challenging for students who are among the best in their year at school, and who will be competitive for admission to the top medical schools in the UK. The UKCAT is not an easy test, in terms of the question formats or the timing, which is brutal. If you have a learning difficulty, one or more sections of the UKCAT may seem like an almost impossible challenge. But it's important to keep in mind that the same section seems just as horrifying to all your fellow test-takers. This is the nature of the exam, and a major source of stress that causes many test-takers to cave under pressure each year. Follow the Kaplan top tips in this book, practise thoroughly and smartly, and be confident in the fact that you have a major advantage over the competition. Keep positive, work efficiently and calmly, and visualise success—you are on your way to a great result and an amazing future.

Score Higher Online

Select extended timing—or untimed mode—when you practise online.

The Mock Online Test and Short Test in your Kaplan Online Centre let you select standard or extended timing.

You can make your own quizzes with the UKCAT Score Higher Question Bank, with three options: Timed, Untimed or Tutor mode.

When building mastery with individual questions or short quizzes, you will likely find it more helpful to work in Untimed mode. Tutor mode is useful if you want to be able to view the explanations as you work through the questions.

APPENDIX B

Diagnostic Test Explanations

Verbal Reasoning

1. (B)

The final sentence of the third paragraph states that brown bears live in a forest and eat a diet that includes meat, plants and berries. Thus, **(B)** cannot be true and is the correct answer.

2. (B)

The ancestry of today's polar bears is explained in the second paragraph. Today's polar bears have the same mitochondrial DNA as prehistoric brown bears that were found in Ireland. Answer **(B)** is therefore correct.

3. (D)

Iceland is never mentioned in the passage, so there is no basis in the passage for inferring anything that must be true about Iceland. Eliminate **(A)** and **(C)**. The first sentence of the final paragraph states that Ireland's climate cooled considerably during the Ice Age; the correct answer is **(D)**.

4. (A)

The passage never states directly that some bears survived the Ice Age. However, it is correct to infer this, based on the fact that today's polar bears share mitochondrial DNA with prehistoric brown bears that lived during the Ice Age. If some bears had not survived the Ice Age, then today's polar bears would not continue to carry the mitochondrial DNA of their Ice Age ancestors. Answer **(A)** is correct.

5. (A)

This is a negative question; the three wrong answers will be supported by the passage, and the one correct answer won't be. Bernhardt's career is discussed throughout the passage, so look for a keyword from each answer choice. Films are mentioned in the passage's first and penultimate sentences, which make

clear that Bernhardt appeared in films. **(A)** contradicts the passage, so it is false—and the correct answer.

6. (C)

The keywords *The Three Musketeers* appear (in very helpful italics) midway through the second paragraph. *The Three Musketeers* was written by the novelist Alexandre Dumas, son of the author Alexandre Dumas (who wrote *Kean*). Scanning the answers quickly, you will likely notice that **(C)** is clearly correct. NB Wrong answer trap **(A)**, as the passage does not say that Dumas the father was a novelist or that *Kean* was a novel.

7. (C)

The keywords 'personal history' are a bit hard to scan for; hopefully, you were able to find the reference to her 'biography and early life' midway through the second paragraph. This part of the passage states that little is known about Bernhardt's personal history, and that her past is largely inscrutable. These details are paraphrased in **(C)**, which is therefore correct. If you were tempted by the other answers, note that Bernhardt's history was not entirely fabricated, and it is relevant to her reputation (given all the rumours about her).

8. (D)

The keywords *French* and *government* appear together in the passage's second sentence, which says that the French Conservatoire was a Government-sponsored school of acting that Bernhardt attended in the mid-1800s. Thus, the correct answer is **(D)**.

9. (B)

The Town and Country Planning Act is mentioned throughout the passage, so check for keywords from each answer. **(A)** is contradicted by the third paragraph, which states that the Act was revised 59 years after it became law. The first paragraph explains that the Act governs construction, while the second paragraph details that it protects existing buildings. **(B)** is correct.

10. (C)

This is a negative question, asking for something that must be false. Thus, the correct answer must contradict the passage; any answers that are supported by the passage will be incorrect. Listed buildings are mentioned in the second paragraph; owners of such buildings are legally required to keep them in good repair, and must get special consent before making any alterations that affect the building's character or appearance. From this, you can infer that listed buildings can be repaired (once consent is obtained). **(C)** contradicts the passage on this point, so **(C)** must be false—and is therefore the correct answer.

11. (A)

Work on a previous question revealed that the Town and Country Planning Act was revised in 2006, and this detail was found in the final paragraph—so check that paragraph for details about the requirements of a UK planning application today. The third sentence of this paragraph indicates what must be included in such an application, such as the extent of public engagement. Thus, **(A)** is correct.

12. (B)

It is safe to infer that the author would agree with anything that is not described negatively in the passage. The question also contains the keywords *town planning*, and the accomplishments of town planning are mentioned in the second paragraph. These include the government achieving objectives for climate control, reduction of carbon emissions and housing access. The only answer that fits these details is **(B)**, which is therefore correct.

13. (B)

The second paragraph states that testimony transcribed in Arabic can only be summarised into French at head office, due to a shortage of Arabic-French translators in the field. From this, it is safe to infer that some translators at head office translate Arabic. On this point, the statement contradicts the passage, so the statement is false.

14. (A)

The first paragraph says that testimony must be transcribed in the language in which it is given, and that testimony can be taken in English. Thus, testimony could be taken and transcribed in English. The second paragraph states that testimony must also be summarised in English or French. Thus, testimony could be taken, transcribed and initially summarised entirely in English. The answer is **(A)**.

15. (B)

The passage's first sentence says that testimony must be transcribed in the language in which it is given, and that testimony may be given in a tribal language. Hence, it is safe to infer that testimony given in a tribal language must be transcribed in the same tribal language. This statement says otherwise; as such, the statement contradicts the passage, and is false.

16. (C)

Strasbourg is mentioned in the second paragraph as the location of the commission's head office; the same paragraph also states that testimony taken and transcribed in Arabic can only be summarised into French at head office. However, the passage does not specify that testimony taken in Arabic can only be summarised into English (the other permissible language for summaries) at head office. The passage likewise does not say that Arabic-language testimony can be summarised into English in the field. Based on information in the passage, there isn't enough information to answer; the correct answer is therefore **(C)**.

17. (B)

The second paragraph states that the United States wanted to protect natural sites in order to preserve them for future citizens of the world. Answer **(B)** is correct.

18. (C)

Liverpool's Maritime Mercantile City was one of the largest trading centres in the 18th and 19th century, it is not stated that this is still the case. Liverpool Waters is being redeveloped, but it is not stated that this is within the Maritime Mercantile City. The last paragraph states that the area made headway in the development of technology, transportation and port management. The correct answer is **(C)**.

19. (D)

This is a negative question, asking for something that is false; the correct answer will contradict the passage. **(A)** is confirmed in the last paragraph, Liverpool Waters would fragment and isolate the distinctive dock area. The World Heritage Trust is discussed in the second paragraph, where **(B)** is confirmed. **(C)** is not discussed in the passage. **(D)** is incorrect, although the first paragraph states that the first World Heritage Site locations were recognised in 1978, but throughout the rest of the passage, UNESCO is referred to at earlier dates, meaning UNESCO must have been formed before 1978. **(D)** is the correct answer.

20. (D)

The number of World Heritage Sites in the US is not mentioned in the passage. Liverpool pioneered modern dock technology in the 18th and 19th century, but is not currently at the forefront of modern technology. Natural sites were not officially recognised until the text came into force in 1975. The last paragraph suggests that the author would agree with **(D)**, the new redevelopment scheme, Liverpool Waters, endangers an existing World Heritage Site.

21. (C)

This is a negative question asking for something the author would be least likely to agree with; thus, any answer that the author would agree with will be incorrect, and the correct answer will most likely contradict the passage. The cost of the storm in 2015 (Storm Desmond) is confirmed in the final sentence. Eliminate **(A)**. **(B)** is supported by the details in the first two sentences of the passage, so eliminate **(B)**. **(C)** does not agree with the first paragraph, which indicates that snow ploughs are used for snowfall of three inches of more. **(C)** is correct.

22. (D)

The keywords *gritting salt* lead to the fourth sentence of the first paragraph, which states the circumstances in which gritting salt is not effective. The previous sentence says that gritting lorries are sufficient for snowfalls of 3 inches or less. Answer **(D)** is thus supported by the passage, and is correct.

23. (B)

Heathrow is mentioned near the end of the passage; a blizzard in 2010 resulted in hundreds of planes at Heathrow having to be dug out by hand, as there was no equipment at Heathrow that could undertake this task. The previous sentence explains that airports in the USA and Canada have mechanised equipment that can do this. Thus, it is correct to infer that Heathrow does not have all the same equipment as Canadian airports, as Heathrow does not have all the same snow-clearing equipment. The correct answer is **(B)**.

24. (C)

This question asks about the passage as a whole, so you must check each answer choice to see if it is mentioned as a consequence of heavy snow in the UK, and then compare those that are to see which is the most severe. The passage states that children sometimes miss a week of school or more, so **(A)** is less severe than the actual detail in the passage. Slippery pavements are not mentioned in the passage. Financial

losses are mentioned in the final sentence, and the detail here is a paraphrase of **(C)**. The passage says nothing about Heathrow hiring American equipment. Answer **(C)** is therefore correct.

25. (C)

Chekhov is mentioned in the second paragraph as a writer who strongly influenced Mansfield, and to whose work she was introduced when she was living in Germany. The sentence that mentions this specifies that Chekhov is 'late', or deceased, so it is not a basis for inferring that Mansfield met Chekhov in Germany, or that he lived there when she became aware of his work in that country. The passage never says whether Chekhov lived in Germany for a time, or if he lived exclusively elsewhere (eg, his native Russia). The answer is can't tell.

26. (B)

The first paragraph states that Mansfield studied cello at Queen's College, but that she was best known for her short stories; her writing continues to be taught today. Thus, it is safe to infer that Mansfield is best known for her achievement in writing, not in music. This statement contradicts the passage, so the statement is false.

27. (C)

The last paragraph gives information about Mansfield's publications; she published more than a dozen short stories in a socialist magazine, *The New Age*. This is the passage's only reference to socialism; no information is provided about Mansfield's political views, so it is impossible to determine on the basis of the passage whether or not she was a socialist. The answer is **(C)**.

28. (A)

The second paragraph describes how Mansfield was married in 1909, and was sent to Germany in the same year, following her divorce. The statement is true.

29. (D)

(A) refers to Foucalt's experiment discussed in the second paragraph, not the use of light-years as a measure of distance. **(B)** cannot be correct as this is still unknown. Eberty was one of the first to understand the implications of a fixed and finite speed of light, but using light-years as a measure of distance is not reliant upon his theory. The second sentence states that knowing the approximate, finite speed of light allows it to be used as a unit of distance. **(D)** is correct.

30. (A)

The final paragraph details how Eberty's theory has been adapted by scientists to discover events during the Big Bang, of the formation of the universe. The answer is **(A)**.

31. (A)

Eberty's theories are discussed in the fourth paragraph, which states that past events could be viewed on Earth if the observer moved away from the Earth at a speed greater than the speed of light, or 299,792,458 metres per second. **(A)** is correct.

32. (B)

Foucalt's experiment is discussed in the second paragraph. **(A)** describes Eberty's theory. **(B)** is confirmed in the final sentence of the second paragraph. **(B)** is correct.

33. (C)

The first sentence of the final paragraph suggests that many football scouts discredit the moneyball method, but it is not clear whether most football scouts do or do not use the moneyball method. **(C)** is correct.

34. (A)

Oakland Athletics are described as underfunded compared to their opponents in the final paragraph. The statement is true.

35. (B)

The final paragraph discusses the issues of applying sabermetrics to football, and suggests that sabermetrics is most successful when used for sports teams with less funding, such as the Oakland Athletics baseball team. The statement is false.

36. (B)

The second paragraph states that Michael L. Lewis wrote a book describing the successful use of sabermetrics by three managers of a baseball team. Michael L. Lewis is not said to have developed the theory himself. The statement is false.

37. (A)

Asteroid 2014 DX110 is described as passing Earth with a 1 in 10 chance of collision in 2014. The statement is true.

38. (B)

Cruithne refers to a quasi-orbital satellite, but the first paragraph describes that the name also refers to a Scottish tribe, in the Old Irish tongue. **(B)** is correct.

39. (C)

Cruithne is described as orbiting Earth as part of its true orbit of the sun, but it is not clear whether HO3 orbits the sun. The answer is can't tell.

40. (C)

An asteroid hitting Earth in 1908 is described in the final paragraph, but it is not stated that this is the last significant asteroid collision on Earth. The answer is can't tell.

41. (B)

The second paragraph describes that there are two Gettier cases, and they describe individuals who have a justified, true belief of a claim but do not know that they one. **(B)** is the answer.

42. (D)

The first paragraph states that Plato was the first to describe the JTB account. The JTB account has three components (justified, true, belief), so **(B)** is correct. The first paragraph gives Socrates' argument for knowledge being prized above true belief. The second paragraph states that Bertrand Russell and Ludwig Wittgenstein questioned the criteria in the early 20th century, while Gettier's paper was published in the second half of the 20th century. **(D)** must be false.

43. (A)

At the end of the second paragraph, the author states that Gettier's paper demonstrated the inadequacy of the JTB theory, and the last paragraph suggests that no adequate responses the Gettier problem have salvaged the JTB theory. **(A)** is correct.

44. (B)

The final paragraph gives counterarguments to the Gettier problem. The second to last sentence of the passage confirms **(B)**, some theorists aim to replace the justification criteria.

Decision Making

1. YES; NO; NO; YES; NO

The first conclusion follows from the first sentence of the text: if it is in the interest of almost all commuters to travel to work by public transport, then necessarily there must be some commuters whose interest is *not* served by travelling to work on public transport. The second conclusion does not follow. The text states that no commuter should travel to work by public transport if they own a bicycle, this does not mean that they should never use public transport, merely that they shouldn't use it to travel to work. The third conclusion does not follow: the text states that it is only in the interest of almost all commuters to travel to work by public transport, not that it is in the interest of all commuters to own bicycles. The fourth conclusion follows from the first and second sentences: almost all (i.e. most) commuters have it in their interest (i.e. should) travel to work by public transport, however if they own a bicycle then they should not (unless is used here to indicate the caveat). The fifth conclusion does not follow as it directly contradiction the second sentence of the text, which states that no commuter should travel to work by public transport if they own a bicycle.

2. NO; YES; NO; NO; YES

The first conclusion does not follow. We are told that some of the indoor wear was made from suede and that none of it was made from fur but we are given no indication as to what materials were used for the outdoor wear. All we know is that some of the winter collection was made from suede. Consequently, no conclusions can be drawn about which materials were used across the collection. The second conclusion does follow. The garment is from the winter collection so must be either indoor wear or outdoor wear. Since it is made from fur, it cannot be indoor wear and so must be outdoor wear. The third conclusion does not follow. We do not know which materials the outdoor wear in the winter collection was made from, so it is possible that a piece of outdoor wear is both hand-stitched and made from fur. The fourth conclusion does not follow either. Only some of the indoor wear was made from suede, which implies that some indoor wear was made from other materials. The fifth conclusion does follow. All items in the winter collection, including indoor wear, were hand-stitched, but no indoor wear was made from fur. Therefore, logically it is true that all indoor wear is either made from fur or hand-stitched (although as it happens, it will always be the case that the indoor wear is hand-stitched and not made from fur).

3. YES; NO; NO; NO; YES

The first conclusion follows: sheep are not horned cows, so they must be brown. The second conclusion does not follow; some of the cows have horns, but this does not mean that none of the sheep have horns. The third conclusion does not follow. All of the animals except the horned cows are brown; because only 'some' of the cows have horns, there could be cows that have no horns, and are therefore brown. The fourth conclusion does not follow; it is not clear that the only animals with horns are cows. The fifth conclusion follows. Since all of the cows with horns are colours other than brown, any animal that is brown and has horns must be a sheep.

4. NO; NO; YES; YES; NO

The question only tells us about where some of the previous principals of schools in Brigg were born; it does not mention anything about where the current principals of schools in Brigg were born, so the first conclusion does not follow. Likewise, the question does not tell us anything about where the previous principals of schools in Astley were born, so the second conclusion also does not follow. The third conclusion does follow because the question tells us that all of the current principals of schools in Astley were born in Brigg—as a result, they cannot have been born in Astley (or anywhere else). The fourth conclusion also follows. The question tells us some of the previous principals of schools in Brigg were born in Astley, which implies that some of them were not born in Astley. The fifth conclusion does not follow for the same reason that the first does not follow: the question tells us nothing about current principals of schools in Brigg, so we cannot draw any conclusions about where they were born.

5. NO; YES; YES; NO; NO

The first conclusion does not follow. The 30% discount on cases of wine does not apply, since sparkling wine cannot be sold by the case and therefore the price increases as more bottles of sparkling wine are bought. The second conclusion follows, as we are told that sparkling wine can only be sold by the bottle. The third conclusion follows: with a 30% discount on 6 bottles of a red wine, they would cost the same as 4.2 individual bottles of the same wine, and thus cheaper than buying 5 individual bottles. The fourth conclusion does not follow. Both red and white non-sparkling wine can be sold by the case. The fifth conclusion does not follow. We do not know the prices of the individual bottles; since they are not clearly the same price (as in the third conclusion), we cannot determine whether this conclusion is true.

6. (B)

The set-up of this Logic Puzzle tells us that all three siblings enrolled at university when they were 19, but that each was born in a different year (i.e. they are all different ages). We are also told that one sibling studied for 3 years, another for 4 years, and a third for 5 years. Start with the third rule, which states that the eldest sibling enrolled in 2009. This means they were born in 1990 (2009 − 19 = 1990). The second rule tells us that Belinda graduated in 2016 and did not take the 5 year course. Therefore, she must have taken either the 4 year or the 3 year course. If she took the 4 year course, then she enrolled in 2012 and was born in 1993 (2016 − 4 = 2012, 2012 − 19 = 1993). If she took the 3 year course then she enrolled in 2013 and was born in 1994 (2016 − 3 = 2013, 2013 − 19 = 1994). Either way, she is not the eldest sibling, meaning either Lawrence or Felix is. The first rule states that Lawrence and Felix graduated in the same year. Since Belinda did not take the 5 year course, either Lawrence or Felix did. Hence we can deduce that Felix and Lawrence graduated in 2014 (2009 + 5). The younger of the pair, who must have taken the four year course, was therefore born in 1991 (2014 − 19 = 1991).

We now know that Belinda was born in either 1993 or 1994, and either Felix was born in 1990 and Lawrence in 1991, or Felix was born in 1991 and Lawrence in 1990. **(A)** must be false; it is impossible for Felix to be any more than one year younger than his brother. **(B)** is the only option which must be true: Felix, regardless of whether he was born in 1990 or 1991, must be at least two years older than Belinda, regardless of whether she was born in 1993 or 1994—in every scenario he is at least two years older than her.

For the record: Both **(C)** and **(D)** could be true, but since there are possible scenarios where they are not the case (e.g. Lawrence have been born in 1990, Felix in 1991 and Belinda in 1993) they are incorrect answers.

7. (D)

This Logic Puzzle includes a diagram which details an aquarium with nine tanks evenly split between three different species. Each tank contains one, two or three creatures. The second rule states that sharks only occupy one-creature tanks, of which there are four in the aquarium, two of which are found in the far right column of the diagram. The third rule states that there are exactly five octopi in the aquarium. Since each species occupies three tanks, the only possible combinations of tanks that the octopi could be held in are either 2 × two-creature tanks and 1 × one creature tank, or 2 × one-creature tanks and 1 × three-creature tanks. The latter is impossible, because three of the four one creature tanks must be occupied by sharks. The two

three-creature tanks then, must be occupied by turtles. (X), then, is occupied by turtles. Eliminate **(B)** and **(C)**.

The first rule states that octopi are never in the same column as sharks. The far right column has two one-creature tanks. Neither can contain octopi, as they only require 1 × one-creature tank and to occupy a tank here would automatically mean they are in the same column as a shark. Therefore, both tanks are occupied by sharks. This means that a shark occupies one of the one-creature tanks in the two middle columns. The two-creature tank in the same column must then be occupied by a turtle. The other middle column must be occupied solely by octopi (1 × one-creature tank and 1 × two-creature tank). This leaves the tank labelled (Y) occupied by octopi (giving five in total). Answer **(D)** is correct.

8. (C)

The following abbreviations will be used in this explanation: Accounts (A), Customer Support (CS), Human Resources (HR), Logistics (L), Marketing (M), Sales (S); Alpha-Section (A-sec), Beta-Section (B-sec), Gamma Section (G-sec), Delta Section (D-sec), Epsilon-Section (E-sec), Zeta-Section (Z-sec).

Start with the third rule, which is the most concrete: S is in D-sec. The fourth rule states that HR is not in E-sec or B-sec, while the fifth tells us that it is not in G-sec either. This means it must be in A-sec or Z-sec. The second rule states that M is also in either A-sec or Z-sec. The first rule tells us that L and CS are not in E-sec. Therefore, they must be in B-sec and G-sec. E-sec, as the only unoccupied section, must house A. This gives us the following sketch:

A-sec	B-sec	G-sec	D-sec	E-sec	Z-sec
M/HR	L/CS	L/CS	S	A	M/HR

The sketch indicates that Accounts is located in Epsilon-Section. **(C)** is the correct answer.

9. (A)

Appliances will be abbreviated as follows in this explanation: hairdryer (aH), ice-cream maker (aI), juicer (aJ), kettle (aK), lamp (aL). Manufacturers will be abbreviated as: Urbit (mU), Vaughn (mV), X-Tech (mX), Yarcol (mY) and Zan (mZ).

Start with the first rule, which tells us that aK requires the least power, which is 3V. Now skip to the fourth rule. The appliance made by mU requires exactly twice the power of aI. The voltages which must be paired in this task are 3V, 5V, 6V, 9V and 12V. Given this set of numbers, it is only possible for an appliance to have exactly double the power if it is either 6V (double 3V) or 12V (double 6V). The former case is not possible, because then mU's appliance would be twice the power of aK. As a result, mU must make the 12V appliance and al must require 6V.

Next consider the third rule: either aH or aJ is made by mY. From this we can deduce that mY must make either the 5V appliance or the 9V appliance: mY cannot make the 3V appliance because this is aK, and it cannot make the 6V appliance because this is al, nor can it make the 12V appliance because the manufacturer of this is mU. This gives us the following sketch, with the uncertainty over mY's exact position indicated by a question mark:

3V	5V	6V	9V	12V
	mY?		mY?	mU
aK		al		

The final rule gives us a relative ordering: mZ requires more power than mV which in turn requires less power than mX. This can be notated as mX ‹ mV ‹ mZ. We also know from the second rule that mV cannot make the 6V appliance, because this is al. Given the sketch above, the only way we can preserve the ordering introduced by the final rule then is if mX is the 3V appliance, mV makes the 5V appliance and mZ makes the 9V appliance. Consequently, mY must make the 6V appliance.

This give us all we need to answer the question:

3V	5V	6V	9V	12V
mX	mV	mZ	mY	mU
aK		al		

The 5V appliance is made by mV, and the 9V by mY. Answer **(A)** is correct.

10. **(A)**

The key terms in the original question are university students, unpaid work, and improve their contribution to the community. **(A)** matches the key terms, verifying the claim in the original question, so **(A)** is the correct answer.

For the record: **(B)** is incorrect because the statement mentions all university students; the fact that some students owe a debt to the community is a weak argument that all students should do voluntary work. **(C)** is incorrect because it shifts the subject from unpaid voluntary work to academic work. **(D)** is incorrect because the fact that some students already do voluntary work is not a reason against making it compulsory; similar to **(B)**, this answer fails to address all students, focusing only on some.

11. **(D)**

The key terms in the original question are electric cars, lower prices, and cut emissions of greenhouse gases. **(A)** is incorrect because it simply asserts the truth of the original statement, in slightly different terms ('good for the environment' is broader and less specific than 'cut emissions of greenhouse gases'), without providing a rationale to justify lowering the price of electric cars. **(B)** is incorrect because it does not mention greenhouse gas emissions, focusing instead on the relative cost of conventional cars. **(C)** is incorrect because it makes an irrelevant prediction about electric cars, again without mentioning greenhouse gases. **(D)** is correct because it includes the key terms of the original question and gives a valid reason not to reduce the price of electric cars.

12. **(B)**

The key terms in the original question are Elgin Marbles, UK Government, and forced to return to Greece. Answer **(B)** addresses these key terms directly, giving a strong reason for the Marbles to be returned to Greece, so it is correct.

For the record: **(A)** is incorrect because it makes a conditional prediction that is not relevant to the key terms of the argument—a possible theft is not the same as the Government returning the Marbles. **(C)** is incorrect as it is a 'slippery slope', shifting to broader terms ('all foreign objects' instead of just the Marbles; 'UK museums' instead of just the British Museum) and potential future dangers. **(D)** mentions the Marbles and the British Museum, but makes an irrelevant claim about the Museum's money-making potential that is quite tangential (at best) to the terms of the original question.

13. **(D)**

There are two key terms in this question: the minimum wage and disabled people's access to employment. The strongest argument will be the one which addresses both. **(A)** makes a claim about the former, arguing that lower rates of pay will increase employment, but says nothing about the latter. **(B)** is the reverse: it talks about the benefits of employment for the disabled, but does not discuss the minimum wage issue. **(C)** is tangential: it argues that paying disabled people less than the minimum wage is discriminatory, but the question asks us whether such a course of action would increase employment opportunities, not whether it is just. **(D)** addresses both elements of the question directly: allowing employers to pay less than the minimum wage, it is argued, may not in fact increase employment among the disabled. **(D)** is therefore correct.

14. (C)

This question asks whether installing televisions in all prisoners cells would prevent rioting. **(A)** mentions neither televisions nor rioting, and instead makes the tangential claim that treating criminals well in prison will encourage them to reform. **(B)** is also somewhat tangential: it discusses the dangers rioting in prison causes but does not relate this to the issue of televisions in cells. **(C)** argues, in effect, that there may be no relationship between the issue of televisions in cells and rioting in prisons. Since it addresses the question directly, it is the strongest argument. **(C)** is correct.

For the record: **(D)** only deals with one half of the question (whether televisions should be installed in all prisoners cells). Since it does not discuss the issue of rioting, it cannot be correct.

15. YES; YES; NO; YES; NO

The first conclusion follows, since the percentage of customers taking a fixed 2 year mortgage was 24% in 2010, and the percentage taking a variable mortgage was 8%. The second conclusion follows as well, since this figure remained at 8% in both years. The third conclusion does not follow; 71% took out a 5 year tracker in 2015, compared to the sum of all types of fixed mortgage (24% plus 51%) in 2010, which totals 75%. The fourth conclusion follows: 9% of customers took out a tracker mortgage compared to 8% with a variable mortgage. The final conclusion does not follow, because we do not know the actual number of customers—only percentages. For example, if the broker had 100 customers who took out mortgages in 2010 and 200 customers in 2015, then she would have had 17 customers that took out a tracker mortgage in 2010 and 18 customers ($0.09 \times 200 = 18$) that took out a tracker mortgage in 2015; in that case, she would have had more customers with a tracker mortgage in 2015 compared to 2010, not fewer. However, it could be that there are fewer customers with these mortgages in 2015—so the answer is no.

16. NO; NO; YES; NO; YES

The first conclusion does not follow. The text describes how lemon ants use formic acid as a form of natural herbicide, but it also states that ants use the same substance as a chemical signal. The first conclusion could be true, but it could also be false—it goes further than the text. The second conclusion does not follow. The text states that lemon ants inject other species with formic acid, but it is not clear whether these species are a threat to lemon ant colonies. The third conclusion follows; it is a paraphrase of the first part of the fourth sentence. The fourth conclusion does not follow, since

we know that lemon ants thrive in *Duroia hirsuta* trees and poison other species of flora in the area. The fifth conclusion follows, paraphrasing the second sentence.

17. NO; YES; YES; NO; NO

The first conclusion does not follow; at 40 mg of citalopram, QTc change is 12.6, which is less than double 6.8, the change at 20 mg escitalopram. The second conclusion follows: according to the table, QTc would prolong by 12.6 ms, giving a total of $430 + 12.6 = 442.6$ ms, which is potentially dangerous as it exceeds 440 ms. The third conclusion also follows: the initial text explains that anything more than a normal QTc (less than 440 ms) is potentially dangerous; it would be dangerous to give a patient with QTc of 450 ms any of the indicated doses of either drug, as these would result in a QTc above 450 ms. The fourth conclusion does not follow: at 10 mg of excitalopram, the QTc increase is 4.2, which is not a third of 10.7, the QTc change at 30 mg. The fifth conclusion does not follow; we do not have data for a 40 mg dose of escitalopram.

18. NO; NO; NO; YES; YES

The first conclusion does not follow; in fact, Liquid A killed more bacteria than Liquid B. Neither does the second conclusion follow; this is true for viruses, not bacteria. The third conclusion does not follow; we are not told the actual percentage of viruses killed by Liquid C. The fourth conclusion follows; we are told Liquid C fared the worst when killing microorganisms. The fifth conclusion follows: Liquid C had the best overall tolerance in those with sensitive skin, causing irritation in only 10% of human test subjects; thus, it must be true that more than 10% of human subjects experienced skin irritation with Liquid A.

19. (A)

The correct answer is **(A)**, as five contestants selected the two combinations mentioned. For the record: Only 2 contestants chose skill at chosen talent as their sole factor, whilst 4 chose evening wear as their sole factor, contrary to **(B)**. A total of 6 contestants selected coaching as a factor, whilst a total of 29 selected quality of makeup as a factor, contrary to **(C)**. Eight contestants chose evening wear (oval) and skill at chosen talent (pentagon) as their sole factors, not nine (which is instead the combination of skill at chosen talent and quality of makeup).

20. (D)

The shapes representing snakes and frogs must be inside the same larger shape (representing cold-blooded), but the frog and snake shapes must not overlap with each other. At the same time, the snake shape must be inside another shape representing reptiles that does not overlap with the frog shape. Answer **(D)** meets these criteria, so it is correct.

21. (C)

A total of 78 students joined the Debate Society, Film Society and Football Club, contrary to **(A)**. **(B)** is incorrect as 76 students joined the Medics Society, whilst 23 joined the Dance Society. All the students who joined Boat Club (pentagon) are inside another shape as well, so it must be true that no students joined Boat Club without joining another society. Answer **(C)** is correct. For the record: 37 students joined only Football Club, whilst 19 joined only the Film Society; 19 is not less than half of 37.

22. (B)

This question asks you to find the correct combination of overlapping shapes from the diagram. **(A)** is incorrect, as the cross (Alaska) and the arrow (Tanzania) never overlap. **(B)** include all the shapes except the cross; these four shapes overlap just inside the top of the D-shape, at the left side of the arrowhead. Answer **(B)** is correct. For the record: **(C)** is incorrect as Alaska and Switzerland (the cross and the D-shape) only overlap outside the octagon (Nepal). Peru and Tanzania (the diamond and the arrow) only overlap inside the D-shape, the octagon or both, so none of the friends has visited only Peru and Tanzania, ruling out **(D)**.

23. (A)

The shapes representing coffee and tea must not overlap with each other, while overlapping with the shape representing milk—which must also be partially outside the coffee and tea shapes. Finally, the shape representing sugar must be entirely within the coffee and tea shapes, overlapping with each individually and in combination with milk. Answer **(A)** is correct.

24. (C)

(A) is incorrect, because there were 35 children with an allergy to each. **(B)** is incorrect, because there were a total of 28 children allergic to shellfish, and exactly half (i.e. not more than half) were also allergic to at least one other allergen listed. **(C)** is correct because there were 8 children with an allergy to just milk and shellfish, and 8 children with allergies to three or four allergens. For the record: **(D)** is incorrect, because of the total 81 children in the survey, only 31 had more than one allergy.

25. (B)

This question asks for the total number of customers that bought novels, but not biographies (the star) or

cookbooks (the crescent). There are three shapes that represent different types of novels: the rectangle, the oval and the triangle. The numbers that are in at least one of those three shapes, but not also in the star or the crescent, add up to $4 + 13 + 14 + 32 + 9 + 16 = 88$ customers. The correct answer is **(B)**.

26. (D)

Each roll of the die is an independent event, so each roll has a 2/3 probability of rolling a 6. The outcome of previous rolls is not relevant to the outcome of the third roll, so **(D)** is correct.

For the record: If you were tempted by **(B)**, remember that in three rolls of this die, the probability of rolling three 6s is $2/3 \times 2/3 \times 2/3 = 8/27$. That is, in 27 sets of 3 rolls, you would expect to get three 6s (with this loaded die) 8 times. That is far more common than **(B)** would allow.

27. (A)

Laptop Q passes the streaming test in 72% of trials and has an average maximum battery life of 8.5 hours. Laptop R fails the streaming test in 56 of 200 cases, which is $56/200 = 28\%$ of the time. That means that Laptop R passes the streaming test $100\% - 28\% = 72\%$ of the time, the same pass rate as Laptop Q. Eliminate **(B)** and **(D)**. Twenty copies of Laptop R have an average maximum battery life of 11 hours, while the other 180 copies have an average maximum battery life of 7 hours. Calculate the weighted average: $((20 \times 11) + (180 \times 7)) \div 200 = (220 + 1260) \div 200 = 1480 \div 200 = 7.4$ hours. Laptop Q's average maximum battery life is more than an hour longer than Laptop R's: 8.5 hours compared to 7.4 hours. The correct answer is **(A)**.

28. (B)

We are not told the exact number of bunnies and sheep in the basket at the start; we only know that there is at least one of each treat remaining in the basket before the last girl selects her treat. Of the children to select prior to the final girl, 6 have selected bunnies and 3 selected sheep. Note that we cannot deduce the claims in **(C)** or **(D)** without assigning some numbers to the starting and finishing amounts of bunnies and sheep, so **(C)** and **(D)** cannot be correct. That leaves two answer choices to test. If there were at least three times as many bunnies as sheep in the basket at the start, and there is at least one of each remaining, then the minimum number of sheep at the start is 4 (1 remaining + the 3 already selected); treble that for 12, the minimum number of bunnies at the start. That makes 16 minimum treats in the basket at the start, with a $12/16 = 3/4$ probability of selecting a bunny. For the final girl, there are $12 - 6 = 6$ bunnies and 1 sheep remaining in the basket, so she has a 6/7 probability of selecting a bunny—the probability has increased from the start. However, note that we still don't know the actual number of each animal at the start or the finish, so **(A)** is not a great answer. Checking **(B)**, we see it gives the exact number of sheep remaining (one) and tells us there were five more bunnies than sheep at the start. Since 3 sheep were selected, we know there were 4 sheep at the start, meaning we started with 9 bunnies. At the start, then, there were 13 treats in the basket, and the first child had a 9/13 (69.2%) probability of selecting a bunny. For the final girl, there are 9 − 6 = 3 bunnies and 1 sheep remaining in the basket, so she has a 3/4 (75%) probability of selecting a bunny. The probability of selecting a bunny now has increased from the start; **(B)** is correct.

29. (C)

Exam X had an average score of 70% in both School A and School B (28/40 × 100 = 70%). Exam Y had an average score of 75% in School A, and of 80% in School B (8 wrong, so 32 correct: 32/40 × 100 = 80%). Across both schools, the average score in Exam Y was higher, so Exam Y is not more difficult. The correct answer is **(C)**.

Quantitative Reasoning

1. (A)

A total of 4768 crimes were committed locally, and 283 of those were thefts of a motor vehicle. Divide to find the percentage: 283 ÷ 4768 = 0.059, or 6%, answer **(A)**.

2. (E)

The table shows that there were 4768 total crimes in Lincoln in 2005/2006, and that Lincoln had a population of 86,547. Divide to find the rate of crimes per person: 4768 ÷ 86547 = 0.055. Since this is more than 1:20 (which equals 0.05), test the two answer choices that are larger in your calculator. 1 ÷ 19 = 0.0526, and 1 ÷ 18 = 0.0556; the correct answer is **(E)**.

3. (C)

The national crime rates are given in figures per 1000 population, so divide the national population by 1000 before multiplying by the rate of violent crimes against a person rate: 60,200,000 ÷ 1000 = 60,200. The national rate of violent crimes against a person was 19.97 per 1000 population, so the total national number of violent crimes against a person was 19.97 × 60,200 = 1,202,194, or approximately 1.2 million. The answer is **(C)**.

4. (B)

The total number of burglaries in the 2005/2006 table is given as 552. 10% of this is 55.2, or approximately 55. Therefore the total number in the 2006/2007 table will be 552 + 55 = 607. The correct answer is **(B)**.

5. (C)

This question requires you to simply look at the chart and find the smallest segment. The smallest segment is the one with 10 percent of the total share, and represents Mathematics. The correct answer is **(C)**.

6. (B)

There are 3 steps to finding the answer to this question. First, find the proportion of total student visitors from the Faculty of Medicine. The chart shows this to be 20%, or $\frac{1}{5}$. To get from 20% to 100%, or $\frac{1}{5}$ to 1, multiply by 5; thus, multiplying the number of student visitors from the Faculty of Medicine by 5 will give the total number of student visitors. 800 × 5 = 4000. The correct answer is therefore **(B)**.

7. (A)

To solve, find the number of Law student visitors, then work out 25% of that number to find the answer. The question gives the number of Mathematics student visitors, and the chart shows that for every 10 Mathematics student visitors, there were 30 Law students visitors; hence, a ratio of 1:3. Thus, multiplying the number of student visitors in Mathematics by 3 will give the number of Law student visitors: 400 × 3 = 1200. The correct answer is 25% of this total, or 300. The correct answer is **(A)**.

8. (B)

To solve, simply subtract the Humanities and the Law percentages from the total (100%) given in the chart. 100 − 25 − 30 = 45. The correct answer is **(B)**.

9. (D)

To solve, add up all the prices of the items in the table: 185 + 45 + 75 + 32 + 19 = 356. The correct answer is **(D)**.

10. (B)

The sales target is 300 tickets at £1.50 each. If Omar hits the sales target exactly, he will make 300 × £1.50 = £450 in income. Subtract the cost of the raffle—the total cost of the prizes—to determine Omar's profit: £450 − £356 = £94. The correct answer is **(B)**.

11. (C)

According to the final bulleted item, there are two electrical prizes in the raffle: the MP3 player and the hair dryer. They have a total cost of £75 + £19 = £94. If they were on sale for 50% off, Omar would save 0.5 × £94 = £47. The correct answer is **(C)**.

12. (C)

To make a profit of £300, Omar will need to make £300 plus the cost of the prizes, which was £356. This total will equal the cost of a ticket (£1.50) times the number of tickets, which is unknown. Substitute x for the unknown number of tickets, and set up an algebraic equation: £300 + £356 = £1.50(x). Add the total on the left: £300 + £356 = £656 = £1.50(x). Then, divide by £1.50 to solve for x: x = £656 ÷ £1.50 = 437.33. Thus, Omar must sell 438 tickets to make a profit of £300. The correct answer is **(C)**.

13. (C)

The total unshaded area is 18 m². Multiply the cost per m² (£70) by the unshaded area to find the total cost: 18 m² × £70 = £1260. The answer is therefore **(C)**.

14. (D)

Russell's vegetable patch is half of the unshaded area, and half of 18 m² is 9m². 1 m = 100 cm, so 1 m² = 1 m × 1 m = 100 cm × 100 cm = 10,000 cm². Thus, the area of Russell's patch in cm² is 9 m² × 10,000 cm² = 90000 cm². The answer is **(D)**.

15. (B)

The total area of shaded land is 8 m × 10 m = 80 m². Pauline buys 30% of the total area of the shaded land, or 0.3 × 80 m² = 24 m². She pays £114 per m², so the total cost is 24 × £114 = £2,736. The correct answer is **(B)**.

16. (C)

Pauline started with half of the unshaded area, or 9 m². She then bought 30% of the shaded area, which was found to be 24 m² in the work for the previous question. Finally, she buys half of Russell's patch, for a further 4.5 m². The total area of Pauline's patch after all these additions is 9 + 24 + 4.5 = 37.5 m². Answer **(C)** is correct.

17. (B)

To calculate how many miles a car can drive on one gallon of fuel, find that particular model on the graph and check for motorway or city driving, as appropriate. In this case, the motorway driving bar on the graph for the Denver car corresponds to 55 miles, so the answer is **(B)**.

18. (E)

There are three steps to answering this question. Firstly, read the graph to find the fuel economy of the Satola car in the city, which is 30 miles per gallon; this means that a 30 mile city journey will use up a gallon of fuel. Next, check the conversion factor under the graph to find that 1 gallon = 4.5 litres. Finally, multiply the price of the fuel to find the cost for 4.5 litres of fuel: £1.10 × 4.5 = £4.95. The correct answer is **(E)**.

19. (C)

The simplest way to tackle this question is by glancing at the graph to see which car provides the best fuel economy. A quick glance shows that Ecogo has the best fuel economy for both motorway and city driving. The correct answer is therefore **(C)**.

20. (D)

First, check how many miles one gallon of fuel allows you to travel on the motorway in a Cruiser. This value is 45 miles, according to the graph. Next, divide 45 by the total miles in the journey to determine how many gallons are required: 405 ÷ 45 = 9. The answer is **(D)**.

21. (E)

In 2016, there were 74 million children in the USA. The information below the table indicates that asthma prevalence in children was 9.4%. Thus there were 74 × 0.094 = 6.96 million children in the USA with asthma in 2016. Next, find how many school days asthma sufferers missed in 2016: 13 million. Finally, divide this by the number of children with asthma in the USA, to find the mean number of school days missed per child suffering from asthma in 2016: 13 ÷ 6.96 = 1.87 days. The answer is **(E)**.

22. (B)

First, calculate the global asthma mortality rate: each year 250,000 people die worldwide from asthma for 300 million asthma sufferers. This is a mortality rate of: 250,000 ÷ 300,000,000 = 0.083, or 8.3%. Next, calculate the mortality rate for asthma in the USA: 3,384 people die for 24.6 million asthma sufferers. Thus, the mortality rate in the USA is 3,384 ÷ 24,600,000 = 0.00014, or 0.014%. Calculate the mean of these two percentages: (8.3 + 0.014) ÷ 2 = 8.314 ÷ 2 = 4.157. Finally, to calculate the percentage difference between USA and worldwide asthma mortality rates, divide the difference between USA and global rates by the mean of the two values: (8.3 − 0.014) ÷ 4.157 = 8.286 ÷ 4.157 = 1.99 = 199%. Answer **(B)** is correct.

23. (A)

The total number of deaths from asthma in 2016 was 3,384. Therefore, there were 3,384 deaths for 323.1 million people. To calculate the number of deaths per 100,000 people, divide the total population number by 100,000. $323,100,000 \div 100,000 = 3,231$. Divide the total number of deaths from asthma in the USA by this value: $3,384 \div 3,231 = 1.05$ deaths per 100,000 people. The correct answer is **(A)**.

24. (D)

The table indicates that there was a 48% increase in asthma cases in the USA during the past 10 years. There were 24.6 million people with asthma in the USA in 2016. Thus, in 2006 there were $24.6 \div 1.48 = 16.62$ million $= 16,620,000$ asthma sufferers. The answer is **(D)**.

25. (C)

Arabella rode Truffles a total of 11 miles, in a ride that took 1 hour, 14 minutes, or 74 minutes. Convert this to hours: $\frac{74}{60}$ hours $= 1.233$ hours. Use the speed formula to find the average trotting speed: Speed $=$ Distance $\div$ Time $= 11$ miles $\div 1.233$ hours $= 8.92$ mph. The answer is therefore **(C)**.

26. (B)

To find Jack of Hearts's average speed on the total ride, find the total distance and total time, and then use the speed formula: Speed $=$ Distance $\div$ Time. The total distance is 11 miles $\times 2 = 22$ miles. The time for the first part of the journey is 44 minutes $\frac{44}{60}$ hours $= 0.733$ hours. Since the speed on the first part of the journey is twice the speed on the second part, use the speed formula to find the speed for the first part of the journey: Speed $= 11$ miles $\div 0.733$ hours $= 15$ mph. The speed on the second part of the journey is half of this, or 7.5 mph. Thus, the time on the second part of the journey must be twice the time on the first part of the journey (since the distance is the same—if unsure, you could confirm this with the speed formula). The time on the second part of the journey is 44 minutes $\times 2 = 88$ minutes, so the total time is $44 + 88 = 132$ minutes, or $\frac{132}{60}$ hours $= 2.2$ hours. Use the speed formula one more time, to calculate the average trotting speed for the total ride: Speed $= 22$ miles $\div 2.2$ hours $= 10$ mph. The correct answer is **(B)**.

27. (D)

Use the speed formula to find Peppermint's trotting speed: Speed $=$ Distance $\div$ Time. The distance is the length of the trail and back again, or 22 miles. The time is 2 hours, 39 minutes, or 159 minutes $= \frac{159}{60}$ hours $= 2.65$ hours. Plug these figures into the speed formula to solve: Speed $= 22$ miles $\div 2.65$ hours $= 8.3$ mph. The answer is therefore **(D)**.

28. (A)

The work required to solve the previous three questions gave average trotting speeds for three horses: Truffles's trotting speed was 8.9 mph, Jack of Hearts's was 7.5 mph and Peppermint's was 8.3 mph. The previous question stated that Dazzle's average trotting speed was 1.4 mph faster than Peppermint's, so calculate: $8.3 + 1.4 = 9.7$ mph. Thus, Dazzle has an average trotting speed that is faster than any of Arabella's other horses—and also faster than Galaxy, her brother's horse, whose average trotting speed is given at the top of the page as 9.2 mph. The correct answer is **(A)**.

29. (E)

The total number of prisoners at the end of 2017 is 819,163. The total number of prisoners 50 or under at the end of 2017 is: $189,447 + 231,701 + 258,312 + 33,387 = 712,487$. Therefore: $712,487 \div 819,163 = 0.87$, or 87%, of prisoners were 50 or under at the end of 2017. The answer is **(E)**.

30. (A)

There are: $3,584 + 663 = 4,247$ prisoners who are 71 years old or older at the end of 2017. The total number of these that were younger than 30 on admission is: $23 + 82 + 82 + 143 = 330$. Thus, the proportion of prisoners 71 years old or older at the end of 2017 that were admitted at age 30 or younger is: $330 \div 4,247 = 0.78 = 7.8\%$. Answer **(A)** is correct.

31. (C)

Raul uses Company II, which has a base rate, an amount per minute and an amount per kilometer. To find the distance, multiply the time by the speed (30 km/hr is equal to 1/2 km/min) $84 \times 0.5 = 42$ km. Now add up the base rate, the time rate and the distance rate, $1.50 + (84 \times 0.7) + (42 \times 1.15) = 1.50 + 58.8 + 48.3) = 108.6$. Raul's journey will cost £108.60. The answer is **(C)**.

32. (B)

First, work out the cost for each journey. Using Taxi Company I costs £7.30 for the first 2 km, then 0.90 for each 250 m after that. There are 3 km remaining in the journey, or 3,000m, so $3,000 \div 250 = 12$ further sets of 250 m travelled, at a cost of $12 \times 0.9 = 10.8$. The total cost of using Company I is $7.3 + 10.8 = £18.10$. The cost of using Company II is 1.5 + (0.7 ×10) + (1.15 × 5) = 1.50 + 7 + 5.75 = £14.25. To find the percentage increase, divide the difference between the two costs by the smaller value, thus (18.1 − 14.25) ÷ 14.25 = 0.27, or 27%. The correct answer is **(B)**.

33. (A)

Because percentage change equals difference divided by original, the band with the greatest percentage rise from Week 2 to Week 3 will have the steepest increase in the slope of the line connecting those two points on the graph; that is, it will have a relatively large difference as compared to its original value in Week 2. The two bands with the steepest increases from Week 2 to Week 3 are Toxic Shock and Cambridge Town Vocal Choir, so compare their figures using the percentage change formula. Toxic Shock has an original value of 15,000 in Week 2 and a final value of 50,000 in Week 3, for a difference of 50,000 − 15,000 = 35,000. The percentage change is 35,000 ÷ 15,000 = 2.33, or 233%. Cambridge Town Vocal Choir has an original value of 2,000 and a final value of 10,000, for a difference of 10,000 − 2,000 = 8,000. The percentage change is 8,000 ÷ 2,000 = 4, or 400%. The answer is therefore **(A)**.

34. (C)

The week with the greatest total sales will have the highest combined values for all five bands, and would likely have the highest sales of any week for some of the bands. The highest individual sales for any band (by 10,000) are the sales for Toxic Shock in Week 3; Cambridge Town Vocal Choir also had their best sales by a significant margin in that week; even though these are the lowest for Week 3, the total of 10,000 is about 8,000 more than the worst-selling band in any other week. The high margin of success for these two bands in Week 3 is more than enough to make up for the difference in the figures for the other three bands, who had their second or third best weeks in Week 3, but by a much narrower margin. Thus, a quick visual estimate shows that the answer must be **(C)**.

35. (E)

Proceed carefully, as this question is not asking for a percentage decrease, but a simple numerical decrease. The biggest drop in sales from one week to the next is the line on the graph with the sharpest decline, which represents the sales for Toxic Shock from Week 3 (50,000) to Week 4 (3,000). None of the other bands recorded sales in excess of 40,000 in a single week, so no other band could have a greater decrease from one week to the next than Toxic Shock. The answer is **(E)**.

36. (D)

MC Einstein's single sold 35,000 in Week 5, and the total sales were approximately 35,000 + 30,500 + 9,000 + 100 + 100 = 74,700. Divide to find the percentage: 35,000 ÷ 74,700 = 0.4685, or 47%. The correct answer is **(D)**. Note that there is a slight shortcut here: once you determine the total, you might have noticed that MC Einstein's sales were not 50% of the total (as this would have required a total of 70,000), but are only slightly less than half of the total. If you were in a rush, this would have been sufficient justification for marking **(D)**.

Abstract Reasoning

1. **(C)**

This pattern involves features of shapes, and also arrangement. In Set A, the arrows are arranged to point at the two shapes that have the same number of sides. In Set B, the arrows are arranged to point at the two shapes that have the same shading. The arrows in the first test shape point at two shapes with 5 sides each, which fits the pattern for Set A. However, the two pentagons are both shaded black, so the test shape also fits the pattern for Set B. Since the test shape can belong to both sets, it fits exclusively into neither. The answer is **(C)**.

2. **(C)**

The arrows in this test shape point at a triangle and a lightning shape, with 11 sides. Since the two shapes do not have the same number of sides, the test shape does not belong to Set A. The triangle is grey and the lightning is white, so the test shape does not belong to Set B. The answer is therefore **(C)**.

3. **(B)**

This test shape has arrows pointing at the two white shapes, a hexagon and a circle. This fits the pattern for Set B.

4. **(A)**

This test shape includes arrows pointing at two quadrilaterals, one white and one grey. This fits the pattern for Set A.

5. **(C)**

The test shape contains a two-headed arrow, which points at two identical grey crosses. Since the crosses have the same number of sides, the test shape belongs to Set A. Since the crosses have identical shading, the test shape belongs to Set B. Since the test shape can belong to both sets, it belongs exclusively to neither. The answer is therefore **(C)**.

6. (D)

In Set A, every box contains a heart, which is positioned according to conditional rules. If the heart is black, it is below a triangle; if the heart is white, it is to the right of a diamond. In Set B, every box contains a hexagon, again with conditional rules. If the hexagon is black, it is above a heart; if the hexagon is white, it is to the left of a triangle.

The first question asks about Set A; check the positioning of the hearts. There are two answers with black hearts, but neither is below a triangle; eliminate **(A)** and **(C)**. There are two answers with white hearts; one is to the left of the diamond, and one—in **(D)**—is to the right of the diamond. **(D)** is correct.

7. (B)

This question is about Set B; check the positioning of the hexagons. Neither black hexagon is above a heart; eliminate **(A)** and **(D)**. Only one white hexagon is to the left of a triangle. The answer is **(B)**.

8. (A)

All the answers include a black heart, which must be positioned below a triangle in Set A. Answer **(A)** is correct.

9. (C)

Two answers include black hexagons, which must be positioned above a heart in Set B. The correct answer is **(C)**. For the record: Note that both white hexagons are to the right of their triangles; in Set B, they must be to the left of the triangle to fit the pattern.

10. (A)

All the answers contain white hearts, which must be positioned to the right of a diamond in Set A. **(A)** is the correct answer.

11. (B)

This pattern involves a feature of the shapes in each box, which appear to form a 'clock' figure, with a short hand and long hand. In Set A, the smaller angle formed by the hands of the clock measures less than 90 degrees; in Set B, the smaller angle formed by the hands of the clock measures larger than 90 degrees. In the first test shape, the smaller angle formed by the hands of the clock is greater than 90 degrees; the test shape therefore belongs to Set B.

12. (C)

The hands on the clock in this test shape form an angle of exactly 90 degrees, meaning that the test shape cannot belong to either set. The answer is **(C)**.

13. (C)

The clock in this test shape has two short hands, rather than a short hand and a long hand. This fits the pattern for neither set. The answer is therefore **(C)**.

14. (A)

The angle formed by the hands of the clock in this test shape measures less than 90 degrees, so the test shape fits into Set A.

15. (B)

This test shape features a clock with hands forming a smaller angle of just under 180 degrees. This angle is larger than 90 degrees, so the test shape fits the pattern for Set B.

16. (C)

This pattern involves two features of shapes: size and colour. Each box in both sets contains a grey shape. In Set A, the grey shape is the largest shape in each box; in Set B, the grey shape is the smallest shape in each box. The first test shape does not include a grey shape, so it belongs to neither set.

17. (A)

The largest shape in this test shape is grey, so it fits the pattern for Set A.

18. (B)

The smallest shape in this test shape is grey, so it fits the pattern for Set B.

19. (B)

This test shape includes more individual shapes than any box in either set; remember, however, that the overall number of shapes in the box is not relevant to the pattern. The smallest shape is grey, so the test shape belongs to Set B.

20. (C)

The grey shape included in this test shape is neither the smallest nor the largest, so it fits into neither set.

21. (A)

This pattern involves arrangement of the shapes in each box. In Set A, each box includes a rectangle that overlaps a square; in Set B, each box includes a rectangle that overlaps a triangle. The exact number of shapes and the exact number of crossover points are distractors.

The first test shape includes a rectangle overlapping a square, so it belongs to Set A.

22. (A)

This test shape includes a rectangle overlapping a square, so the answer is **(A)**.

23. (C)

The test shape includes a rectangle overlapping both a square and a triangle. The test shape fits both patterns, so it belongs exclusively to neither.

24. (B)

This test shape includes a rectangle overlapping a triangle, and thus fits the pattern for Set B.

25. (B)

The test shape contains a rectangle overlapping a triangle, so the answer is **(B)**.

26. (A)

This pattern involves a particular type of shape in each set. In Set A, each box contains an isosceles triangle (a triangle in which two of the sides are of equal length). In Set B, each box contains a right triangle. The triangle in the first test shape has two equal sides, so it fits the pattern for Set A.

27. (C)

The triangle in this test shape has three sides of equal length, so it does not fit the pattern for Set A. Because it is an equilateral triangle, all its angles measure 60 degrees; as such, it does not fit the pattern for Set B. Thus, the test shape belongs to neither set, and the answer is **(C)**.

28. (C)

The test shape contains a triangle with two sides of equal length, so it belongs to Set A. However, the triangle also features a right angle, so it also belongs to Set B. Since the test shape can fit into both sets, it belongs exclusively to neither. The answer is therefore **(C)**.

29. (A)

This test shape includes a triangle with two equal sides and no right angle. Thus, the test shape fits into Set A.

30. (B)

The final test shape contains a triangle with a right angle and sides of varying length. As such, the test shape belongs to Set B.

31. (B)

All the boxes in both sets contain two or three black shapes. Whilst the type of shape varies, there is always

a black shape in the centre of the box. In Set A, the shape in the centre of the box has the fewest sides of any shape in the box. In Set B, the shape in the centre of the box has the greatest number of sides of any shape in the box.

The centre shape in the first test shape is a pentagon, which has more sides than the other shape, the heart. This fits the pattern for Set B.

32. (C)

The centre shape in this box is a parallelogram, with more sides than the triangle but the same number of sides as the diamond. This test shape belongs to neither set.

33. (B)

The centre shape, an octagon, has more sides than the pentagon or the quadrilateral. The answer is **(B)**.

34. (C)

The centre shape here is a triangle; there are shapes with more sides (the hexagon) and fewer sides (the heart) than the centre shape, so the test shape cannot belong to Set A or Set B. The answer is **(C)**.

35. (A)

The centre shape in this box is a cross with 12 sides; the other shape, a 3-headed arrow, has 17 sides. This fits the pattern for Set A.

36. (C)

All the boxes in both sets contain the same 9 shapes in a 3x3 grid. In each box, there are 3 black shapes, 3 white shapes and 3 striped shapes. The pattern is all about the arrangement of these colours, in a single row or column. In Set A, there is one row in each box where the shapes are striped, black and white; in Set B, there is one column in each box where the shapes are white, black and striped. Note that this order must apply left-to-right in Set A and top-to-bottom in Set B.

The first test shape does not have any striped-black-white rows, so it cannot belong to Set A. There are no white shapes in the top row, so it cannot belong to Set B. It belongs to neither set.

37. (A)

The middle row follows the striped-black-white arrangement, so it fits the pattern for Set A. There isn't a column with the white-black-striped arrangement, so it does not fit the pattern for Set B.

38. (C)

The only row that starts with a striped shape is striped-white-black, which does not match Set A. The only column that starts with a white shape is white-striped-black, which does not match Set B. The test shape fits neither pattern.

39. (B)

The right column follows the white-black-striped arrangement, so it fits the pattern for Set B. There isn't a row with the striped-black-white arrangement, so it does not fit the pattern for Set A.

40. (C)

The shapes across the middle row are striped, black and white, fitting the pattern for Set A. The shapes down the middle column are white, black and striped, fitting the pattern for Set B. Since the test shape fits both patterns, the answer is **(C)**.

41. (C)

The boxes in these sets each appear to contain a letter, which has been broken down into the line segments that make up the letter. In Set A, each box contains a total of three line segments. In Set B, each box contains a total of two line segments. The first test shape contains four line segments, so it does not fit into the pattern for either set. The answer is therefore **(C)**.

42. (A)

This test shape includes three line segments, so it fits the pattern for Set A.

43. (C)

The test shape consists of a single line segment, forming an 'O'. As such, it belongs to neither set.

44. (B)

Two line segments make up this test shape, which therefore fits the pattern for Set B.

45. (A)

The final test shape includes a total of three line segments, so it belongs to Set A.

46. (D)

The first box includes a small triangle atop a medium-sized diamond atop a large square. In the second box, each shape has moved down the stack—and thus increased in size—except for the large square, which is now the topmost, smallest shape. The triangle also flips vertically with each subsequent box, so that it points up, then down, then up, then down. The triangle must be pointing up in the final shape; eliminate **(A)** and **(B)**.

The stack of shapes is the same in **(C)** and **(D)**, so check the shading. In the original boxes, the large shape always has vertical stripes, and the smallest shape has horizontal stripes. Answer **(D)** is correct.

47. (A)

Check each shape to see how many rotations it makes in the first four boxes. The white arrow rotates through four positions, and the black arrow rotates through three positions. Thus, in the correct answer, the white arrow will be in the first position and the black arrow will be in the second position. The correct answer is **(A)**.

48. (B)

In the first progression, the circles move from the bottom to the top; there is one fewer circle, and the remaining circles become wider. Thus, the four hexagons in the bottom of the second progression must move to the top, with one fewer, and the remaining hexagons wider; eliminate **(A)** and **(C)**. In the first progression, the diamonds at the top move to the bottom, there is one more, and they become shorter. Hence, there must be one more triangle in the bottom of the answer. **(B)** is correct.

49. (D)

In the first progression, each shape is replaced by a shape that has exactly half as many sides as the original. In the second progression, the two shapes at the left in the first box have eight sides each, so they must each be replaced by a shape with exactly four sides. Answer **(D)** is therefore correct.

50. (C)

In the first progression, the shape originally on the left moves to the right, and the shape that was on the right moves diagonally into the original position of the shape that was on the left. Thus, the heart must move to the right; eliminate **(A)** and **(B)**. In the first progression, the black arrow—the inner shape that was originally on the left—flips vertically in the second box. Hence, the white chevron must flip vertically in the answer. The correct answer is **(C)**.

51. (A)

All boxes in both sets contain a star and a circle with an arc around it. The difference in the patterns involves the arrangement of the star and the arc. In Set A, if the star is below the circle, the arc opens downwards; if the star is above the circle, then the arc opens upwards. This conditional pattern is reversed in Set B: if the star is below the circle, the arc opens upwards; if the star is above the circle, the arc opens down. In the first test shape, the star is below the circle, and the arc opens downwards. This fits the pattern for Set A.

52. (C)

There is no star in this test shape, so it belongs to neither set.

53. (B)

The star is above the circle and the arc opens downwards, so this test shape belongs to Set B.

54. (C)

The test shape includes a circle, a star and an arc, but the circle isn't arranged within the arc. As such, the test shape fits the pattern for neither set.

55. (B)

The star is below the circle, and the arc opens upwards; thus, this test shape belongs to Set B.

Situational Judgement

1. (D)

This would be inappropriate, as Samia has not attempted a local solution to the problem by asking Hayley what has been going on. Also, Samia does not know for sure that Hayley has been lying.

2. (B)

Whilst this option is good in that it offers Hayley a chance to explain her actions, the wording is somewhat confrontational and may hinder a successful conversation about the problems that she may be having.

3. (A)

This open question allows Hayley to open up about the previous day without fear of condemnation or judgement. If she denies being out of the house, then Samia has a reason to challenge this and also a lead-in to doing so.

4. (A)

Since Shaun is Tameka's student and his remark was well out of order, it is very appropriate for Tameka to apologise to the patient on his behalf.

5. (A)

Since Shaun is Tameka's student and his remark was well out of order, it is very appropriate for Tameka to ask Shaun to apologise.

6. (A)

This response allows Tameka to address the patient's underlying concerns while also ensuring that the critical surgery can go ahead, so it is a highly appropriate response.

7. (B)

It is appropriate for Tameka to tell Shaun to keep his personal views to himself, and he will need to learn to do so if he is to have a career as a doctor. However, this response is not ideal, as it does not directly address why Shaun's views are inappropriate or the patient's underlying concern, which are the two main issues in this scenario.

8. (B)

Whilst this is an acceptable course of action, it is not ideal, as Lisa may still be able to complete the coursework once she learns the details of the task involved. This would ensure there is no delay in her work. The most appropriate action would involve finding out the details of the coursework before requesting any extension if necessary, and enquiring if there have been any other emails she has not received and making sure she is on the correct mailing list for future emails.

9. (D)

Whilst her exams are extremely important, ignoring other pieces of work could compromise Lisa successfully qualifying from medical school. By ignoring the coursework, she would also be demonstrating lack of integrity, a trait paramount to students and doctors, who also have a responsibility for their own learning. Thus, this response is highly inappropriate.

10. (A)

Addressing the issue locally, immediately and discreetly is a very appropriate course of action, and would ensure Lisa has completed all the necessary coursework to qualify from medical school.

11. (C)

While it is the job of a porter to assist patients in the hospital, this response is inappropriate as the patient seems extremely agitated and has directed his anger at the consultant, so a better response would be for the consultant to do something to help address the patient's agitation. However, this response is not awful, as a porter would have some role in helping a patient in this context.

12. (A)

This response would give the consultant a chance to understand the patient's exact concerns, and to do so immediately, discreetly and calmly. It is a very appropriate thing to do.

13. (A)

This is an immediate response, and a relatively calm and discreet one, so it is highly appropriate.

14. (A)

This response is somewhat forceful, however it is highly appropriate, as Haroon can see that the receptionist is not working, and this is an immediate solution that will ensure the patients are attended to quickly while also avoiding any comments on the receptionist's professionalism in the presence of the patients.

15. (D)

The receptionist's behaviour is clearly unacceptable; however, addressing it in front of patients in this way is very inappropriate, particularly as the more pressing concerns are the ringing phone and the queue of patients waiting to speak to the receptionist.

16. (C)

This response is inappropriate, as the practice will not run more smoothly if Haroon helps the receptionist by answering the phone. However, this approach is not awful, as it does seem there are quite a lot of patients that need to be spoken to, and the patients will appreciate Haroon's intervention.

17. (A)

This is a very appropriate thing to do, as it will allow Haroon to address Mrs Rahman's concern in discreetly, locally and immediately.

18. (D)

The patient has to come first in this situation and it would be very rude to keep the patient waiting, especially for that long. The patient would not even know where they were if they did not call the patient. The duo should go and see the patient together without Kyle and he should join them when he gets there.

19. (C)

This is not going to solve the current issue, which is that the students would be late to meet the patient. Whilst it is important that Kyle knows that he is letting the group down, telling him how the rest of the group feel is not going to get Kyle there any quicker. Thus, this response is inappropriate, but not awful.

20. (D)

This response will keep the patient waiting, and given the fact that the group has been late on all their previous visits, notifying the patient in advance of their tardiness will not reassure the patient. This response

does not address the unprofessionalism of the group, and does nothing to avoid inconveniencing the patient, so it is highly inappropriate.

21. (A)

This option does not inconvenience the patient in any way, and the patient must be their first priority. It will also address the issue so that hopefully the situation will not happen again.

22. (D)

Katie's consultant appears to be a patient, and as such, he would expect a certain level of privacy and discretion. It would therefore be very inappropriate for Katie to ask him why he is here.

23. (A)

Given that it seems clear to Katie that the consultant is likely to be visiting the hospital as a patient, and that he does not seem to have seen her, it is best to pretend she didn't see him, unless he brings it up later.

24. (D)

If her consultant is attending the hospital as a patient, then asking if her friend who works there knows the consultant is highly inappropriate, as her friend is required to maintain patient confidentiality.

25. (D)

This is not appropriate because it is not a local solution, and it does not deal with the situation immediately. Asking Tom to take off his watch would solve the problem quickly and prevent the spread of infection.

26. (D)

This does not address the issue straightaway, and therefore puts the patients at risk of catching infections. Since patient safety is of paramount importance, this is very inappropriate response, even though it is a local solution.

27. (A)

This is an ideal solution, as it is local and addresses the problem immediately and discreetly.

28. (A)

This is an ideal solution as it ensures the patient's questions will be answered, and does not undermine the consultant in any way by disclosing that she is on holiday.

29. (D)

This would be an inappropriate thing to do since Eoghan is only a medical student and is unlikely to be able to answer all of the patient's questions correctly or satisfactorily. Also, the patient has requested to speak to the consultant, so it would be appropriate to arrange for the patient to speak to a doctor.

30. (D)

This is very appropriate, as Eoghan can deal with the questions that he feels he can answer straightaway so that the patient does not have to wait for answers. By getting a doctor to come and talk to the patient as well, Eoghan would maintain confidence in the profession and continuity of care, and ensure that no incorrect information is given to the patient.

31. (B)

This is appropriate, as Esme would likely be endangering herself if she tried to drive to the hospital whilst feeling dizzy. However, it is not an ideal response, as it does not supply alternative sources of help for the junior colleague.

32. (D)

This option would ensure that Esme gets to the hospital safely without the risk of causing an accident. However, if she is too unwell to drive for even 5 minutes, then Esme should realise that she will not be able to give effective assistance to a patient in her condition. Reporting to the hospital to see patients in her current condition would thus be highly inappropriate.

33. (A)

This is the best response to the problem. It allows Esme to take responsibility for finding appropriate cover when she is unable to fulfil her duties.

34. (A)

This is a highly appropriate response, since Ellen does not seem confident in being able to help Rupa as she is only a medical student. In any event, it would not be appropriate for Ellen to treat Rupa even if she were a fully qualified doctor, since the GMC recommend that doctors do not treat friends.

35. (D)

Ellen clearly does not think she is qualified to help Rupa, and she is not yet a fully qualified doctor. For these reasons, it would be highly inappropriate for Ellen to conduct a patient examination of Rupa.

36. (D)

This response is very inappropriate, as Luke does not actually know that the treatment is new; furthermore, telling the patient that he does not know about the treatment will undermine patient confidence in the medical profession.

37. (A)

This is a very appropriate thing to do, as it maintains patient confidence in the profession and continuity of patient care, while also allowing Luke to take some time to look into the treatment and ensure he can provide the patient with the information requested.

38. (C)

This response is factually correct; however, it is inappropriate, as the fact that the prescribing doctor is away (and that Luke is unaware of the treatment) should not impact on patient care. However, this response is not awful, as it gives Luke an opening to provide the patient with the requested information.

39. (D)

This is not important; the public perceive medical students as doctors in training, so they should behave as such. It is highly inappropriate for medical students or doctors to use such language to talk about patients, and even more so in a public area.

40. (A)

This factor is of the utmost importance. Doctors and medical students should always be mindful of how they talk about patients in a public area; any indiscretion could be very damaging to the public's perception of the medical profession.

41. (D)

Regardless of the reason that Rob is leaving, it is wrong to leave Jitesh to do his work for him, especially as Jitesh is only a medical student and is not being paid for his work.

42. (D)

Although Jitesh is doing tasks that are expected of him by his medical school, he is not there to replace the junior doctors. He is not qualified to do so, and he should not be doing the doctor's job for him.

43. (B)

This is important, since this is the time when the ward is in most need of a junior doctor and by not being there Rob is putting his patients at risk. However, this is not of highest important to Jitesh in deciding how to respond because Rob should be there on the ward anyway, whether it is the busiest time or not.

44. (B)

This is an important factor to consider, as if there is a suitably private location for Lauren to change clothes, then her behaviour in the supply cupboard is highly unusual and must be addressed as such.

45. (D)

Nima's religious beliefs are entirely irrelevant to her response to Lauren's behaviour.

46. (A)

This is a very important factor, as it suggests that Lauren is not changing clothes, but undressing in the supply cupboard for some other reason, which must be addressed urgently.

47. (A)

This is extremely important, as it would mean that Lauren is lying about her reason for undressing in the supply cupboard, and thus it would be all the more urgent for Nima to address this with her.

48. (B)

This is an important factor, as it would indicate some other factor—such as an intoxicant or a psychiatric condition—that could play a role in Lauren's bizarre behaviour.

49. (D)

This is unimportant—he may have excellent hearing with his aids, or he may be able to lip read. Even if the elderly man cannot hear the junior doctors, it would be important to challenge the doctors to ensure that their behaviour is not repeated in front of an audience who can hear every word

50. (C)

This mitigates the behaviour of the doctors slightly, but is mostly unimportant as the patient may be recognisable from other details. In addition, the public would not like to think of their own personal details being discussed in such a forum, even if they were not specifically mentioned by name.

51. (D)

This should not outweigh Abiola's responsibility to protect patient confidentiality and the public's opinon of the hospital and its staff. It is thus entirely unimportant.

52. (D)

This is unimportant, as the principles of medical professionalism and patient confidentiality must apply in all circumstances, regardless of whether the patient is known to others.

53. (A)

This is an important factor, as the tutor will expect Violet to behave professionally and notify him of the reason for her absence before the tutor group meets. If she has a phone number where she can reach the tutor, then she can be sure of having an opportunity to explain the situation with her grandmother, and make arrangements for making up anything she misses in the tutor group.

54. (C)

This factor is of minor importance, since Violet should only ask Uma to explain her absence as a last resort. She would do better to email or phone the tutor before the tutor group meets, so that she can explain her absence herself.

55. (A)

This is an important consideration, as if she will be able to email the tutor from the train, then she can proceed immediately to the train station and get to her grandmother as quickly as possible.

56. (A)

The fact that the medical school has made it clear that the students are expected to be presentable when on the wards is very important, as these are the rules that the students must obey. It reflects badly on the medical school and also on the hospital if the students are not smartly presented.

57. (D)

This is not at all important, as Adam needs to maintain a professional appearance in hospital, no matter what his situation is at home. It will reflect poorly on him, the hospital and the medical school if he appears scruffy and not smartly dressed.

58. (D)

This is not important, as you can still make yourself look presentable and not scruffy without spending money. If Adam was having financial difficulties that meant that he could not afford to buy suitable smart clothes for the wards, then he could approach his university for a hardship grant. Maintaining a professional appearance is important to help gain the respect and trust of patients.

59. (A)

The fact that Adam has signed an agreement means that he has no excuse for not knowing the rules and what is expected of him whilst in hospital. He has also agreed to follow those rules, especially if it is only his first week on the wards.

60. (D)

Doctors are required to be honest and trustworthy when giving evidence in court or before a tribunal. Thus, Fraser and the consultant each have an obligation to disclose that the consultant was told about the painkiller before the operation. The fact that the consultant has a great deal of influence over Fraser's career is entirely irrelevant to the ethical issues at hand. Given that the consultant appears to have behaved poorly twice—first, in disregarding Fraser's warning, leading to a patient's death, and second, in lying to the investigating committee—makes it all the more important for Fraser to tell the truth, setting aside any potential negative consequences for his career.

61. (C)

The scenario only mentions that Fraser told the consultant who was leading the operation; the consultant should have told the anaesthetist. However, the anaesthetist should also have checked the patient's notes, so there is a strong probability that the anaesthetist also bears some responsibility for the patient's death. Even so, Fraser's responsibility is to testify honestly about what he does know. He cannot testify about what he doesn't know, so the fact that he doesn't know about the anaesthetist's knowledge is of minor importance.

62. (A)

This factor is very important. Fraser must testify honestly about what happened, so that the adverse event investigation committee can reach a fair and complete conclusion about the patient's death.

63. (A)

This factor is especially important. Sienna has only seen one message from a patient that might be inappropriate; however, it could also have an entirely innocent explanation—for example, Lexi may have been checking on the patient the night before, or perhaps it's the patient that is pursuing Lexi without her encouraging him or returning his interest. Sienna should discuss carefully with Lexi, since she doesn't know for sure that Lexi has done anything wrong. It does seem odd for hospital patients to be texting doctors on their mobiles, so it is an issue for Sienna to raise with Lexi.

64. (B)

This factor complicates the situation, as it means that Lexi has a prior history of forming inappropriate romantic relationships with a patient's close family member. The GMC explicitly prohibits doctors from pursuing sexual or improper emotional relationships with close family members of patients, as well as patients themselves; it's a vulnerable time for anyone when your parent or child is in hospital, so it was wrong of Lexi to pursue a relationship with her previous boyfriend at that time. That does not mean that she is pursuing an improper relationship with this patient, but it is all the more reason to raise the issue, and to tread carefully. This factor is therefore important to consider.

65. (D)

This factor is not at all important. At minimum, it appears that the patient is pursuing an improper relationship with Lexi; there's a chance that she may have either encouraged him, or given the appearance of encouraging him, since he has her mobile number and is texting her a quite personal message. The patient's behaviour, and the fact that he has Lexi's mobile number, need to be discussed with Lexi as a matter of urgency. The fact that Lexi is responsible for assessing Sienna's work should not be a consideration in responding to this situation.

66. (C)

It seems that something is different in the consultant's treatment of the all-female intake of new junior doctors. It could be because they are women, or because there is some other stress in the consultant's life, or a combination of the two. The fact that there have been no similar complaints from male junior doctors is of minor importance, because it indicates that something is different now. Thomas might want to mention the lack of prior complaints in his conversation with the consultant. However, this factor is not of greater importance since it is a relatively minor point, and describes past behaviour, rather than what is currently going on.

67. (A)

This factor makes it all the more likely that the consultant will appreciate Thomas's intervention in this matter, or at the very least, that he is likely to give Thomas a fair hearing when he airs the junior doctors' concerns. This factor is therefore very important to consider.

68. (C)

There is really no need to submit a formal complaint, since Thomas is well-positioned to pass on the junior doctors' concerns to the consultant; he can do so informally, as this would be a direct, local solution. You might wonder why this factor is of minor importance, rather than no importance—it's because the fact that the consultant is serving as acting hospital chairman could go some way to explaining his particularly rude treatment of the new junior doctors. The scenario suggests that he was generally rude to junior doctors in the past, but this has worsened with the new, all-female intake. It could well be because of the pressures of doing double duty, as a consultant and hospital chairman. His responsibility for training junior doctors would only add to the stress, though the consultant does have an obligation to support their training, and to consider the way that his behaviour affects the team. Thus, this factor is of minor importance.

Mock Test Explanations

Verbal Reasoning

1. (B)

The third paragraph describes the negative impact of radiation on humans and animals. Acute radiation in humans, cataracts in voles, and an initial decrease in population sizes are all mentioned here, but infertility in animals is not mentioned. **(B)** is correct.

2. (D)

(A) is contradicted by the long-term effects of radiation described in the third paragraph, such as partial albinism in swallows, and cataracts in voles. **(B)** is disproved in the second paragraph, which describes the methods used to determine population size without entering the exclusion zone. **(C)** is not confirmed in the passage, though long-term effects of radiation still exist, it is not clear that these issues outweigh the benefits of population growth. **(D)** is confirmed in the final paragraph, the author believes that living on irradiated land has a less harmful impact on population size than living near humans. **(D)** is correct.

3. (B)

Wolves in the exclusion zone are discussed in the second paragraph. **(A)** is not correct, in one case, the population of wolves was seven times greater, but it is not confirmed that the overall wolf population grew by a factor of seven. The beginning of the second paragraph details that the wolves left tracks while hunting for prey after dark. **(B)** is the correct answer.

4. (A)

The first paragraph explains that those living within the 4,200 kilometre area worst effected were permanently evacuated from their homes. **(A)** is correct.

5. (C)

The second paragraph states the carbon nanotubes have a diameter which measures on the nanoscale, but it is not stated that they have an average diameter of one nanometer. The answer is can't tell.

6. (A)

The first paragraph confirms that the darkest man-made substance is made from carbon nanotubes. The statement is true.

7. (B)

The second half of the final paragraph states that carbon nanotubes cannot currently be used for clothing, as the surface is too brittle. The statement must be false.

8. (C)

The second paragraph describes carbon nanotubes as being *grown* by humans, but it is not clear whether or not carbon nanotubes grow naturally, or can only be created by humans. The answer is **(C)**.

9. (D)

The question asks for the statement which must be false. **(A)** is confirmed in the second paragraph, which states that menageries in Europe were used to demonstrate scholarly advancement. **(B)** is not stated, as the zoo mentioned in Vienna is the oldest still in existence, but it is not directly contradicted by the passage, so it could be true. The first paragraph states that animals in Babylonia were infrequently trained to perform in parades, so **(C)** could be true. This leaves **(D)**, which is confirmed as the first menagerie in Britain at the Tower of London included lions, and animals brought home by explorers. The menagerie cannot have only contained native animals. **(D)** is the answer.

10. (C)

The zoo in Regent's Park is discussed in the final paragraph. The zoo was created for scholarly use, not to display wealth and prowess. White pelicans are stated to be inhabitants of St James's Park, not Regent's Park. **(C)** is correct; the zoo was used only by scholars when it first opened.

11. (A)

Britain's first scientific zoo was London Zoo in Regent's Park, which was given public access in 1847. **(A)** is correct.

12. (A)

The last sentence of the passage states that zoos have come full circle, as they are once again flashy political status symbols. This compares modern zoos to European menageries of the 16th and 17th century. **(A)** is the correct answer.

13. (A)

The keyword Durham appears in the second paragraph, which states that students at Durham no longer had to pass a religious test for admissions after the 1871 Universities Test Act. From this information, you can infer that students at Durham did have to pass a religious admissions test before 1871; this statement is therefore supported by the passage. The answer is **(A)**.

14. (B)

The keyword smallest leads to the first paragraph, which states that Mansfield is Oxford's smallest college, except for Harris Manchester. This statement contradicts the passage, so it is false.

15. (C)

The keyword 'Chapel' occurs in the final paragraph, which explains that the Mansfield College Chapel continues to perform services and employ chaplains in the Nonconformist tradition. None of this indicates whether or not the chapel has been consecrated, so the answer is **(C)**.

16. (B)

The keywords 'Oliver Cromwell' and '1662 dissenters' appear in the same sentence of the final paragraph. However, the first part of this sentence states that Cromwell died in 1658, four years before the dissenters separated from the Church of England. The answer is **(B)**.

17. (C)

The author would least likely agree with the answer that contradicts the passage; any answer that is supported by the passage will be incorrect. The first sentence of the second paragraph states the author's opinion that the problem of water usage is much bigger than the current conservation efforts in the UK, which are detailed in the first paragraph. Thus, the author would agree with **(A)** and **(D)**, and would disagree with **(C)**. **(C)** is therefore correct.

18. (A)

The keywords England and Wales appear in the second sentence; the next sentence says that most water used daily by people in England and Wales is used in washing and toilet flushing. The correct answer is (A).

19. (C)

Examples of embedded water are given in the second paragraph. These include a pint of beer, a cup of coffee and a cotton t-shirt; there is also a mention of water used to grow crops that are exported to developed nations. There is, however, no example of livestock; the answer is **(C)**.

20. (A)

The keyword is *embedded water*, which is discussed in the second paragraph. 3% is mentioned here, but it describes the amount of water usage that consumers see, not the percentage of embedded water. A cup of coffee embeds 140 litres of water, which is almost twice as much as the water embedded by a pint of beer (74 litres). The answer is **(A)**.

21. (A)

The keywords 'non-professional players' lead to the end of the passage, where the final sentence explains that amateur players will often play a table tennis game under the old rules, either due to nostalgia or because they are unaware that the rules have changed. Answer **(A)** corresponds precisely with the second of these reasons, so it is correct.

22. (C)

Numbers make for great keywords, and scanning for 11 and 10 leads to the first sentence of the second paragraph, which explains that a player wins a game by scoring 11 points under ITTF rules, unless both are tied on 10, in which case a win requires a 2-point lead. Thus, a game could not be won by a score of 11-10 or 12-11, as once both players have reached 10 points, the winner must have a margin of 2. Thus, the correct answer is **(C)**.

23. (D)

This question asks for something that must be false, so the correct answer must contradict the passage regarding the Chinese National Team. The Chinese players are mentioned in the fourth sentence of the passage; they unsuccessfully challenged an increase in the diameter of table tennis balls, as the larger balls had less speed and spin, which were essential to the Chinese playing style. Thus, the first three answers are supported by the passage, and thus are incorrect; **(D)** contradicts the passage, and is correct.

24. (D)

The colours of ITTF-sanctioned table tennis balls are indicated in the first paragraph. Stars may be black or blue, and may also include a second colour: red, green or purple. The balls themselves must be orange or white. The combinations given for **(D)** would not work, as none of the balls have white stars. **(D)** is correct.

25. (A)

Scan for 'Second Empire', which is included in the title of Zola's cycle of novels set during that time period. The first paragraph does not specify the years of the Second Empire; however, the final paragraph indicates that Zola's cycle of novels were set in Paris from 1852 to 1870. Thus, it is safe to infer that the Second Empire took place during these years, and therefore during the 19th century. The statement is true.

26. (A)

Scan for the keywords Zola and naturalist; these appear together in the last sentence of the first paragraph, which states that Zola's cycle of novels established his reputation as a preeminent proponent of the literary movement of naturalism. This statement is a close paraphrase of this detail from the passage, and is therefore true.

27. (C)

The keyword Paris is found in brackets, midway through the final paragraph, indicating that Zola's novels in the cycle *Les Rougon-Macquart* are set in Paris. However, the passage does not clarify whether the novels in this cycle are the only novels that Zola wrote. If they are, the statement is true; if they are not, then the existence of any other novel he wrote that was not set in Paris would make it false. Since it is impossible to tell from the passage whether Zola wrote novels beyond this cycle, the answer is **(C)**.

28. (B)

The keyword Balzac appears in the first paragraph; the second sentence contrasts *La Comedie Humaine*, Balzac's cycle of novels, with Zola's cycle, which was to focus on a single family. Thus, it is safe to infer that Balzac's cycle involved more than one family. However, the passage does not indicate the exact number of novels in Balzac's cycle. The final sentence of the passage mentions that *La Comedie Humaine* included more than 90 works, some of which were novels, and represented the only cycle of novels that Balzac wrote. Thus, it is safe to infer from the passage that Balzac did not write a cycle of 20 novels; this statement says otherwise, so it is false.

29. (C)

The keywords *full access to all levels of education* appear in the second paragraph, which states that women did not achieve this access in the UK until the late 1980s. The correct answer is **(C)**.

30. (D)

This question is somewhat vaguely worded, but it's asking for something that the author would agree with. Scan for keywords from each answer, and eliminate those that are not supported by the passage. In the second paragraph, the author cites research that students who are most struggling when they start a single-sex school are most likely to benefit; **(A)** contradicts this point, so it is incorrect. The second paragraph lists several benefits to women students at single-sex schools, so **(B)** is incorrect. The final paragraph includes information that suggests that socioeconomic factors are tied to student performance in school. Hence, the author does not seem open to **(C)**, and **(D)** is supported by the passage and thus correct.

31. (D)

(A) can be inferred as in 1944 an Act was passed which guaranteed free education to all students, so it can be inferred that prior to this, not all students were entitled to free education. **(B)** can be inferred, as the final paragraph suggests economic differences between parents of mixed and same sex school students. **(C)** can be inferred from the information in the first paragraph. **(D)** cannot be inferred, as graduates of all-girls schools only earn more than girls from mixed schools, it is not stated that they earn more than both boys and girls. **(D)** is the answer.

32. (B)

The keywords *at their peak* and *secondary schools* lead to the first paragraph, where it is explained that there was a historical UK high of about 2,500 all-women's secondary schools in the 1960s. The answer is therefore **(B)**.

33. (D)

Scanning for the keywords 'world's food supply' leads to the first paragraph, where the final sentence states that more than four-fifths of the world's food crops that require pollination are pollinated by honey bees. Answer **(D)** is a very close paraphrase of this detail from the passage, and is therefore correct. Hopefully, you weren't tempted by wrong answer **(A)**, which is broader than the passage; there's no way to know from the passage whether most of the world's crops – which would include cotton, tobacco and other crops not grown for food – depend on bees for pollination.

34. (C)

The third paragraph states that the number of hives deaths was greater in the winter of 2007-2008 than 2014–2015, but this is not specific to the US. The following sentence states that the population of bees in the US increased in 2017 from the population size of the previous year. **(C)** is correct.

35. (B)

The keywords IIV and 'sole cause' lead to the second paragraph; the fourth sentence states that IIV are found in 100% of collapsed hives in a study of CCD, but that IIV are often found in strong colonies; as such, IIV alone cannot be the cause of CCD. Answer **(B)** matches this detail from the passage, so it is correct.

36. (B)

Recent studies on the effects of pesticides are covered in the second half of the final paragraph. Clothiandin, the pesticide used on corn, can be toxic and present a risk to bees, but its effect on reproduction is not discussed. The next study mentioned in the passage is funded by the makers of clothiandin, linking another pesticide with detrimental effects on bee health and population. This suggests that the research is not funded by an impartial party, as clothiandin is also linked to detrimental effects on bee health. **(B)** is correct.

37. (C)

The Imperial War Museum appears in the final paragraph, which states that the first Imperial War Museum was at Crystal Palace. The passage does not specify where the current Imperial War Museum is located, so there is no way of knowing based on the passage whether or not it is still at Crystal Palace. The answer is Can't tell.

38. (A)

Scanning the passage for information about the original Crystal Palace from the 1851 Great Exhibition should lead you to the second paragraph. This is also where you will find the passage's only mention of public toilets. The third sentence states that public toilets made their debut in the Crystal Palace during the Great Exhibition. This statement is true.

39. (A)

This statement may sound a bit unusual, but scanning for the keywords 'Hyde Park' leads to the first sentence of the second paragraph. The building destroyed in 1936, referred to in the previous paragraph sentence as Crystal Palace, was erected in Hyde Park for the Great Exhibition of 1851. This statement is supported by the passage, and is therefore true.

40. (B)

The fire that destroyed Crystal Palace is mentioned in both the first and the last paragraphs, but most of the key information is in the first paragraph. The final sentence gives us the details – the fire began as a small office fire and quickly expanded. Don't mix and match details. The final paragraph does state that the Crystal Palace was the site of regular fireworks shows in the early twentieth century, but these were not responsible for the fire. The answer is **(B)**.

41. (D)

The second paragraph states that a charity may work towards advancing religion. Salaries for employees within a charity are discussed in the first paragraph. If a charity is not benefitting the public or relieving poverty, it could be advancing education, but it could also be advancing religion. The final two sentences discuss why a charity may not seek to change the law. The last sentence describes that if a charity sought to change the law, this might prevent charities from working towards benefitting the public. **(D)** is correct.

42. (C)

Note that the question asks for the statement that must be false. **(A)** is confirmed in the third paragraph. **(B)** is correct; a trustee may be removed if they do not make sure a charity's funds are used appropriately. **(C)** is not correct, the second paragraph states that charities are regulated by the Charity Commission and the High Court of Justice. The correct answer is **(C)**.

43. (C)

The Charitable Uses Act is discussed at the beginning of the second paragraph. Political campaigning is discussed later on in this paragraph, but this is not described as being part of the Charitable Uses Act. The passage does not mention that the Act has been revised. The passage states that the definition of the Act was derived from case law, as is typically done in English law, so the Act can be said to conform to the traditions of English law. **(C)** is correct.

44. (A)

The trustees of a charity are discussed at the beginning of the third paragraph. The Memorandum of Understanding is defined in the first paragraph as the mission of the charity. As one of the trustee's responsibilities is fulfilling the charity's mission, a trustee must ensure the Memorandum of understanding is followed. The answer is **(A)**.

Decision Making

1. YES; NO; YES; NO; NO

The first conclusion does follow. If not all the rides at the fair were deemed unsafe, then some of the rides at the fair were not deemed unsafe. The second conclusion does not follow because some of the rides must not have been deemed unsafe. The third conclusion follows. 'Not all the rides at the fair were deemed unsafe except for those visited by the health inspector' implies that all the rides at the fair which were visited by the health inspector were deemed unsafe, but not all the rides at the fair as a whole. Hence the third, fourth and fifth conclusions do not follow. The fourth conclusion does not follow because, although all the rides visited by the health inspector were deemed unsafe, it is possible that there were other rides at the fair not visited by the health inspector but which were deemed unsafe nonetheless. The fifth conclusion cannot follow, because all the rides visited by the health inspector were deemed unsafe, and yet we know that some rides at the fair were also not deemed unsafe

2. NO; YES; NO; YES; NO

The first conclusion does not follow. Although some of the students going to university are studying abroad, there is no information stating that none of those going into full-time employment will be going abroad. The second conclusion follows. Since fewer than half of the students going to university will study abroad, the remainder must study in the UK. The third conclusion does not follow. Although all of the students are going to study or into employment, it is possible that some of the students could be employed by the sixth-form college. The fourth conclusion follows. If 70% of students are studying at university, then the remaining 30% will be going into full-time employment. If fewer than half of those going to university are studying abroad, then at least 35% of the total students will be studying in the UK. The fifth conclusion does not follow. All of the students are going straight to university or into full-time employment.

3. YES; NO; NO; YES; NO

The first conclusion follows: Pearton employees work in either manufacturing or the service sector, since Sheila is employed by Pearton and does not work in the service sector, she must work in manufacturing. The second conclusion does not follow: the text only tells us that 35% of Dizon employees work in the service sector; it does not tell us what kind of work the other 65% do. The third conclusion does not follow: someone might work for any of DTP's three arms and be employed in the service sector since each corporation has some service sector workers. The fourth conclusion follows: all of Transmet's employees work in the service sector, therefore anyone who does not work in that sector cannot be employed by them. The fifth conclusion does not follow: the text does not indicate, as this option seems to imply, that DTP have a monopoly on the service sector.

4. NO; NO; YES; NO; YES

The first conclusion does not follow. Although the majority of restaurants are Italian, and there are therefore more Italian restaurants than Indian restaurants, we have no information about the number of Indian takeaways. The second conclusion does not follow. Only some of the takeaways offer Chinese food; the remainder serve Indian food. The third conclusion follows. All of the Italian food is sold from restaurants; there are no Italian takeaways. The fourth conclusion does not follow. Without knowing the relative numbers of restaurants and takeaways, it is impossible to determine whether this is true or not. The fifth conclusion follows. Since some of the takeaways sell Chinese food and the majority of the restaurants sell Italian food, there could be some takeaways and restaurants selling Indian food.

5. NO; YES; NO; NO; YES

All clowns are unhappy (i.e. not happy) and all morticians are happy. The person in question is either a mortician or a clown. Therefore the first conclusion does not follow: the person is either happy and a mortician or unhappy and a clown; they cannot be either happy *or* a mortician. The second conclusion follows. Happy people always attend funerals, so we know that people who never attend funerals are unhappy. Meanwhile, since all morticians are happy, we know that unhappy people are not morticians. Taken together, these two deductions tell us that people who never attend funerals are not morticians. The person in question is either a mortician or a clown, so if they never attend funerals, then they are not a mortician and therefore must be a clown. The third conclusion does not follow: all morticians are happy and happy people always attend funerals, therefore if this person is a mortician, then they always attend funerals. The fourth conclusion does not follow, but the fifth does: the third statement tells us that people who never attend funerals are not happy (i.e. unhappy). So the fifth conclusion is valid. We cannot, however, deduce anything about people who always attend funerals from any of the statements, so the fourth conclusion does not follow.

6. (D)

Solving this Logic Puzzle requires some basic arithmetic. The set-up involves three flagpoles, each constructed from four steel tubes, of which there are three different types (distinguished by their length). Before doing any calculations, take heed of the fourth rule: no flagpole has been constructed with more than 2 R-type tubes. This immediately places a limit on the number of potential configurations for any given flagpole.

Flagpole III, the third rule tells us, is constructed from 4 tubes of the same length (4 P-type, 4 Q-type or 4 R-type). Since no flagpole is made from more than 2 R-type tubes, flagpole III must be constructed from either 4 P-type ($120 \times 4 = 480$ cm) or 4 Q-type ($80 \times 4 = 320$ cm). Now consider flagpole II, which the second rule tells us is constructed from only P-type and R-type steel tubes. This means that flagpole II is constructed from either 2 P-type ($120 \times 2 = 240$) and 2 R-type ($160 \times 2 = 320$) or 3 P-type ($120 \times 3 = 360$) and 1 R-type (160). Due to the fourth rule, 1 P-type and 3 R-type is an inadmissible combination. Therefore, flagpole II is either $240 + 320 = 560$ cm, or $360 +$

$160 = 520$ cm. Therefore whichever of the two possible combination of tubes flagpole II and flagpole III are constructed from, flagpole II (either 560 cm or 520 cm) will always be longer than flagpole III (either 480 cm or 320 cm). Therefore **(D)** is the correct answer.

For the record: We could calculate the possible lengths of flagpole I. The first rule tells us flagpole I has been constructed with all three types of tube. This means flagpole I must be constructed from either 2 P-type, 1 Q-type and 1 R-type, or 1 P-type, 2 Q-type, and 1 R-type, or 1 P-type, 1 Q-type and 2 R-type. That gives us the following possible lengths: 2P ($120 \times 2 = 240$) + 1Q (80) + 1R (160) = 480 cm; 1P (120) + 2Q ($80 \times 2 = 160$) + 1R (160) = 440 cm; 1P (120) + 1Q (80) + 2R ($160 \times 2 = 320$) = 520 cm. Flagpole I has a length of either 440 cm, 480 cm or 520 cm then. Answer **(C)** could be true if both flagpole I and II are 520 cm long; since they could be other lengths and still be consistent with the rules, **(C)** could also be false. Answer **(B)** could likewise be false if flagpole III was 480 cm and flagpole I was 440 cm. Finally, answer **(A)**: at best, flagpole I could be tied for longest length with flagpole II if both were 520cm long. Since we have no reason to suppose that both are in fact this length rather than any of the alternative possibilities, **(A)** cannot be correct.

7. (A)

The key to solving this Logic Puzzle is in the initial set-up: the publisher only releases works in two genres (science fiction and historical novels), and alternates between them each quarter. The third rule tells us that a work of science fiction is being released in Q2. Therefore, a historical novel must be being published in Q1 and Q3, and another work of science fiction will be published in Q4. The second rule tells us that neither Prandesh nor Gordell writes historical novels. Therefore, Prandesh and Gordell must write science fiction and either Prandesh is being published in Q2 and Gordell in Q4, or vice versa. This leaves Wilkins and Levi writing the two historical novels. The first rule tells us that Levi's novel will be published after Wilkins's. So Wilkins's work is being published in Q1, and Levi's in Q3. Taken together, this gives us the following sketch:

Q1	Q2	Q3	Q4
Hist.	Sci.	Hist.	Sci.
Wilkins	Prandesh or Gordell	Levi	Prandesh or Gordell

Clearly then, **(A)** must be true, making it the correct answer.

For the record: **(C)** and **(D)** must be false, while **(B)** could be false (i.e. Prandesh's work could be being published in Q2).

8. (B)

The key to solving this puzzle is to unearth the identity of the person in the middle seat. We know from the first rule that this not Artemis. The third rule states that there are two people between Roxie and Charlie. Since there are only five seats, either Roxie or Charlie must take one of the window seats. The other, due to the second rule, is taken by Deandre. This means the middle seat must be occupied by Frank. Abbreviating the people by their first initials, we can deduce from the three rules that there are four possible seating arrangements: DCFAR, CAFRD, DRFAC, and RAFCD. As can be seen, regardless of the seating arrangement the friends take, Frank is always sat next to Artemis. Answer **(B)** is correct.

9. (C)

This Logic Puzzle requires you to match the colours of shirts and socks worn by the five sales reps. We are told that each sales rep is wearing a different colour combination – so you can't have one in blue shirt and pink socks and another in pink shirt and blue socks. We also know that no one is wearing shirt and socks of the same colour, and no one is wearing shirt and socks of colours that start with the same letter. These rules are worth bearing in mind as we get to the rules with more concrete information.

The third rule is the most concrete, since it specifies the exact colour for one sales rep – the one with blue socks is sitting between the two wearing pink. We also know (from the final rules) that one of those in pink is wearing blue, meaning that person must have a blue shirt and pink socks (since blue socks are already taken by the sales rep between the two in pink). The fourth rule is a bit more complicated, but bear in mind that the pink-blue socks-pink group means that the person in green (a socks colour) cannot be between the two people in pink (since that person has blue socks). That means one of the three individuals mentioned in the fourth rule must be the blue socks person, with the other two on either side of the pink people. The only shirt colour covered in the fourth rule is white, so we know that the person in blue socks has a white shirt. Eliminate **(D)**.

At this point, it would be helpful to make a quick sketch (if you haven't done so already):

Shirt:	???	Pink	White	Blue	???
Socks:	White	???	Blue	Pink	Green

Note that the two individuals in pink could swap places, and the two outer individuals (white and green socks) could also swap places. At this point, however, the key issue is filling in the blanks. There is only one remaining colour of socks – black – so the person in the pink shirt wears black socks. The correct answer is **(C)**.

For the record: Since the person in the green socks cannot wear a grey shirt (as the colours start with the same letter), you could fill in the remaining colours:

Shirt:	Grey	Pink	White	Blue	Purple
Socks:	White	Black	Blue	Pink	Green

Note that **(A)** is a wrong answer trap for anyone who worked a bit too quickly, as if you rushed you might have noted that white and blue were a colour combination – but **(A)** inverts the correct pairing. Someone must wear a white shirt and blue socks, not the inverse as indicated in **(A)**.

10. (C)

The key terms in the original question are tourists, denied access to cultural sites, and protect for future generations. **(A)** is incorrect because it only argues against the current level of tourism, whereas the original question suggests stopping tourism completely. **(B)** makes an interesting and important point, but it does not address the impact of denying tourist access on the condition of these sites. **(C)** is correct: it links tourism to the funding needed to maintain the sites, which also sustains local communities.

For the record: **(D)** is incorrect because it makes an argument against itself; if everyone should be able to appreciate these sites then this implies it is important to protect them for future generations. It does not also explicitly state whether or not cessation of tourist visits to these places would impact their survival.

11. (B)

The key terms in the original question are schools, gardens and fields, students growing vegetables, and health of students. **(A)** does not address whether using school land to grow vegetables will improve the health of their students. **(B)** cites evidence that being involved in growing food will improve the health of their students, so **(B)** is correct.

For the record: **(C)** is incorrect because it does not state whether using some of the space in gardens and fields to grow vegetables would stop students from using these spaces to play sports. **(D)** is incorrect because it does not address whether using school land to grow vegetables would impact the health of students.

12. (D)

The issue at hand in this question is whether the NHS should stop prescribing gluten-free foods because they are now available in most supermarkets. **(A)** and **(B)** both make claims to the effect that gluten intolerance is not a serious illness. The question however is not about gluten intolerance, or indeed about whether it is a serious condition, so **(A)** and **(B)** are too tangential to be correct. **(C)** discusses gluten-free foods and argues that not everyone can afford them. This is slightly too broad, because the question asks whether the wider availability of gluten-free foods in supermarkets is a good reason for the NHS to stop prescribing them. **(D)** addresses the issue of supermarket availability more directly, asserting that in some parts of the country, gluten-free foods are not available in supermarkets. In effect then, the argument is that the wider availability of gluten-free foodstuffs is not a good reason for the NHS to stop prescribing them. Since this option bears the greatest relation to the particulars of the question, **(D)** is the correct answer.

13. (A)

The key terms in the original question are compulsory, students taking GCSEs and modern foreign language. **(A)** addresses the benefits of studying a foreign language for these students, so it directly addresses the key terms. For this reason, **(A)** is correct.

For the record: **(B)** is incorrect because if taking a language was compulsory for all students, then all students would have studied a language and this would not be a way of differentiating between job candidates. **(B)** is not logically sound, so it cannot be correct. **(C)** is incorrect because the fact that some students can already speak more than one language is not an argument against making all students learn at least one language. **(D)** is incorrect because it implies that the only use of studying a foreign language is to be able to understand others who speak that language; **(D)** is also 'strong but wrong' because it focuses on translation technology instead of the benefits (or problems) of studying a foreign language for GCSE students. Be suspicious of any answer that sounds good but omits several key terms from the original question, as these are unlikely to be correct on Test Day.

14. (B)

This question asks whether being made to pay a small charge for disposable cups at coffee shops would encourage people to bring their own mugs. The strongest argument must address the specific issue of customers bringing their own mugs, rather than any assumed broader implication. Both **(A)** and **(C)** neglect the mug aspect, and make claims about the environmental-friendliness of coffee cups instead. This is too broad, and so does not address the question directly. **(D)** makes an assertion about the potential effect the measure proposed might have on the coffee shop business. This is tangential, and so is not a strong argument. **(B)** argues that, if such a system were in place, people would be encouraged to bring mugs to the coffee shop, because doing so would provide them

with a small saving (i.e. they would not have to pay the charge for a disposable cup). Of the four options, it addresses the question most directly; **(B)** is the strongest argument.

15. NO; YES; NO; YES; NO

The first conclusion does not follow; asparagus and grapefruit both contain 0.03 mg of vitamin B6 per 100 g. The second conclusion follows, since 17 is less than half of 40. The third conclusion does not follow; it could be true, but we don't know as we only have information for these six fruits and vegetables. The fourth conclusion follows: 100 g of grapefruit contain 0.07 mg of vitamin B1, so there would be $0.07 \times 10 = 0.7$ mg in a kilogram of grapefruit; 100 g of kiwi contains 1/7 as much vitamin B1, so multiplying the weight of kiwi by a factor 7 would make the amount of vitamin B1 equal. The fifth conclusion does not follow; avocado has more vitamin B2 than kiwi.

16. NO; NO; YES; YES; YES

The first conclusion does not follow; we are told of two known species of coelacanth, but we don't know whether there could be more to be discovered. The second conclusion does not follow: coelacanths are normally found 150 m to 250 m underwater, where they feed on squid and other animals; this does not mean that squid do not live any deeper in the sea. The third conclusion follows: the first sentence of the second paragraph explains that some researchers believe the coelacanth's unique features could mark a step in the evolution from water-based to land-based animals. The fourth conclusion follows; the discovery of a living coelacanth in 1938 overturned a scientific consensus that the animal went extinct at around the same time as the dinosaurs. The fifth conclusion follows; coelacanths area typically found 150 m to 250 m underwater.

17. YES; NO; NO; NO; YES

The first conclusion follows: brushing your teeth twice a day reduces tooth decay by a third compared to brushing your teeth once a day, so brushing once a day is not the most effective way to reduce tooth decay. The second conclusion does not follow; fewer English people (61%) said they visit the dentist regularly compared to people in the rest of the UK (65%). The third conclusion does not follow; a lower rate of tooth decay is seen with regular brushing. The fourth conclusion does not follow; it misinterprets the percentages from the third sentence of the passage: The passage states that 25% of people in the UK haven't seen a dentist for more than two years, leaving the remaining 75% of people who have seen a dentist. This detail matches the fifth conclusion, which therefore follows.

18. YES; NO; YES; NO; NO

The first conclusion follows: Medium A resulted in approximately 20 male flies with red (wild type) eyes and 5 with white eyes, so males with white eyes are $5/25 = 1/5$ of males from Medium A; Medium B resulted in approximately the same number of males with red and white eyes (about 15 of each), so males with white eyes are $15/30 = 1/2$ of males from Medium B. One-fifth doubled is two-fifths, and one-half is more than two-fifths. The second conclusion does not follow; since there are 20 wild type (red eye) males in Medium A, compared to approximately 15 in Medium B. The third conclusion follows: the total number of males in Medium B is clearly no more than 30, whilst the number of females is closer to 35. The fourth conclusion does not follow; the difference in medium is actually seen least in wild type females, with almost equal numbers. The fifth conclusion does not follow; there are about 40 females, compared to roughly 35 males.

19. (D)

The omega overlaps the circle (rich), the hexagon (happy) and the triangle (a doctor), but not the trapezium (married) or the star (famous). The correct answer is **(D)**.

20. (B)

(A) is incorrect because of a total of 58 competitors, only 26 compete in the javelin. **(B)** is correct, because there are 28 competitors for both events. For the record: **(C)** is incorrect because there are a total of 58 competitors, but 28 discus competitors. **(D)** is incorrect because there are 36 people competing in exactly two events, and only 5 competitors in exactly three events.

21. (C)

(A) is incorrect because there are a total of 34 teachers who speak both French and Spanish, and only 10 of these (less than half) can speak Hindi also. **(B)** is incorrect because there are 22 teachers who speak only Hindi and Spanish, and 15 teachers who speak only Mandarin and Spanish. **(C)** is correct because there are a total of 90 teachers who speak Spanish, and a total of 45 teachers who speak Mandarin. For the record: **(D)** is incorrect because there are a total of 36 teachers who can speak a combination of 3 or more languages, and only 9 of these (1/4) cannot speak Mandarin.

22. (A)

(A) is correct: there are a total of 102 dishes, of which 56 contain orange. For the record: **(B)** is incorrect, because there are 6 dishes which only used caramel, but there were 8 dishes that contained caramel and at least two other flavours. **(C)** is incorrect, because there were 18

dishes containing three or more of these ingredients and 9 (half, so not a majority) used chocolate. **(D)** is incorrect, because there were 47 dishes containing chocolate and 43 dishes containing pistachio.

23. (C)

This question asks for a combination of instruments that are not played by musicians in the orchestra. Viola (the oval) overlaps with two groupings of shapes that do not overlap with each other: the lower grouping, with the triangle and pentagon (flute and piccolo) and the upper grouping, with the square, hexagon and arrow (violin, oboe and cello, respectively). Thus, there are no musicians who play both the violin (square) and flute (triangle), as these shapes do not overlap. The correct answer is **(C)**.

24. (D)

There are two types of halfwiches containing cheese – Brie and grape and cheddar and pickle – and one type containing bacon. These halfwiches are represented by the quadrilateral, hexagon and star, respectively. Just be careful not to add the same figures to your total twice as you work out the sum. The quadrilateral includes a total of $48 + 4 + 16 + 52 + 27 + 14 + 9 + 33 + 17 = 220$ customers. There are a further $35 + 18 = 53$ customers in the star that are not also in the quadrilateral, and another $23 + 21 = 44$ customers in the hexagon that are not in the star or the quadrilateral. This yields a total of $220 + 53 + 44 = 317$ customers. Answer **(D)** is correct.

25. (A)

The shape representing coyotes must be entirely inside the shape representing dogs, which must be entirely inside the shape representing mammals. The shape representing pets must partially include the shape representing dogs, but must also include a region that does not overlap with mammals. Answer **(A)** is correct. For the record: **(B)** is incorrect because some dogs are pets, and not all pets are mammals. **(C)** is incorrect because all coyotes are dogs. **(D)** is incorrect because not all pets are mammals.

26. (D)

In Class A, 95% of students passed the Biology exam. In the same class, 10% of students failed the Chemistry exam, so the remaining 90% passed. In Class B, 7% of students failed the Biology exam, so 93% passed. 90% of the students in Class B passed the Chemistry exam. Hence, the pass/fail performance of the two classes was the same in the Chemistry exam, but a higher proportion of Class A passed the Biology exam. Answer **(D)** is correct.

27. (C)

(C) is correct because there are 36 possible combinations (6 × 6) in total. Since a sum of 7 can be result from 6 possible combinations: (1 + 6, 2 + 5, 3 + 4, 4 + 3, 5 + 2, 6 + 1), the probability of rolling a sum of 7 with the two dice is 6/36, which is reduces to 1/6, which is greater than 1/11.

28. (D)

Medication I is effective at treating the condition in 100% − 36% = 64% of patients. Of these, 12.5% experience a relapse; 12.5% = 1/8, so 8% of those treated with Medication I experience a relapse, meaning that 64% − 8% = 56% are treated successfully without relapse. Medication II is effective at treating the condition in 76% of patients. Of these, 75% do not experience a relapse; 75% = 3/4, so 75% of 76% = 57%. That means that Medication II is more successful than Medication I at treating the condition without relapse: 1% more patients treated successfully (57% versus 56%) will not relapse with Medication II, as compared to Medication I. The correct answer is **(D)**.

29. (A)

At the start, the probability of selecting a white counter is 1/2. The probability of selecting a black counter is the same, since there is an equal number of white and black counters. After the first two draws, the counters selected are not replaced, so the probability of selecting a white counter on the third draw will have decreased from the start if both counters already selected are white. Answer **(A)** is correct.

For the record: If one counter of each colour is selected on the first and second draws, then the probability of a white counter being selected on the third draw is 1/2, since at that point there would be an equal number of white and black counters in the bag (as one of each had been removed), ruling out **(B)**. If both counters selected on the first two draws were black, then the probability of selecting a white counter on the third draw would have increased, as there would be more white counters than black in the bag. If there were four white counters in the bag at the start, there were also four black counters, so this detail would not help you to answer the question. As long as there are an equal number of white and black counters at the start, **(A)** must be the correct answer.

Quantitative Reasoning

1. (B)

First calculate the total number of hours worked from home by the couple: 6 + 4.5 + 11 + 4.5 = 26 hours per week. Sandra works an extra three hours from home on Wednesday and 9 hours on Friday: 3 + 9 = 12 hours. Thus the percentage increase in hours worked from home for the couple is: 12 ÷ 26 = 0.462 = 46.2%. The answer is **(B)**.

2. (C)

John is taxed 21% on his income, therefore his pay after tax is: 15.17 × (1 − 0.21) = 15.17 × 0.79 = £11.98 per hour. John works a total of 11 hours per week at home, all on Thursday. Thus John makes: 11.98 × 11 = £131.78 per week after tax while working from home. Answer **(C)** is correct.

3. (A)

Sandra pays £7.50 per week for her gym membership; she uses the gym 2 hours per week. John pays £8.99 per week for his gym membership and uses the gym 8 hours per week. Thus, the two pay a total of: 7.50 + 8.99 = £16.49 per week for gym membership and use it for 10 hours. Therefore the cost per hour for gym membership is: £16.49 ÷ 10 = £1.649 = £1.65 per hour. The correct answer is **(A)**.

4. (E)

The information below the timetable states that Sandra's office is 16.2 km away from her gym. If she leaves at 08:00 and arrives 22 minutes early the journey takes 38 minutes, To calculate her speed use this information and convert minutes to hours: 16.2 ÷ (38 ÷ 60) = 25.58 km/h. The answer is **(E)**.

5. (B)

The combined area of the director's office and conference room ($D + C$) has dimensions of 40 ft × 18 ft, so the combined area is $40 \times 18 = 720 \text{ ft}^2 = D + C$. The area of the director's office equals the area of the conference room minus 108 square feet, or $D = C - 108$. Substitute this for the area of the director's office, and solve for the area of the conference room:

$$C + C - 108 = 720 \text{ ft}^2$$
$$2C - 108 = 720 \text{ ft}^2$$
$$2C = 828 \text{ ft}^2$$
$$C = 414 \text{ ft}^2$$

Thus, the area of the conference room is 414 ft², and the answer is **(B)**.

6. (D)

Divide the conference room's area by its known dimension (18 ft), which represents the wall shared with the director's office, to find its other dimension, representing the wall shared with the reception/front office room: $414 \text{ ft}^2 \div 18 \text{ ft} = 23 \text{ ft}$. The other dimension of the reception/front office room is the combined length of both the conference room and the reception/front office room (56 ft) minus the length of the conference room (18 ft): $56 \text{ ft} - 18 \text{ ft} = 38 \text{ ft}$. Multiply for the total area of the reception/front office room: $23 \text{ ft} \times 38 \text{ ft} = 874 \text{ ft}^2$. The correct answer is **(D)**.

7. (E)

According to the bulleted info, the reception area is 35% of the combined reception/front office room, or $0.35 \times 874 \text{ ft}^2 = 306 \text{ ft}^2$. If the width of the reception area is 12 ft, then the length is $306 \div 12 = 25.5 \text{ ft}$. The dimensions of the reception area are 12 ft × 25.5 ft. The correct answer is **(E)**.

8. (A)

First, calculate the total area to be carpeted. The combined area of the director's office and conference room is $18 \text{ ft} \times 40 \text{ ft} = 720 \text{ ft}^2$. The area of the front office, not including the reception area, is 65% of the combined reception/front office area: $0.65 \times 874 \text{ ft}^2 = 568.1 \text{ ft}^2$. Add these for the total area to be carpeted: $720 \text{ ft}^2 + 568.1 \text{ ft}^2 = 1{,}288.1 \text{ ft}^2$. Next, multiply by the cost of carpeting per sq ft for the total cost: $1{,}288.1 \text{ ft}^2 \times £2.99/\text{ft}^2 = £3{,}851.42$. The answer is **(A)**.

9. (E)

The initial starter requires 1 cup of sugar. In growing the starter, you add one cup of sugar on Day 5 and again on Day 10, for a total of 2 cups of sugar in each cycle. The cake requires a further 2 cups of sugar. Thus, each cycle of growing the starter and baking a cake uses 4 cups of sugar. If you complete the cycle and bake a cake 3 times, then you would use $4 \times 13 = 12$ cups of sugar, plus the cup from the initial starter, for 13 cups total. Multiply to convert to grams: $13 \times 240 = 3.120 \text{ g}$, or 3.12 kg. Answer **(E)** is correct.

10. (B)

A total of 39.7 billion text messages were sent over mobile phone networks in the UK in 2011, yet only 21 billion such messages were sent in 2014, a difference of 39.7 billion − 21 billion = 18.7 billion text messages. To solve for percentage decrease, divide the difference by the original: 18.7 billion ÷ 39.7 billion = 0.471, or 47.1%. The answer is **(B)**.

11. (D)

The male pigs – Horatio, Otto and Sebastian – have a total weight of $46.1 + 25.4 + 38.1 = 109.6 \text{ kg}$ in March, and a total weight of $62.4 + 36.8 + 54.5 = 153.7 \text{ kg}$ in August. This results in an average weight of $109.6 \div 3 = 36.53$ in March, and an average weight of $153.7 \div 3 = 51.23 \text{ kg}$ in August. The difference in the average weights is $51.23 - 36.53 = 14.7 \text{ kg}$; dividing the difference by the original gives 0.4024, or 40.2%. The answer is **(D)**.

12. (E)

To find the amount of espresso in each drink, turn the ratio into fractions for espresso content. For each drink, cappuccino is 1/3 espresso; latte is 1/6, espresso is 1/1, macchiato is 8/9 and breve is 2/5 . Calculating the amount of espresso in ml for each drink: for cappuccino, $200 \div 3 = 66.7 \text{ ml}$; for latte $250 \div 6 = 41.7 \text{ ml}$; for espresso 40 ml; for macchiato $(80 \div 9) \times 8 = 71.1 \text{ ml}$; for breve, $(180 \div 5) \times 2 = 72 \text{ ml}$. Breve contains the largest amount of espresso. **(E)** is correct.

13. (B)

The information needed to answer is found in the graph, which gives a figure of 2.6 for Retail in 2016. The figures on the bars represent millions of pounds, so 2.6 equals a value of £2.6 million. Answer **(B)** is correct.

14. (C)

Again, find the relevant information in the graph, which gives a figure of 1.7 for Leisure in 2017. This is the equivalent of £1,700,000, so the correct answer is **(C)**.

15. (D)

The Commercial sector made £2.4 million in profit in 2015, which increased to £3.2 million in profit in 2016. The difference is £3,200,000 − £2,400,000 = £800,000. Use the percentage change formula (difference ÷ original) to solve: 800,000 ÷ 2,400,000 = 0.333, or 33.3%. The answer is therefore **(D)**.

16. (C)

To find the total 2016 profits of all the different business sectors, add up the relevant figures from the graph: $1.6 + 2.6 + 3.2 + 2.2 = 9.6$ million. The correct answer is **(C)**.

17. (B)

The wholesalers sell fillet steak, rump steak and belly pork in the ratio of 4:3:2. The total number of parts = $4 + 3 + 2 = 9$. The total amount of meat sold is 120 kg. Each part is equal to $120 \div 9 = 13.33 \text{ kg}$. The amount of fillet steak sold is $13.33 \times 4 = 53.33 \text{ kg}$. The cost of fillet steak is 53.33 × 44 = £2346.52. The amount of rump steak sold is 13.33 × 3 = 39.99 kg. Thus, the cost of rump steak is 39.99 × 19.50 = £779.81. The amount of belly pork sold = 13.33 × 2 = 26.66 kg. The cost of belly pork = 26.66 × 8.50 = £226.61. The total amount of money made by the wholesaler = 2346.52 + 779.81 + 226.61 = £3353. The answer is **(B)**.

18. (D)

On average, the restaurant sells 55 servings of fillet steak, 47 servings of belly pork and 42 servings of gammon joint per week. The total amount of fillet steak that needs to be purchased is therefore 55 × 0.2 = 11 kg. The amount spent on fillet steak is 11 × 44 = £484. The total amount of belly pork that needs to be purchased is 47 × 0.325 = 15.28 kg. The amount spent on belly pork is 15.38 × 8.50 = £130.73. The total amount of gammon that needs to be purchased is 42 × 0.250 = 10.5 kg. The amount spent on gammon is 10.5 × 11 = £115.50. The total amount spent at the wholesalers is therefore 484 + 130.73 + 115.50 = £730.23. The answer is **(D)**.

19. (C)

The wholesale price of a portion of fillet steak is 0.2 × 44 = £8.80. The wholesale price of a portion of rump steak is 0.310 × 19.50 = £6.05. The wholesale price of a portion of lamb is 0.225 × 17 = £3.83. The wholesale price of a portion of pork belly is 0.325 × 8.50 = £2.76. The wholesale price of a portion of gammon is 0.25 × 11 = £2.75. The profit made for each serving of fillet steak is 24.95 − 8.80 = £16.15. The profit made for each serving of rump steak = 18.00 − 6.05 = £11.95. The profit made for each serving of lamb = 21.00 − 3.83 = £17.17. The profit made for each serving of pork = 19.95 − 2.76 = £17.19. The profit made for each serving of gammon = 14.95 − 2.75 = £12.20. The total profit is therefore 16.15 + 11.95 + 17.17 + 17.19 + 12.20 = £74.66. The correct answer is **(C)**.

20. (A)

The wholesale prices of rump steak and belly pork increase by 3% and 5% respectively. The new wholesale price of rump steak is 19.50 × 1.03 = £20.09 per kg. The new wholesale price of belly pork = 8.50 × 1.05 = £8.93 per kg. Prior to the price rise, the profit made when 1 serving of rump steak and belly pork were sold was (19.95 − (0.325 × 8.50)) + (18.00 − (0.310 × 19.50)) = 17.19 + 11.96 = £29.15. After the price rise the profit made is (19.95 − (0.325 × 8.93)) + (18.00 − (0.310 × 20.09)) = 17.05 + 11.77 = £28.82. The percentage decrease in the profit is

therefore (29.15 − 28.82) ÷ 29.15 = 0.011, or 1.1%. The answer is **(A)**.

21. (D)

The question provides Christos's speed (45 mph) and time (1 hour, 12 minutes), and asks you to find Christos's distance, so use the speed formula: Distance = Speed × Time. Since the speed is in mph, convert the time into hours: 1 hour, 12 minutes = 72 minutes = $\frac{72}{60}$ hours = 1.2 hours. Use this figure to calculate his distance: Distance = 45 mph × 1.2 hours = 54 miles. Answer **(D)** is correct.

22. (C)

Use the speed formula to solve for Vasilis's speed: Speed = Distance ÷ Time. The distance is 16 miles more than Christos's, or 54 + 16 = 70 miles. The time is 75 minutes = $\frac{75}{60}$ = 1.25 hours. Calculate using the speed formula: Speed = 70 miles ÷ 1.25 hours = 56 mph. The answer is **(C)**.

23. (A)

The previous question indicates that Vasilis travels 16 miles further than Christos. This question does not mention the top speed of the jet skis, but this speed is given in the information above the set as 60 mph. Since Christos would travel a mile a minute at top speed, he would need 16 minutes to travel the 16 miles needed to catch up to Vasilis. The answer is therefore **(A)**.

24. (B)

This question requires the percentage change formula: Percentage change = Difference ÷ Original. The original time is 75 minutes, and the new time is 2 hours, or 120 minutes. The difference is therefore 120 − 75 = 45 minutes. Divide to find the percentage change: 45 ÷ 75 = 0.6, or 60%. The correct answer is **(B)**.

25. (C)

To find the cost of lawn turf for the entire circular garden, find the area of the garden and then multiply by the cost of lawn turf. The garden is a circle, so use the equation $A = \pi r^2$. The radius is 5 metres, so $A = \pi(5)^2 = 3.14 × 25 = 78.5$ m². Lawn turf costs £2 per m², so multiply to find the cost of lawn turf for the circular garden: 78.5 m² × £2/m² = 157. The correct answer is **(C)**.

26. (B)

This question requires the same approach as the previous one, so simply multiply the area of the circular garden by the cost of paving slabs, which is £6 per m^2: 78.5 m^2 × £6/ m^2 = £471. The answer is therefore **(B)**.

27. (C)

Work on the previous questions gave the area of the circular garden (78.5 m^2) and the cost of paving slabs for the garden (£471). The labour cost for installing paving slabs is £2 per m^2, which is the same as the charge for lawn turf, so the labour cost is the same as the answer to the first question: £157. Subtract the cost of the paving slabs and the labour from the budget figure of £750 to find how much Mr Singh will have left over: £750 − £471 − £157 = £122. The answer is **(C)**.

28. (E)

To solve, subtract the area of the fountain from the area of the entire garden (78.5 m^2). The fountain has a diameter of 2 m, which means it has a radius of 1 m. Use the area formula to solve for the fountain's area: $A = \pi(1)^2 = 3.14 \times 1 = 3.14$ m^2. Subtract the area of the fountain from the area of the entire garden to find the area that is not covered by the fountain: 78.5 m^2 − 3.14 m^2 = 75.36 m^2. The correct answer is **(E)**.

29. (C)

The price of gold in dollars per ounce is indicated by the dashed line and the figures on the Y-axis on the left-hand side of the graph. The price of gold in 2007 is just above the line for $600 per ounce, which is equivalent to a value of $610 per ounce. The correct answer is **(C)**.

30. (E)

The scale of the labels for gold and silver prices make this question a lot more straightforward than it might initially seem. Since the labels for the price of gold increase by $100 for each line, those for silver increase by only $2 for each dash, and both start at $0 at the bottom of the graph, the year with the greatest difference in price per ounce between gold and silver will simply be the year with the greatest price per ounce for gold. In 2010, gold was approximately $1150 per ounce – a few hundred dollars above its price per ounce in the next highest year, and well above the price of silver in any year. The answer is therefore **(E)**.

31. (B)

To find the percentage increase in the price of silver per ounce, use the percentage change formula: Percentage change = Difference ÷ Original. The price of silver was approximately $5 per ounce in 2000 and $17 per ounce in 2010, for a difference of $12. Calculate the percentage change: 12 ÷ 5 = 2.4, or 240%. Answer **(B)** is correct.

32. (D)

Gold was $1150 per ounce in 2010, so 100 ounces of gold would have a value of 100 × $1150 = $115,000. Silver was $17 per ounce in 2010, so divide to find the ounces of silver you could buy with this value: $115,000 ÷ $17 per ounce = 6765 ounces, answer **(D)**.

33. (E)

First, we need to work out the total number of incorrect answers for both Amna and Joel, so subtract the correct answers from the total in each test, and add the numbers. For Amna, (60 − 29) + (80 − 74) + (100 − 54) + (100 − 42) = 141 incorrect answers. For Joel, (60 − 41) + (80 − 28) + (100 − 96) + (100 − 74) = 101 incorrect answers. To find the percentage difference, divide the difference by the smaller value: 40 ÷ 101 = 0.396, or 39.6%. The correct answer is **(E)**.

34. (C)

On questions like this, try to answer by comparing the data in the table, rather than making any calculations, which could be very time-consuming. The first step is to see if anyone scored the highest in more than one subject. The only student who did so was Emily. She scored the highest mark in English, Maths and French, and the second-highest mark in Science. The only student that scored higher than her is Joel, but his result in Maths is the lowest of all 6 friends, and he is in the bottom half in the results for English. Thus, it is clear from looking at the data that Emily scored the best across all subjects, out of all her friends. The answer is therefore **(C)**.

35. (D)

Percentage change equals difference divided by original. The difference between David's old score and his new score from his resit is 36 − 4 = 32; his old (original) score is 4. Plug these values into the formula and divide to solve: 32 ÷ 4 = 8, or 800%, answer **(D)**.

36. (B)

To solve, add up the Science scores for all 6 friends and divide by 6, the number of friends. The sum of all 6 scores is 84 + 78 + 54 + 47 + 89 + 96 = 450. The mean score of the six friends is 450 ÷ 6 = 75. Answer **(B)** is correct.

Abstract Reasoning

1. (B)

This pattern involves a feature of the shapes in each box: the number of sides. In Set A, the shapes in each box have a total of 12 sides. In Set B, the shapes in each box have a total of 8 sides. The first test shape has two rainbow shapes with 4 sides each, for a total of 8 sides; as such, it belongs to Set B.

2. (B)

The pentagon and triangle in this test shape have a total of 8 sides, so the answer is **(B)**.

3. (C)

The two triangles and diamond in this test shape have a total of 10 sides. Since this does not fit the pattern for either set, the answer is **(C)**.

4. (C)

This double-headed arrow has a total of 10 sides, so it fits into neither set.

5. (A)

The test shape contains an octagon and a diamond, with a total of 12 sides; as such, the test shape belongs to Set A.

6. (A)

All the boxes in Set A and B contain a shape made up of 3 line segments, so the difference in this shape must be key to both patterns. In Set A, all the angles in the 3-segment shapes are obtuse (greater than 90 degrees); in Set B, all the angles in the 3-segment shapes are acute (less than 90 degress). The first test shape contains a 3-segment shape with obtuse angles, so it belongs to Set A.

7. (B)

The 3-segment line in this test shape contains only acute angles, so it belongs to Set B,

8. (C)

This line shape consists of only 2 segments, so it fits neither pattern.

9. (C)

This 3-segmented shape has an acute and an obtuse angle, so it belongs to neither set.

10. (B)

The 3-segment line in this test shape has only acute angles, so it fits into Set B.

11. (C)

In Set A, each box has 4 black circles in a row. In Set B, each box has 4 white circles in a row. Note that in both sets, the row could be horizontal, vertical or diagonal, but it's the only occurrence of 4 circles of the same colour in a row in each box.

This question asks about Set A. There are 4 black circles arranged vertically in **(B)**, which is therefore correct.

12. (D)

This question asks for the test shape that belongs to Set A. There are 4 black circles on a diagonal in **(D)**. Answer **(D)** is correct.

13. (C)

This question relates to Set B. There are 4 white circles arranged vertically in **(C)**, which is therefore correct.

14. (A)

This question relates to Set A. Answer **(A)** has 4 black circles on a diagonal, so it is correct.

15. (D)

There are 4 white circles arranged horizontally in **(D)**, which fits the pattern for Set B.

16. (B)

This pattern involves a feature of the shapes: whether their sides are curved or straight. In Set A, all the shapes have curved sides. In Set B, all the shapes have straight sides. The first test shape includes three stars, with entirely straight sides; this fits the pattern for Set B.

17. (B)

The three triangles in this test shape have straight sides, so it belongs to Set B.

18. (C)

The test shape contains a rainbow shape, consisting of two curved sides and two straight sides. The curved sides fit the pattern for Set A, and the straight sides fit the pattern for Set B. Since the test shape fits the pattern for both sets, it belongs exclusively to neither. The answer is therefore **(C)**.

19. (A)

This test shape includes three crescents, consisting entirely of curved sides. As such, it fits the pattern for Set A.

20. (C)

The test shape contains a cross and a crescent. The cross has straight sides, so it fits the pattern for Set A. The crescent has curved sides, so it fits the pattern for Set B. Since the test shape fits the pattern for both sets, it belongs exclusively to neither. The answer is **(C)**.

21. (C)

All the boxes in both sets feature four white shapes of approximately the same size, so the colour and number of the shapes cannot be the key to the patterns. Check each set to see whether any of the same types of shape appear in each box in the set. In Set A, each box includes a pentagon and a crescent, arranged diagonally opposite each other; in Set B, each box contains a hexagon and a circle, arranged diagonally opposite each other. The first test shape includes a hexagon diagonally opposite a pentagon, and a circle diagonally opposite a crescent. As such, the test shape fits the pattern for neither set. The answer is **(C)**.

22. (C)

This test shape contains a pentagon diagonally opposite a crescent, so it fits the pattern for Set A. However, the test shape also includes a hexagon diagonally opposite a circle, so it also fits the pattern for Set B. Since the test shape fits the patterns for both sets, it belongs exclusively to neither.

23. (A)

The test shape contains a pentagon diagonally opposite a crescent, and therefore belongs to Set A.

24. (C)

This test shape includes a triangle diagonally opposite a diamond, and a heart opposite a 'D' shape. As such, the test shape fits the pattern for neither set.

25. (B)

The test shape contains a hexagon diagonally opposite a circle, so it fits the pattern for Set B. Since the crescent in the test shape is diagonally opposite a 'D' shape, the test shape does not fit the pattern for Set A. The answer is therefore **(B)**.

26. (C)

This pattern involves the arrangement of colours or shapes in the box. In Set A, all the black shapes are in the left half of the box, and all the white shapes are in the right half of the box. In Set B, all the stars are in the right half of the box. Any shapes that are not stars are distractors in Set B. In the first test shape, the black trapezium is to the left of the two white stars. Note,

however, that the larger white star straddles both sides of the box – it crosses the vertical centre line; as such, the larger white star violates both patterns, with a white shape in the left half of the box (contrary to Set A) and a star in the left half of the box (contrary to Set B). The answer is **(C)**.

27. (A)

The black shapes are in the left half of the box and the white shapes in the right half, so the test shape belongs to Set A.

28. (A)

The black crescent is in the left half of the box; the white shapes are in the right half of the box. The test shape fits the pattern for Set A.

29. (B)

All the stars are in the right half of the box, so the test shape fits the pattern for Set B.

30. (A)

The black shapes are in the left half of the box, with the white shape in the right half of the box. The test shape belongs to Set A.

31. (B)

At first glance, the patterns in both sets appear to be very similar, as all boxes in both sets include two shapes, one large and one small, one black and one white. The type of shape does not appear to be relevant to the pattern, as some boxes have the same type of shape, but most have two shapes of different types. When the boxes appear to be very similar, check for an arrangement pattern – these can be subtle, and less obvious than patterns involving size and colour. In both patterns, the arrangement pattern is based on the colour of the shapes, irrespective of their size: in Set A, the white shape is arranged to the left of the black shape; in Set B, the black shape is arranged above the white shape. In the first test shape, the black oval is to the left of the white parallelogram; as a result, the test shape does not fit into Set A. The black shape is above the white shape, so the test shape fits into Set B.

32. (A)

In this test shape, the white arrow is to the left of the black triangle; the test shape fits the pattern for Set A. The arrow is also above the triangle, so the test shape does not fit the pattern for Set B. The answer is therefore **(A)**.

33. (C)

The white shape is to the left of the black shape, so this test shape belongs to Set A. However, the black shape is also above the white shape, so the test shape also belongs to Set B. Since the test shape belongs to both sets, it belongs exclusively to neither. The answer is therefore **(C)**.

34. (B)

This test shape includes a black cross above a white triangle, fitting the pattern for Set B. The black shape is to the left of the white shape, so the test shape does not also belong to Set A. Thus, the answer is **(B)**.

35. (C)

This test shape includes a white parallelogram above, and to the left of, a black oval. However, both shapes are medium-sized, rather than the one large and one small required in both Set A and Set B. As a result, the test shape cannot fit into either set. The answer is **(C)**.

36. (A)

All the boxes in both sets feature the same seven shapes, with the same shading. This is a great hint to look for an arrangement pattern, as the only difference can be in how the identical shapes are arranged. In Set A, the black donut is always positioned directly above the white cross; in Set B, the black square is always positioned directly above the white triangle. There is no other aspect of the pattern involving the arrangement of the other shapes. In the first test shape, the black donut is directly above the white cross; thus, the test shape belongs to Set A.

37. (C)

This test shape includes all seven shapes, and the black donut is directly above the white cross, which fits the pattern for Set A. However, the black square is directly above the white triangle as well, which fits the pattern for Set B. Since the test shape fits into both sets, it belongs exclusively to neither. The answer is therefore **(C)**.

38. (A)

The test shape features the black donut above the white cross, so it belongs to Set A. The black square is not above the white triangle, so it cannot belong to Set B. The answer is **(A)**.

39. (C)

This test shape includes the seven required shapes; however, the black donut is not above the white cross,

and the black square is not above the white triangle. Thus, the test shape fits into neither set.

40. (B)

The test shape has its black square positioned above its white triangle, so it fits the pattern for Set B. Since the black donut is not positioned above the white cross, it does not fit the pattern for Set A. The answer is therefore **(B)**.

41. (A)

Each box in Set A contains a triangle formed by other shapes. Each box in Set B contains a rectangle formed by other shapes. The first test shape contains a pentagon and octagon, which overlap to form a triangle in the lower-right portion of the figure. The answer is **(A)**.

42. (C)

The intersection of the arrows creates both a triangle and a rectangle. This test shape fits both patterns, so it belongs exclusively to neither. The answer is **(C)**.

43. (B)

This test shape includes rectangles formed by other shapes, so it fits the pattern for Set B.

44. (A)

This test shape contains a triangle formed by other shapes, so it fits the pattern for Set A.

45. (B)

The pentagons overlap with the parallelogram to form a rectangle. The test shape belongs to Set B.

46. (B)

All the boxes in both sets include an arrow, a large shape, a small shape and a medium-sized shape; only one of the shapes in each box is white, and the others are black. Since the boxes are so similar, check for an arrangement pattern. In Set A, the arrow points at the largest shape; in Set B, the arrow points at the white shape. In the first test shape, the arrow points at the white shape; since it is not also the largest shape, the answer is **(B)**.

47. (C)

The arrow in this test shape points at the largest shape, which fits the pattern for Set A. However, the largest shape is also the white shape; thus, the test shape also fits the pattern for Set B. Since the test shape can belong to both sets, it fits exclusively into neither. The answer is **(C)**.

48. (A)

The test shape contains an arrow pointing at the largest shape, which fits the pattern for Set A. The largest shape is black, so the test shape does not fit the pattern for Set B. Thus, the answer is **(A)**.

49. (C)

This test shape includes an arrow pointing at the largest shape, which fits the pattern for Set A. However, the largest shape is also the white shape; the test shape thus also fits the pattern for Set B. Because it fits the pattern for both sets, the test shape belongs exclusively to neither set.

50. (C)

The arrow in this test shape is pointing at the medium-sized shape, not the largest, so it does not belong to Set A. The arrow is pointing at a black shape, so the test shape does not belong to Set B. The answer is therefore **(C)**.

51. (B)

The colour of the shapes changes between white and black, so the correct answer will have white shapes; eliminate **(C)** and **(D)**. The key to the pattern is the total number of sides in each box, which doubles with each subsequent box. Thus, the first box has a total of 3 sides, the second a total of 6 sides, followed by boxes with totals of 12 and 24 sides. The final box must have a total of 48 sides; the correct answer is **(B)**.

52. (C)

The parallelogram progresses through three types of shading: white, grey and chequered. It is white in the fourth box, so it will be grey in the correct answer; eliminate **(B)** and **(D)**. The grey triangle is in the same position in the remaining answers, so it will not help in determining which is correct. The black triangle alternates between two positions, adjacent and outside the parallelogram, or just inside the upper-left corner. It is inside in the fourth box, so it must be outside in the correct answer. **(C)** is therefore correct.

53. (A)

It's quickest to start with the simplest part of the progression. In the first row of boxes, the bottom shapes are simplest. The two trapeziums switch positions from left to right, but retain their original colours. Thus, the white chevron must be on the left in the correct answer; eliminate **(C)** and **(D)**. In the first boxes, the colour of the stars shifts by one position to the left, with the leftmost colour moving to the rightmost position; thus, the white circle –which is

leftmost in the third box – will be in the rightmost position in the answer. **(A)** is correct.

54. (D)

In the first progression, the pentagon – the large outer shape – switches places and sizes with the parallelogram – the smaller inner shape – but both retain their original colour; the final parallelogram has also been flipped, but the final pentagon hasn't. In the second progression, then, the large trapezium will become the smaller inner shape and retain its original orientation. Eliminate **(A)** and **(C)**, which incorrectly flip the final trapezium. It's the final, large arrow that must be flipped from its original orientation, so **(D)** is correct.

55. (A)

Each box includes a large figure made up of three stacked shapes, with a multi-pointed star on top. There is a second small shape in a corner of the box. In the first box of the first row, the multi-pointed star has 7 points, and the shapes in the stacked figure are black, grey and white (from front to back); the small triangle is grey. In the second box, the multi-pointed star has 10 points, and the shapes in the stacked figure are white, black and grey (front to back); the small shape is now a white hexagon. The large figure has moved to the opposite corner of the box - taking the position of the small shape in the first box, which moves to the opposite side of the box. The number of sides on the first small shape (3) equals the number of extra points on the star in the second box; the number of sides on the small shape increases by the same amount – or you could say the number of sides on the small shape doubles. In the second row, the first box includes a star with 4 points and a parallelogram. The second box should therefore have a star with 8 points and an octagon. Eliminate **(C)** and **(D)**. The small shape moves to the wrong place in **(B)** – it should be in the lower-left corner, directly opposite the upper-left corner in its original position. Answer **(A)** is correct.

For the record: The colour of the small shape matches the colour of the middle shape in the large figure in the first box; the colour changes to match the front shape in the second box. The colours in the large figure move one position to the back, with the back colour moving to the front. Note that if you had started with the colours, you would have eliminated **(B)** and **(C)**, leaving only two answers to test against the counting rules. It doesn't matter which details you start with – the key is to eliminate answers as you work. Don't try to memorise all the details from the first row – compare to the second row (and the answers) as you find them. Otherwise, you will waste valuable time.

Situational Judgement

1. (C)

Telling a peer would allow Adam to leave without disrupting the class, so it is not an awful response. However, leaving the classroom without planning to catch up on what will be missed means Adam will miss part of his training. Thus, this response is inappropriate.

2. (C)

Walking out of the classroom is not an appropriate course of action if Adam is beginning to feel sick. He needs to inform someone, before simply leaving for what may appear to be no good reason. However, Adam does feel sick, so this response is not awful.

3. (A)

This option provides an excellent response to the immediate problem, since Adam would be informing the instructor that he feels sick before leaving the class and would be making up what has been missed later.

4. (D)

Being dishonest is an inappropriate course of action in any context. This option also demonstrates Adam would not be admitting his need for help which may have further consequences to his training and to becoming a good doctor. This is therefore highly inappropriate.

5. (A)

This response is neutral and supportive, and is thus highly appropriate.

6. (A)

This response addresses one of the underlying issues: Darryl is not in a fit state to encounter patients at the hospital. As such, the response is very appropriate.

7. (D)

This is a highly inappropriate response, as it is not a local solution, and also because it is not likely that anonymous complaint that does not specify which doctor has a drinking problem would lead to any help for Darryl.

8. (A)

Darryl may require additional support as he gets his professional and personal life in order, so it would be very appropriate to encourage him to discuss matters with his consultant.

9. (D)

This is a very inappropriate response, as it is unprofessional for Saba to socialise with a patient. Accepting the request in order to explain why she cannot socialise would send the patient a mixed message, and would also begin a conversation on the social networking site, which could lead to serious professional consequences for Saba, despite her best intentions.

10. (A)

This would be a highly appropriate response, since it will not escalate the situation further, and it will ensure that Saba does not engage in any inappropriate social contact with a patient.

11. (C)

It is inappropriate for a doctor to speak to nurses in such a manner; however, the nurses are behaving unprofessionally, so this response is not awful.

12. (C)

Clearing her throat will not ensure that the nurses notice her presence or stop their gossiping, so it is not an effective or appropriate response. However, there are no negative consequences from doing so, other than potentially having to wait a bit longer for help from the nurses – so it is not an awful response.

13. (A)

This response is quick and direct, and is thus highly appropriate.

14. (D)

Rescheduling all the patients would be very inconvenient for them; it's not at all appropriate in these circumstances. Anwen should not let the training courses affect patient care, if at all possible.

15. (A)

It is always appropriate for a junior doctor to ask a senior colleague for advice.

16. (A)

This response would be a highly appropriate solution, as it would allow Anwen to attend the mandatory training courses without affecting patient care.

17. (A)

Whilst this would be a difficult action for Ian to pursue, it is a very appropriate response that deals with the situation immediately, discreetly and locally. No student under any circumstances should be allowed to cheat, and this response ensures that Ben must face with the consequences of his actions.

18. (C)

This response is inappropriate, as it does not deal with the situation as swiftly as possible. However, it does deal with the situation, so it is not awful.

19. (D)

This may save Ian from a difficult conversation with his best friend; however, this response is neither immediate nor local. By the time the medical school investigates further, it will be hard to prove that Ben cheated. This means it is likely that Ben will not have to face consequences for having cheated, and that he will be able to maintain an unfair advantage over their fellow medical students. Thus, this is a highly inappropriate response.

20. (D)

There are a number of reasons that the patient is not responding to Arissa. Perhaps Arissa is not speaking loudly or clearly enough, or the patient may have trouble hearing, or may not speak English well or at all. The patient's name will not help in addressing the exact cause of the problem, as a patient with a foreign name could speak English well but could also have a hearing problem. Thus, this is a very inappropriate response.

21. (D)

The patient has not given consent for the treatment, so it would be highly unprofessional for Arissa to proceed with the treatment. This would be a highly inappropriate thing to do, and could result in serious professional consequences for Arissa.

22. (A)

It is always very appropriate for a doctor to seek advice from a senior colleague.

23. (D)

This is not a local solution to the problem, and Freddie should talk to Joanna herself first before risking damaging her reputation their consultant. Thus, it is a highly inappropriate response.

24. (A)

This would be a very appropriate thing to do, since it would give them both equal opportunities to teach and to help complete the paperwork.

25. (C)

This response is inappropriate, as it focuses on Freddie's preferences, rather than a fair and professional balance of their responsibilities. However, it is not awful, as it would open a discussion of the division of their responsibilities, which has been made based on Joanna's preferences.

26. (D)

Olubayo is right to be concerned that the power may go out again, and patient health and safety could be compromised if this were to happen once Olubayo starts treatment. However, this is a decision that must be taken by the dentist on behalf of the patient; asking whether the patient is comfortable with proceeding is therefore very inappropriate.

27. (A)

This is a very appropriate response, given that Olubayo cannot be assured of being able to complete the treatement without disruption due to the storm, which could place the patient's health at risk.

28. (A)

This is a highly appropriate thing to do, as many treatments at the dental surgery would require the use of electricity. Given that the backup generator has already failed once today, proceeding with any treatment as another storm approaches would be reckless and unprofessional.

29. (A)

This is a very appropriate response, as Emmanuel may need some support if the patient has said anything to make him feel uncomfortable. This will also inform Simone's decision as to whether to take over the patient's care.

30. (D)

This is a very inappropriate response, as there is no indication from what Emmanuel has said that he has behaved inappropriately towards the patient. Approaching the patient in this manner implies that Emmanuel may have done something wrong, which is not at all appropriate for Simone to do.

31. (B)

This response is appropriate, and Simone would be correct to remind Emmanuel of his duty to treat all patients, even when their beliefs differ from his own. However, this response is not ideal, as Emmanuel does seem unsettled by this patient; a more appropriate response would allow Simone to assess whether Emmanuel requires any support from her, and inform a decision as to whether to take over the care of this patient.

32. (A)

This is a highly appropriate response, as it is an open and neutral question, with no possible negative consequences for Alfie.

33. (A)

If Hannah wants to examine Alfie's injuries, then it would be highly appropriate to get consent from his carer before doing so.

34. (A)

This is a very appropriate thing to do, as it will help to calm Alfie and make it easier for Hannah to treat him.

35. (D)

It is not clear that Alfie has been abused, though his injuries are worrying and would justify further investigation by Hannah before making a report to children's services. The next step would be to examine the injuries, ideally after obtaining consent from Alfie's carer. Phoning in a report before checking the injuries would be highly inappropriate.

36. (D)

This is a very inappropriate thing to do, as the patient has given consent for his family to be informed of his condition, and it's likely that his niece has come to the hospital for this very purpose. The doctor should make some time to speak with her, even if to briefly explain that she must wait to speak with the consultant.

37. (D)

This response is very inappropriate, and it is also inaccurate, as the patient has given consent for his condition to be explained to his family.

38. (A)

This is a very appropriate thing to do, as it defers to the patient's wish to have the consultant explain his condition to his family. It also allows Dr Miller to guide the woman to a more appropriate place to wait for the consultant.

39. (A)

The fact that the junior doctor has tried to schedule meetings, only to have these cancelled at the last minute by Dr Khavari, suggests that the fault may lie with Dr Khavari. This is a very important factor to consider; it should prompt Dr Zaghari to speak to her colleague and find out why he is not doing more to support the junior doctor he is meant to be supervising.

40. (D)

The consultants agreed to share the responsibility of supervising the junior doctor, so the fact that they have other duties is not an important factor.

41. (D)

This is not at all important, as Jackson should not be stealing the supplies for any reason.

42. (B)

The reason that Jackson is stealing the supplies is irrelevant to how Zakariyah responds to the situation. However, if Jackson has talked about putting up drips on himself and his friends, this is an important factor to consider, as the fact that Jackson is taking drips and bags of intravenous fluids makes it more likely that Jackson is actually engaging in an illegal and potentially dangerous misuse of medical equipment, and Zakariyah should take this into account when dealing with the situation.

43. (D)

Jackson should not be stealing medical supplies from the hospital. The fact that the medical supplies are not safe to use at the hospital is not at all important in responding to Jackson's behaviour.

44. (D)

Whilst it may be tempting for Zakariyah to 'let this one go' in support of his friend, stealing hospital supplies is completely against all regulations and also calls into question a doctor's probity; therefore, it is important that Zakariyah raise this through the appropriate channels without placing any importance at all on the consequences for Jackson's medical career.

45. (D)

This factor is not at all important, as it does not mitigate Liam's unprofessional comments about this patient in any way.

46. (A)

This is a very important factor to consider, as Conor will need to decide whether to respond to Liam immediately, or to move the conversation to a more private space where they can speak freely.

47. (D)

This is not at all important, as Liam's comments are so extreme that Conor must address them with Liam immediately, directly and discreetly, even if this is the first time that Liam has made them.

48. (A)

This is a very important factor, as it means that it will be simple and direct for Conor to get support in addressing Liam's behaviour effectively. Given the nature of Liam's remarks about not being able to deal with 'another one of these people,' it is likely that there are serious issues that need to be addressed, and Conor may need help from a senior member of staff to do so effectively. This factor makes it more likely that Conor could get such help, so it is very important.

49. (C)

This factor is of minor importance. It makes it more likely that Conor would want to be sensitive yet effective in responding to Liam's remarks, but it does not mitigate the need to address Liam's behaviour in any way.

50. (A)

This is a very important factor, since the consultant obviously had a good reason for requesting the x-ray, and patient health and the professionalism of the team may be compromised if it is not completed on time.

51. (A)

This is very important to consider, since the safety of patients has to come first. If there was a very sick patient on the ward who urgently needed medical care, then they should have taken priority over other non-urgent jobs, such as organising this x-ray.

52. (B)

This is an important factor, as it means that there is sufficient time remaining to organise this non-urgent x-ray before the patient leaves the hospital.

53. (D)

Patients must always come first, so this factor is not at all important. The fact that Dr O'Keefe had this news a few days ago means that she had time to organise someone to cover for her if she needed to take a few days off.

54. (A)

This is a very important factor, as it would allow for Maisie to ring Catriona and encourage her to make every effort to come to the meeting before it starts. If Catriona will be delayed, then the group could delay the start of the meeting. This is something best explained directly, rather than in a text message, so a private spot for this conversation would be very important.

55. (B)

This is an important consideration, as it would give Catriona a likelihood of arriving relatively soon, although she would be likely to arrive late. This would be preferable to Catriona skipping the meeting due to car trouble, so Maisie would be right to encourage Catriona to consider other transport options.

56. (A)

This factor is of utmost importance. If they have been clearly assigned a project that must be completed as a group, then it is inappropriate for Catriona to ask Maisie to cover for her.

57. (A)

This factor is extremely important, as it is fundamental to the matter at hand, and Addison must disclose what he observed to the hospital administrator.

58. (D)

This is not at all important, as Addison remembers noticing something an error during the procedure and thus has a professional obligation to disclose it to the hospital, even if he is not directly asked about it.

59. (C)

This factor is of minor importance. It does not mitigate Addison's responsibility to disclose Petra's error to the hospital, though it makes it more urgent that he do so, as the other staff may have lacked the training to understand that it was an error, or to comprehend its implications.

60. (A)

This factor is very important to consider. Medical students are not sent on hospital placements to 'just get stuck in,' but in order to complete specific criteria that are relevant at that stage of their medical education. If Rhiannon is to help mentor the students, she needs to be aware of these criteria to ensure she gives the students appropriate tasks on the ward and that she guides them sufficiently and appropriately as they complete these tasks.

61. (A)

This factor is extremely important. The hospital would not want medical students wandering the ward and 'just getting stuck in' wherever they like – that would be quite chaotic, not to mention the risk to patient health and safety. Rhiannon is a junior doctor, so she could potentially help in supervising the medical students; however, this does not seem to have been one of her responsibilities prior to the consultant telling her to 'just come up with something'; she would do well to discuss her concerns with the consultant, including the fact that she likely has a very full shift without having several medical students to mentor and supervise.

62. (B)

This factor does not excuse the consultant's failure to mentor and supervise the medical students, but it would explain why the consultant is so overrun and why he has failed so far in his duties to the medical students. This factor is important, as it must be addressed urgently to ensure that there is adequate cover for patients as well as for supporting the medical students on their placement. It is not the main issue here, but it is a contributing factor that Rhiannon should address with the consultant. A hospital should provide adequate cover, for example, bringing in locum consultants or arranging for support from consultants at nearby hospitals, while staff are away on medical or annual leave.

63. (C)

It is clear from the scenario that the consultant does not speak Spanish very well; it also seems clear that the consultant's attempts at speaking Spanish have confused and agitated the patient. The failure to communicate with the patient, and the distress that this causes the patient, are the main issues in this scenario. The consultant's lack of fluency in Spanish is of minor importance – it needs to be acknowledged, but only so that they can move on to calming the patient and resolving the language barrier.

64. (D)

If the patient's injury were life-threatening, then it would be all the more urgent to resolve the language barrier, as they would need to be able to communicate with her in a language she understands in order for her to consent to treatment. However, the consultant's inept attempt at speaking Spanish has created a new problem – the patient is confused and agitated. This is the pressing issue at the end of the scenario, more so than her injury. Thus, the fact that her injury is not life-threatening is of no importance.

65. (A)

This is one of the main problems in this scenario, so it is an extremely important factor to consider in responding to the situation. The consultant has assumed that the woman speaks Spanish because she appears to be Latin American. Perhaps she is Brazilian, in which case she would speak Portuguese; in any case, it's not advisable to try to guess a patient's nationality based on their appearance. They need to determine what

language she speaks, so they can calm her down and give her the chance to consent to treatment.

66. (D)

This factor is not important. The young patient is clearly distressed, and she needs someone to talk to her and listen to her. The consultant paediatrician should take a few minutes to do so before heading home.

67. (A)

This factor is very important, as it would explain a likely reason why Alice is so distressed. A chat with her consultant paediatrician would make her feel ever so much better.

68. (C)

This factor is important to Alice's physical health, but it would not make much of a difference to her emotional well-being at the moment; she's a young girl on her own in hospital, and clearly feeling lonely and distressed. Thus, the factor is of minor importance; if Alice says that she really wants to go home, for example, then the doctor might mention the fact that she is due to go home tomorrow.

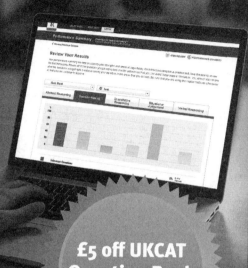

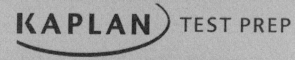